Overcoming
Estrogen
Dominance

MAGDALENA WSZELAKI, CH, HHC

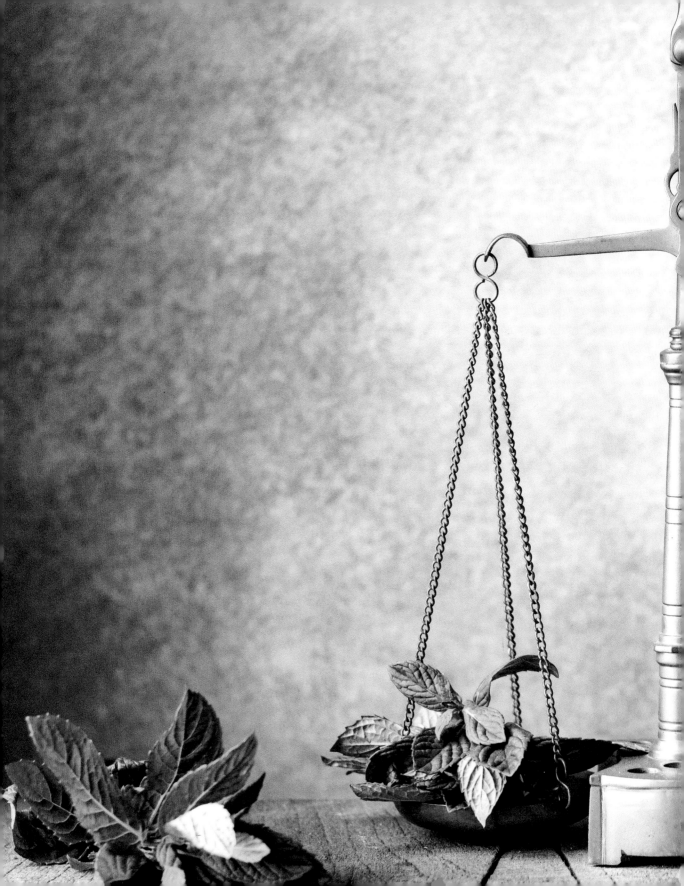

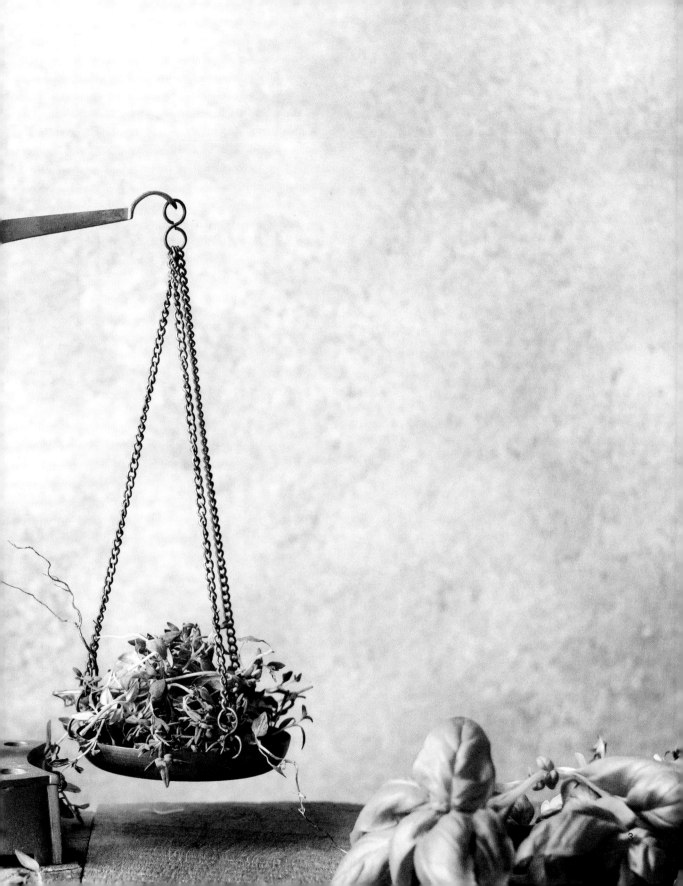

To request permissions, contact team@hormonesbalance.com

Hardcover: ISBN 978-0-578-82243-3

First edition: January 2021

Written by: Magdalena Wszelaki and Julia Pastore
Edited by: Terry Walsh
Graphic Design by: Ryan Long, Bill Callahan, and David Kinzel
Watercolors by: Heather Good, Kate Ferry
Recipes & Photographs by: Jennafer Mostowski
Personality Photos: Photography by Jitka Perez
Author Photos: Photography by Jitka Perez

Printed by: New Type Publishing

Dedicated to all women with an inner whisper that healing is our invincible superpower.

Table of Contents

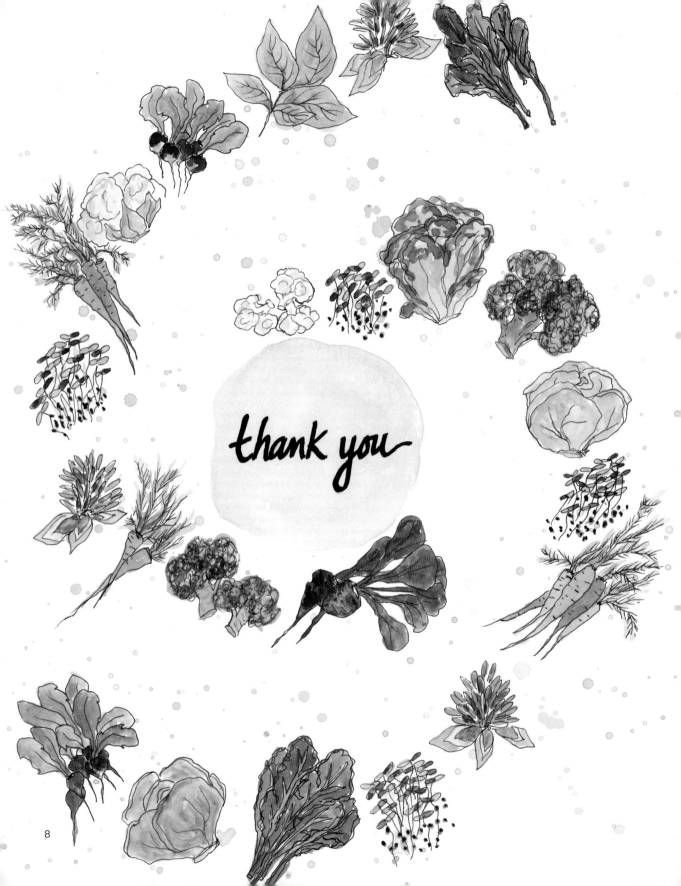

thank you

Acknowledgments

It takes a village to raise an author.

As I jotted down the names of the people who have been instrumental in my life and in creating this book, I choked up. I didn't realize how much help, dedication, and unconditional support have fed the creation of this resource.

As a creative business owner with countless ideas and ongoing projects, this book wouldn't be possible without the help of Julia Pastore. Julia was the executive editor at HarperCollins and we worked together on my first book, *Cooking for Hormone Balance*. She subsequently left and created her own writing agency; this is when we got to work together again—to birth this book. Julia's wit, strategic mind, and attention to details have turned the much scattered material into the cohesive book and resource you are now reading.

Born into a Polish family, I am blessed with parents who shielded my sister and me from processed foods and unnecessary rounds of antibiotics, and who kept things "natural" at home before it became fashionable and declared "healthy." We never spent our weekends in front of a television; camping, hiking, and city tours were the order of the day. My sister, Patrycja, has been a stellar catalyst of our family's unity.

I would have blown my health (a common problem with many book writers!) while working on this project if it were not for the outstanding Hormones Balance team: Courtney Webster, Astrid Kihl, Charisma Madarang, Deanna Shank, Jennifer Colletti, Jeanne Geroux, Taylor Hurry, and Courtney Hamilton. And my great design team: photography by Jennafer Mostowski, watercolors by Heather Good and Kate Ferry, and graphic design by WLxJS. Most importantly, they never stopped showing deep care and concern for our readers and their health.

This book is deeply rooted in the Hormones Balance and Hormone Thrivers communities, as well as our Thriver Mentors; your experiences, questions, concerns, and stories have provided priceless input for this book. You have helped me become a better practitioner.

It is through my very dear friend Dr. Izabella Wentz that I got pulled into the mighty Mindshare community, helmed by JJ Virgin and Karl Krummenacher. I owe the growth of my business, the strength to persevere, and the blessing of new friendships to this community. Not only do I feel like am I no longer alone, but I have the support and wisdom of people who thrive on seeing others grow and prosper. Much love goes to Dr. Marisol Teijeiro and Dr. Anna Cabeca, my mastermind sisters whom I so look forward to connecting with each Friday to bounce ideas, brainstorm, rant, and laugh.

I want to recognize practitioners in this space who do outstanding work in the women's health and hormone space, namely Dr. Izabella Wentz, Dr. Jolene Brighten, Dr. Mariza Snyder, Dr. Shawn Tassone, Ari Whitten, Dr. Alan Hopkins and Amy Beth Hopkins, Dr. Anna Cabeca, Dr Sara Gottfried, Dr. Marisol Teijeiro, Lara Adler, Dr. Erika Gray, Wendy Myers, Razi Berry, Dr. Beth O'Hara, Amy Medling, Kevin and Annmarie Gianni, Nicole Jardim, Christa Orecchio, Trudy Scott, Leanne Ely, Dr. Elisa Song, Steve Wright, and Dr. Jill Carnahan, Jessica Drummond, Julie Matthews,

Dr. Marcelle Pick, Dr. Veronique Desaulniers, Dr. Doni Wilson, Dr. Fiona McCulloch, Dr. Tom O'Bryan, Dr. Kelly Brogan, and Jon Gabriel.

This book wouldn't be what it is if it weren't for the courses by Andrea Nakayama, the creator of the Functional Nutrition Lab, which taught me how to think like a true functional nutrition practitioner with an eye for broader concepts and subtle, revealing details.

Deep gratitude goes to the Colorado School of Clinical Herbalism programs which are as equally rooted in herbal traditions as they are in science. They were the inspiration and wisdom behind the herbal recipes in this book. Much love goes to Lisa Ganora for her smarts and kindness, as well as formulating some of the supplements and tinctures at the Wellena store.

I would not have left advertising and Shanghai when I got sick in 2008 had it not been for my then boss, Steve Hsia. He made sure my wish to recover my health and live in the United States materialized, even though the U.S. economy was tanking and he was losing me as a key resource in the fast-growing China market. That's selflessness and love.

I love this work. I love food and herbs. Let them guide you and show you the way.

I love you all,

Magdalena

Medical Disclaimer

The publisher and the author are providing this book and its contents on an "as is" basis and make no representations or warranties of any kind with respect to this book or its content. The publisher and the author disclaim all such representations and warranties, including but not limited to warranties of healthcare for a particular purpose. In addition, the publisher and the author assume no responsibility for errors, inaccuracies, omissions, or any other inconsistencies herein.

The content of this book is for informational purposes only and is not intended to diagnose, treat, cure, or prevent any condition or disease. You understand this book is not intended as a substitute for consultation with a licensed practitioner. Please consult with your own physician or healthcare specialist regarding the suggestions and recommendations made in this book. The use of this book implies your acceptance of this disclaimer.

The publisher and the author make no guarantees concerning the level of success you may experience by following the advice and strategies contained in this book, and you accept the risk that results will differ for each individual. The testimonials and examples provided in this book show exceptional results, which may not apply to the average reader and are not intended to represent or guarantee you will achieve the same or similar results.

OVERCOMING ESTROGEN DOMINANCE

Introduction

Heavy, clotty, debilitating periods. Mood swings damaging relationships to the point I don't recognize myself. Limbs so swollen that I can't take off my rings or put on shoes. Thyroid nodules. Breast lumps ("Is it cancer?"). Hair loss in spite of having fixed my thyroid.

I've struggled with estrogen dominance as far back as I can remember. Perhaps you can relate. If so, you are in the right place to get help to reverse these symptoms naturally, live a symptom-free life, and never fear this hormonal imbalance wreaking havoc on your health again. Fear is a powerful emotion I've grown to respect and eventually like—it pushes me to take action and take care of myself the way I wouldn't otherwise. Maybe that's you, too.

The first thing I want you to know is that estrogen dominance, like all hormonal imbalances, doesn't come out of nowhere or occur for no reason. It's also not "natural" because you are aging or because your mother had it. Estrogen dominance happens because underlying health issues have gone unresolved. It could be that you've struggled for years with nutrient deficiencies, chronic stress, toxic relationships, frequent and persistent infections, poor sleep, a sluggish liver, erratic blood sugar, or the use of the birth control pill or conventional (but toxic) skincare and cleaning products. These are just a few examples of what can fuel estrogen dominance.

My start in life set me up for hormonal challenges. I was not breastfed as a baby, and we know now this contributes to highly compromised gut health and a very weak immune system. I had pneumonia in the first month of my life and was put on broad-spectrum antibiotics. As a child, I suffered with chronic ear infections and eczema and numerous food sensitivities that left me in constant digestive discomfort. In adulthood, my symptoms transformed into severe cystic acne spread across my face, chest, back, and buttocks, debilitating migraines (the type that prevent you from even opening your eyes), terrible PMS, and excessive bloating in my fingers and feet. I've also had lumpy and fibrocystic breasts on and off for most of my young adult life. Quitting gluten, dairy, and eggs cleared up the acne, but my other symptoms—clear signs of estrogen dominance—persisted.

In my late 20s, I developed Graves' disease, an autoimmune condition that causes the thyroid to produce too much thyroid hormone. The thyroid blockers I was prescribed quieted my overactive thyroid but did nothing to address the autoimmune component of this condition. It was no surprise a few years later when I developed another autoimmune disease, this time involving an underactive thyroid: Hashimoto's Thyroiditis. Meanwhile, I was pumping more and more of my energy and drive into my career and competitive sports, working 80-hour weeks and pushing hard at the gym. Fatigue, anxiety, insomnia, and foul mood swings became everyday occurrences. I was maxed out and my symptoms of estrogen dominance were raging. I also began to experience hair loss and lumpy breasts. I may have looked ripped on the outside, but on the inside I was a wreck. Scared, I realized I needed to make a total life change. The founders sold the company and I got a significant earnout, the majority of which I decided to forego by leaving earlier than was expected—to save my health and sanity.

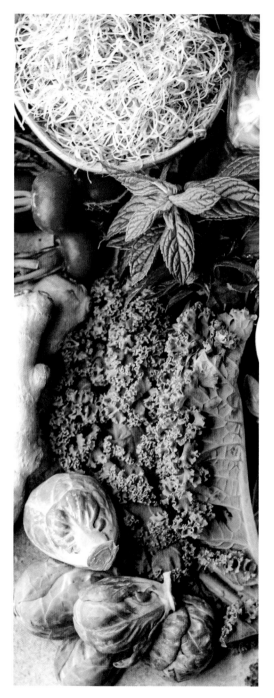

I left my stressful, unsatisfying job in advertising in Shanghai, moved from environmentally polluted China to the United States, and enrolled in nutrition school to understand what was really going on in my body and how to heal it naturally.

I learned there's no one pill that will reset your hormones, but you can give your body what it needs to restore balance. With organic food, clean air, less stress, and more sleep I was able to get my thyroid, nervous system, and estrogen dominance issues under control. I developed a new way of eating that repaired and kept my hormones running smoothly. In 2009 I started my nutrition practice, Hormones Balance, to help other women use food to do the same. Since getting certified as a nutrition coach, I've also become an herbalist, speaker, educator, and author of *Cooking for Hormone Balance*, a cookbook published by HarperCollins.

The Estrogen Reset Foundation Protocol grew out of my own experience and the work I've done with thousands of women to balance their hormones. It is based on the principles of functional medicine, emphasizing the importance of uncovering, and treating the root causes of disease rather than just the symptoms. This is done alongside your bio-individuality (one person's food is another's poison), including your biochemistry, genetics, current health status, and living environment. While there are some universal truths (such as processed foods, alcohol, drugs, and excessive sugar are bad for all of us), so much of healing is subjective. A food that supports your health may cause an allergic reaction in your friend. In this book, you'll learn how to eat what is right for you to manage your estrogen dominance, keep you healthy and satisfied, and prevent future diseases.

> At 48, I feel more vibrant and energetic than I did at 28. I am thriving—and I hope that this book will help you get here, too.

My health journey continues. Keeping my estrogen dominance in check is ongoing. As much as I feel and look great for my age (I'm 48 years old at the time of writing this book), I need to keep things in check to feel at my best. I sometimes envy women who can live on coffee, gluten, and dairy yet feel amazing (I think of that every time I'm in Italy). And I remind myself that I was put on this planet for a higher purpose: to pass this hard-won knowledge on to you so that you can benefit from it. Without my fragile hormonal balance I wouldn't know all that I do about the peculiarity of our hormones.

Lastly, I discovered that I have several genetic mutations that predispose me to estrogen dominance. In fact, when I first met my functional doctor, she asked me if I had ever had breast cancer. I said no and asked her why she would say that. Her response was: "Because women with your genetics and this age would typically have this issue." Clearly, genes are not destiny. Nutrition and lifestyle play a major role in whether or not we develop disease. Rest assured, you can resolve your estrogen dominance with the Estrogen Reset protocols in spite of your genetics, like I have.

At 48, I feel more vibrant and energetic than I did at 28. I am thriving—and I hope that this book will help you get here, too.

Who This Book Is For

Estrogen dominance is very common. About 70% of the women I work with have some form of it, experiencing many of the most common symptoms: lumpy and fibrocystic breasts, fibroids, thyroid nodules, painful periods, PMS, heavy bleeding, absent periods, mid-cycle spotting, uterine polyps, infertility and miscarriages, endometriosis, brain fog, mood swings, insomnia, fatigue, bloating, and weight gain (especially around the hips and thighs), among others. It's at an all-time high in women in their 40s on up. This is when many women enter peri-menopause, the period lasting an average of four to eight years before menopause (average age 51) and the end of their period. Hormones go haywire during this time, setting you up for imbalance. In menopause and post-menopause, low levels of the reproductive hormone progesterone increase your likelihood of developing estrogen dominance.

No matter what your age or phase of life, if you are struggling with any of the symptoms mentioned here or have been diagnosed with estrogen dominance (see Recommended Lab Tests), you will benefit from the Estrogen Reset protocol.

Those of you with a thyroid condition or autoimmune disease, such as Hashimoto's Thyroiditis, should also see improvement by following this protocol. Excess estrogen lowers the amount of thyroid hormone available in your body, causing all of the issues associated with hypothyroidism.

It's also highly inflammatory, and inflammation is one of the main drivers of an autoimmune flare-up.

My biggest wish for you is to shift your energy from confusion, resignation, fear, or anger to empowerment and a strong sense of control of your health. If you follow the protocols in this book, you will gain the tools needed to get there and feel like yourself again.

My Approach to Healing

Managing your estrogen dominance is not about balancing estrogen only or any one hormone; it's about balancing *all* of your hormones. This may sound impossible, but it really isn't that complicated. You can balance most hormones with a healthy gut, well-functioning liver, and stable blood sugar. I've found over the years that taking care of these three bodily systems will have a profoundly positive impact on all your hormones.

Fix the Three-Legged Stool

The foundation of your hormonal health is your digestive health, liver health, and blood sugar levels.

Think of these three as forming the legs of a stool. If each leg is even and stable, the stool will remain firmly in place when you sit down. But if one leg is shorter than the others or missing entirely, the stool will wobble—and you will fall. Your hormonal health works the same way: If one aspect of your foundation is unsteady, you'll fall into imbalance.

The goal of this book and the protocols is to fix and maintain a healthy foundation by restoring your gut, detoxing your liver, and balancing your

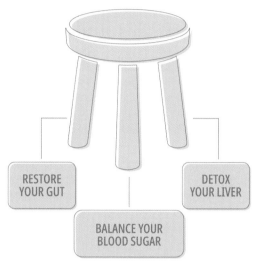

HORMONAL BALANCE

RESTORE YOUR GUT

DETOX YOUR LIVER

BALANCE YOUR BLOOD SUGAR

blood sugar. Once your three-legged stool is in good shape, your hormones will start fixing themselves. So much so the majority of your symptoms will probably go away—including symptoms you never thought were hormone related.

Follow the Pyramid

There are several tools in our toolbox for building a healthy foundation. Food is your best one and the reason the Foundation Protocol includes a meal plan with recipes. Food is the majority of what you put in your body each and every day; eating clean is paramount.

Herbs are often made part of your daily diet, and if not, they can easily be incorporated. Supplements are sometimes part of a daily routine, too. Both herbs and supplements will support, as well as amplify healing, but they aren't magic bullets. If your digestion is in disarray, your liver is toxic and overloaded, and/or your blood sugar is spiking or crashing regularly, there is only so much herbs and supplements can do for you.

Medications (and surgery) are called for only when absolutely necessary and all other options have been exhausted.

If your food is not dialed in, herbs, supplements, and medications won't be nearly as effective.

Stop Chasing Symptoms

Too often, we spin our wheels chasing after our symptoms, trying to find a fix for each individual ache and/or dysfunction. What herb should I take for my hot flashes? What cream should I use for the skin rash? Round and round we go, taking one supplement for hair loss, another to induce sleep, and yet another to boost our energy or libido. We seek out creams, potions, and pills to relieve our symptoms, yet all we get is more frustrated and

tired. If you had to do 12 different things to ease 12 different symptoms, you'd be tired, too!

Well, guess what? When you stop chasing symptoms and start fixing your foundation—healing your digestion, supporting your liver, and balancing your blood sugar levels—your symptoms will begin to disappear. After a few weeks, five of the 12 issues you were dealing with will drop off. The next month, another three will drop off. And so on. When you stop playing whack-a-mole with your symptoms and give yourself the chance to rebuild your foundation, you'll notice amazing changes to your health and well-being.

I've used the image of a three-legged stool to describe your hormonal foundation, but you can also think of it as rich, fertile soil. If you have ever gardened, you know that a vibrant and lush garden can only grow in nutrient-dense soil. Without nourishment, your health cannot thrive and

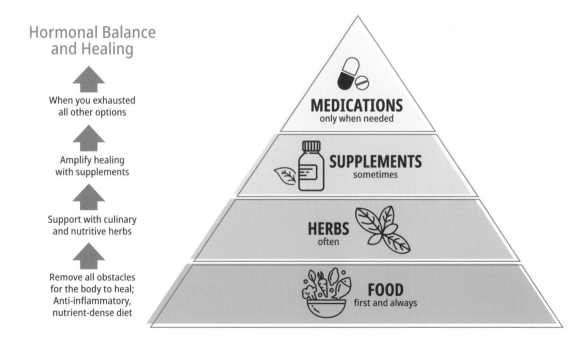

Hormonal Balance and Healing

When you exhausted all other options

Amplify healing with supplements

Support with culinary and nutritive herbs

Remove all obstacles for the body to heal; Anti-inflammatory, nutrient-dense diet

MEDICATIONS only when needed

SUPPLEMENTS sometimes

HERBS often

FOOD first and always

flower either. Taking care of your gut, liver health, and maintaining steady blood sugar levels fertilizes the soil. And when you do that, you often have to do very little else for a healthy garden to bloom and thrive.

It's Okay Not
to Be Perfect

It's more than okay; it's completely normal! The reality is, work, school, partners, kids, travel, holidays, and so on will make it challenging to implement the Foundation Protocol. Don't get discouraged or beat yourself up if you slip up or take more time. I want you to think "positive change" and "one step at a time," not perfection. Use these strategies to troubleshoot some of the most common challenges I hear from our community:

YOU SHOULD KNOW . . .

Too much estrogen isn't the problem. Estrogen dominance can happen for a few different reasons. The problem could be that you have *too much of a specific type of estrogen*, are *breaking down estrogen* in an unfavorable way, or *don't have enough of the hormone progesterone* to balance out your estrogen. Another problem? A poor hormonal foundation. A weak gut, toxic liver, and erratic blood sugar levels all can contribute to estrogen dominance. We need to look beyond an oversimplified definition of estrogen dominance as "too much estrogen" and understand the nuances—this knowledge is power and will help you navigate what is or isn't right for you. More on this later in the book.

Estrogenic foods aren't driving up your estrogen dominance. Foods such as flax seeds and soy are called phytoestrogens because they contain a naturally occurring compound similar to the estrogen made by your body. You'd be inclined to think that adding more estrogens to your diet when you are already grappling with estrogen dominance would be a bad idea. But remember, estrogen dominance isn't about too much estrogen. It's important to keep two things in mind:

1. Not all estrogens are the same. Natural, minimally processed phytoestrogens such as flax seeds, tempeh, edamame, and soy sauce (fermented soy) are okay. Phytoestrogens are much weaker than our own estrogen and can block more potent forms of estrogen, reducing the symptoms of estrogen dominance in some women. Avoid the highly processed, rubbish kinds of soy: soy milk, tofu, and tofu meats. You should also avoid xenoestrogens, man-made chemicals that mimic estrogen and are found in plastic bottles, personal care products, perfumes, and household cleaning supplies. These include BPA, phthalates, and parabens.

2. How you break down and excrete excess estrogen matters more than the amount of phytoestrogens you are consuming. Those processes depend on a strong hormonal foundation, especially a healthy gut and liver.

1. "I can't implement the Foundation Protocol 100% perfectly. I give up!"

Reframe: Every small change matters. Do what you can.

Practical tip: Try doing one new practice each week and don't worry about the rest.

2. "My family will never get on board with this."

Reframe: Do it for yourself. A happy mom is a better mom; a happy partner is a better partner.

Practical tip: Ask for their support; explain why it matters to you.

3. "I don't have time to do this."

Reframe: You're worth the time. Do what you can, little by little, you don't have to do it all.

Practical tip: Identify one change you'd like to implement for the week and schedule a few minutes each day to make it happen.

4. "There are too many things to keep track of and remember."

Reframe: Your health deserves the effort. What is your quality of life without your health?

Practical tip: Use organizational/scheduling tools and technology to assist you; smartphones have a ton of these.

5. "I'm a lousy cook. I'll never be able to follow the recipes for the meal plan."

Reframe: You do not need to be a gourmet chef. With an open mind, a willingness to learn, and a sharp knife you can make the recipes in this book.

Practical tip: Pick one recipe from the meal plan that appeals to you, read the directions carefully, and give it a try. We kept the recipes intentionally simple.

6. "I can't afford to eat this way. It's too expensive."

Reframe: The cost is an investment in your health and good preventative care. Spending a little more money now will save you money—maybe thousands of dollars—in healthcare costs down the road. It's more expensive to deal with cancer, surgeries, and rehab.

Practical tip: Eating local and in-season, buying in bulk, using coupons, and shopping online are just a few of the many ways to eat organic, non-GMO foods on a budget.

7. "I don't deserve to feel better and be healthy."

Reframe: Every single one of us, including you, deserves to feel absolutely amazing.

Practical tip: Consider therapy to address the trauma that may be underlying these feelings of unworthiness and any self-sabotaging behaviors preventing you from reaching your full potential.

My Wish for You

My life's mission is to help you heal and feel your absolute best. I'm so grateful you're here, ready to join the thousands of other women who have regained hormone balance, and restored their health with my programs.

My wish for you: Don't let anyone dim your fire and desire to heal. You can naturally reverse estrogen dominance. You can shrink your thyroid nodules and fibroids. You can reverse endometriosis. You can get rid of lumpy breasts. Skeptics and the word *impossible* are banned as you embark on the Estrogen Reset and transform your health.

How to Use This Book

Drawing on my more than 10 years of research and experience, this book is rich in information. I don't want you to feel the least bit intimidated or overwhelmed by it. I've organized the material to make it easy for you to find exactly what you need to heal and feel better.

Parts I and II will help you understand what's happening in your body and why the Foundation Protocol is so powerful.

If you're thinking, "I don't need to know the why. Just tell me what to do to start feeling better *right now!*" head directly to Part IV. These chapters show you how to implement the specific practices of the protocol in straight-forward, easy-to-follow formats, including a quick-start chart of what to add or remove, and a 28-day meal plan based on simple recipes. Turn to Part IV and you'll have everything you need to get started on the Foundation Protocol today.

Keep in mind it takes most women longer than four weeks to get comfortable with the Foundation Protocol and that's okay. It might be a lot of change to undertake, after all, you're juggling work, family, friends, and a long list of demands on your time. Go easy on yourself. If you are able to implement the protocol 100% for four weeks and see results, great! But if you need more time, take it whether that's two, three, or six months.

The good news is that after doing the Foundation Protocol many women find their symptoms have gone away and they feel like a million bucks. You may not even need the symptom-specific add-on protocols in Part III. But, if you've been following the Foundation Protocol and still have some specific symptoms you'd like to target, such as fibroids, hot flashes, or irregular periods, go to Part IV and implement the tactics.

If you're struggling with a specific symptom, it may be tempting to skip straight to the relevant chapter in Part III. You'll immediately see that the first step in every one of those individualized protocols is to do the Foundation Protocol. Starting off with the Foundation Protocol to restore your gut, detox your liver, and balance your blood sugar is the best way to manage your estrogen dominance long-term (and most of your other ailments, to be honest!). It's likely you'll see such incredible improvements you may not even need to use the personalized protocols.

To recap:

If you are an "I like to understand everything" kind of person, a geek, or a practitioner:

1. Read Part I to understand estrogen dominance.

2. Read Part II to know what you'll be doing on the Foundation Protocol and why.

3. Read Part IV for tools that pull together all of the elements of the Foundation Protocol into a clear, organized program, and implement them the best you can.

4. Once you are comfortable and have implemented the Foundation Protocol, consider adding

a personalized protocol from Part III, if needed, and put that into practice the best you can.

If you want to start the Estrogen Reset Foundation Protocol immediately:

1. Skip to Part IV for the specifics of what to do to get going.

2. Once you are comfortable with the Foundation Protocol, consider adding a personalized protocol from Part III.

3. As time or interest allow, read Parts I and II.

No matter which approach you choose, you will nurture the rich, fertile soil necessary for your health to bloom. Welcome to *Overcoming Estrogen Dominance*. I'm so excited you're here and wish you all the best on this incredible journey.

A common question I get is: "How long will it take for me to feel better?" I hate to give you an inconclusive and vague answer of "It depends," but it really does depend on the current state of your health, how committed are you to following my protocols, how well do you sleep, etc. Most women start feeling better in one to two weeks. I've seen women saving their uteruses because their fibroids had shrunk in weeks. Some women manage to normalize their menses in one cycle and others need three. Women have emailed us and say they could sleep again after following the protocol for just a week. When you remove rigid expectations, surrender to nourishing and honoring your body, marvelous things will start to happen.

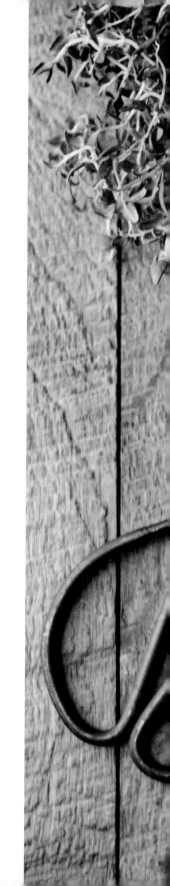

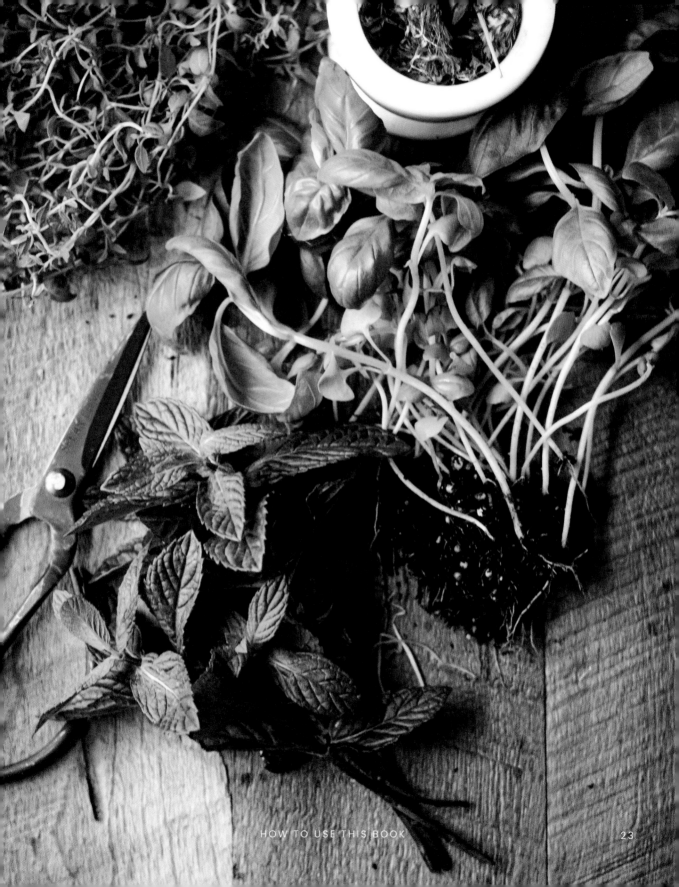

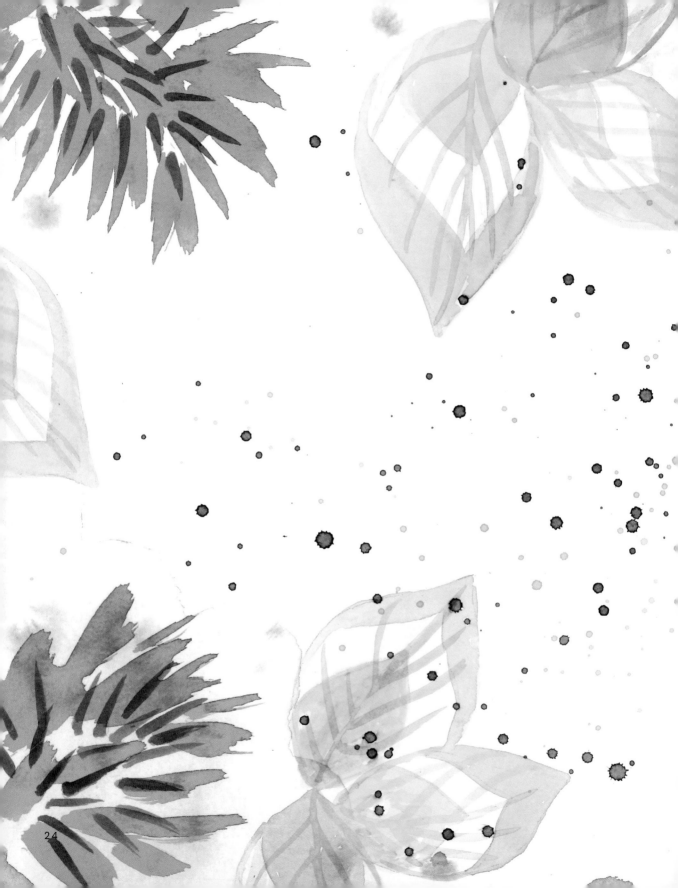

Part I

Understanding Estrogen Dominance

Chapter 1

What's Going on in Your Body

The Signs of Estrogen Dominance

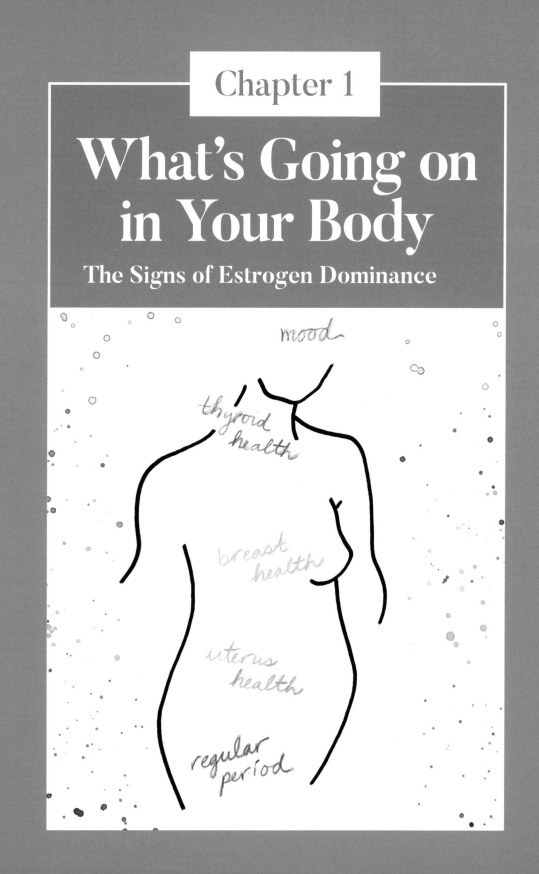

As you'd expect, we're going to cover a lot about estrogen in this book. It's so important that you don't demonize it or fear it. We need estrogen, the right kind and in the right amount, to be healthy, happy women. The trouble arises when we don't have the right balance and we experience estrogen dominance. But estrogen isn't the only hormone we should be paying attention to as we restore balance.

A Fun Way to Understand Estrogen Dominance

Dealing with hormonal problems is a lot like dealing with a bad romantic relationship so let me use this metaphor to illustrate how things can go wrong with estrogens. It is logical to think that since you show symptoms of estrogen dominance, you may have too much estrogen. This, however, is incorrect and overly simplistic. Estrogen dominance can manifest in three different ways. The problem is one, two, or all of the following three scenarios.

Scenario 1: Too Much of a Bad Guy (too much estradiol, or E2)

This one is pretty straightforward: You have too much estradiol, the "antagonistic" estrogen. Estradiol can do us a lot of good, preparing our body for pregnancy, supporting a positive mood, and protecting against bone loss. But too much of a good thing is a bad thing. Estradiol is just too powerful in high doses-just like when there is too much of a bad guy.

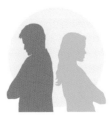

Scenario 2: An Ugly Breakup (the unfavorable breakdown of estrogen results in too many harmful metabolites or "dirty" estrogens)

Most of us have gone through a romantic or professional breakup that was less than ideal and the consequences lingered on. In the context of hormones, the liver is responsible for breaking down estradiol and estrone into smaller pieces as the first step in the process of eliminating metabolized or "used up" estrogen. There are three different smaller pieces estrogen can be broken down into:

- 2-hydroxyestrone (2-OH): a "good" estrogen that does not stimulate cell growth and can block the action of stronger, potentially cancer-causing estrogens.
- 4-hydroxyestrone (4-OH): potentially harmful, with increased estrogenic activity. A "dirty" estrogen.
- 16-alpha-hydroxyestrone (16-OH): potentially harmful, associated with an increased risk of breast cancer. A "dirty" estrogen.

We want more 2-OH with limited amounts of 4-OH and 16-OH. If that's not happening because your liver is already taxed and therefore not able to break down the estrogens to eliminate them properly, it will generate too many "dirty" estrogens, so you'll experience estrogen dominance. This is why the health of the liver is so vital when you're experiencing estrogen dominance.

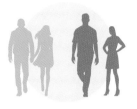

Scenario 3: Unbalanced Partners (not enough progesterone to balance estrogen)

You know that couple where she's overly timid and he's loud and obnoxious? Or, another couple who seem to be in a lovely flow and harmony? Estrogen and progesterone are the perfect couple when they are balanced. We

can't function without them and can only function well when they even each other out. This chart illustrates how well these two hormones complement each other.

As in any relationship, when one partner dominates, the delicate balance is destroyed. In the case of estrogen dominance, there's not enough progesterone to balance out the more aggressive estrogen.

If you're experiencing the symptoms of estrogen dominance, you have one or possibly all of these scenarios underway in your body.

Estrogen	Progesterone
• creates endometrium	• maintains endometrium
• stimulates breast cells (fibrocystic breasts*)	• protects against breast cysts
• increases body fat and causes weight gain*	• helps use fat for energy
• causes retention of salt and fluid	• promotes urination, a natural diuretic
• promotes depression, anxiety, and headaches*	• calms anxiety, a natural antidepressant
• promotes cyclical migraines*	• prevents cyclical migraines
• disturbs sleep patterns*	• promotes normal sleep patterns
• interferes with thyroid hormone function*	• facilitates thyroid hormone function
• impairs blood sugar control*	• helps normalize blood sugar levels
• lowers libido*	• restores normal libido
• increases risk of breast cancer*	• stimulates new bone formation
• restrains bone loss	• prevents autoimmune diseases
• triggers autoimmune diseases*	• increases sleepiness, depression**
• relieves hot flashes***	• promotes digestive problems**
	*with estrogen dominance
	**excess of progesterone
	***low estrogen

ESTROGEN

Causes endometrium to proliferate

Causes breast stimulation that
can lead to breast cancer

Increases body fat

Increases endometrial cancer risk

Increases gallbladder disease risk

Reduces vascular tone

Restrains osteoclast function slightly

Increases blood clot risk

PROGESTERONE

Maintains secretory endometrium

Protects against fibrocystic breast
and prevents breast cancer

Helps use fat for energy

Prevents endometrial cancer

Promotes osteoclast function,
leading to bone growth

Restores vascular tone

Normalizes blood clots

The Symptoms of Estrogen Dominance

Estrogen plays a major role in many aspects of our physical, mental, and emotional health; therefore, symptoms of estrogen dominance are many, as well as varied. Symptoms may range from cellulite and heavy bleeding to irritability and thyroid nodules.

Another issue is that estrogen is highly inflammatory. Inflammation is an essential part of a healthy immune system, indicating damaged tissues that need repair or a threat (infection, foreign invader) to be fought. As the body heals, the inflammation subsides. But if the irritant persists, the inflammation doesn't subside. It continues unchecked, becoming a chronic problem that has been linked to autoimmune diseases, cancer, heart disease, diabetes, asthma, and Alzheimer's. Women with estrogen dominance suffer from chronic systemic inflammation; the whole body is inflamed.

In turn, the inflammation caused by estrogen dominance leads to poor estrogen metabolism, perpetuating a vicious cycle. It also compromises hormone receptors throughout the body, making it hard for hormones to get into the cells and do their job. This applies to *all* hormones, not just estrogen. For example, your hair follicles have receptors for thyroid hormone. If that receptor is inflamed, it is unable to accept thyroid hormone and your hair will fall out. So, even if you have enough of the hormone in your bloodstream, it can't get into the cell to be used. It's as if inflammation has blocked the door. You have receptors for estrogen pretty much everywhere, including your bones, brain, and breasts. If inflammation is blocking the door to those receptors and estrogen can't get to work in the cell, you'll start experiencing symptoms.

Symptoms of estrogen dominance include:

- breast lumps
- fibrocystic breasts
- ER+ (estrogen receptor-positive) breast cancer
- fibroids
- hot flashes
- PMS and PMDD
- heavy bleeding or postmenopausal bleeding
- spider or varicose veins
- fat and/or cellulite (especially around butt and thighs)
- heavy periods
- absent periods
- irregular or sporadic periods
- ovarian cysts
- uterine polyps
- irritability, mood, swings, or anxiety
- headaches or migraines, particularly before your period or mid-cycle
- thyroid nodules and thyroid cancer
- bloating, puffiness, or water retention
- endometriosis
- gallbladder problems
- melasma, brown facial discolorations or spots above your lips, on the side of your face and forehead
- allergies, due to estrogen's highly inflammatory nature
- estrogen-fueled cancers, such as ovarian, uterine, and lung cancer (in nonsmokers)

Inflammation increases your risk for the chronic health issues mentioned above

CAN I BE IN MENOPAUSE AND LOW IN ESTROGEN AND HAVE ESTROGEN DOMINANCE AT THE SAME TIME? YES!

You are probably thinking, *Well, I'm in menopause. My estrogen is at its lowest ever. How can I be experiencing the symptoms of estrogen dominance?* There are a few ways. Think back to the scenarios outlined earlier.

You could be experiencing Scenario 1, where you have too much of the aggressive "bad guy" estradiol compared to the other two estrogens.

Or, you could be in Scenario 2 and what little estrogen you do have is being broken down in an unfavorable way into too many of the potentially harmful "dirty" estrogens.

Scenario 3 is also a possibility. Even though your estrogen levels are low, your progesterone levels are even lower, and not enough to adequately oppose estrogen. Notice in the graph on page 225 how at age 35 estrogen and progesterone are balanced. In your 50s, both hormones drop (and go a little haywire during peri-menopause), but progesterone drops so much more than estrogen. At age 55, there is no balance; there is much less progesterone compared to estrogen, setting the stage for estrogen dominance.

So yes, it's absolutely possible to have estrogen dominance in menopause, and that's why the Estrogen Reset Foundation Protocol will benefit peri-menopausal, menopausal, even postmenopausal women.

and estrogen dominance is also linked with an increased cancer risk. Thyroid, ovarian, uterine, and estrogen receptor positive (ER+) breast cancer are common symptoms of estrogen dominance.

The Symptoms of Low Progesterone

Low progesterone may be one cause of estrogen dominance (Scenario 3) so it's worth familiarizing yourself with the symptoms of low progesterone, too. Women with low progesterone will have issues with falling and staying asleep, feel anxious a lot of the time, experience irregular menstrual cycles, and may struggle to conceive. Low progesterone also puts you at higher risk for miscarriage or pre-term delivery, because the hormone helps maintain the pregnancy. The symptoms are the same as estrogen dominance, plus:

- insomnia
- waking in the middle of the night
- infertility
- miscarriages in the first trimester
- mid-cycle spotting
- anxiety and restlessness
- mood swings

Estrogen Dominance and Autoimmune Diseases

Women are more likely to develop an autoimmune disease. There is a hypothesis that this is due to the fluctuations in our hormones. Excess estrogen is inflammatory

It's as if inflammation has blocked the door

_____

and can aggravate an autoimmune condition. If you have an autoimmune condition, it's another good reason to address estrogen dominance and lower your inflammation.

The Estrogen Dominance Quiz

To help you tune into your symptoms and determine if you have estrogen dominance or low progesterone, I've created the following quiz.

Part 1. Which symptoms are you currently experiencing?

Y   N
☐   ☐   Headaches, especially around your period?

Y   N
☐   ☐   Ovarian cysts or polyps?

Y   N
☐   ☐   Fibroids?

Y   N
☐   ☐   Breast lumps or fibrocystic breasts?

Y   N
☐   ☐   Endometriosis?

Y   N
☐   ☐   Itchy or restless legs, especially at night?

Y   N
☐   ☐   Heavy or painful periods?

Y   N
☐   ☐   Bloating, especially in the belly and ankle area and/or water retention?

Y N
☐ ☐ Irregular periods and/or cycles that became more frequent as you age?

Y N
☐ ☐ Hot flashes?

Y N
☐ ☐ Irritability and/or anxiety?

Y N
☐ ☐ Difficulty falling and/or staying asleep?

Y N
☐ ☐ Dry skin or skin that has lost its fullness?

Y N
☐ ☐ Spider or varicose veins?

Y N
☐ ☐ Cellulite?

Y N
☐ ☐ Fat around your hips?

Y N
☐ ☐ Melasma (facial brown skin discoloration)?

Part 2. Which symptoms are you currently experiencing?

Y N
☐ ☐ Heavy menstrual bleeding?

Y N
☐ ☐ Irritability and mood swings?

Y N
☐ ☐ Anxiety?

Y N
☐ ☐ Feeling unsettled?

Y N
☐ ☐ Heavy bleeding or postmenopausal bleeding?

Y N
☐ ☐ Crying spells for no good reason?

Y N
☐ ☐ Can't fall asleep or stay asleep?

Y N
☐ ☐ Infertility or subfertility?

Y N
☐ ☐ Miscarriages in the first trimester?

Y N
☐ ☐ Mid-cycle spotting?

Reading Your Results

Part 1. If you answered yes to more than three questions, there is a good chance that you have estrogen dominance.

Part 2. If you answered yes to more than three questions, there is a good chance that you have low progesterone.

Lab Testing

Do you need to order labs? Only you can decide whether or not lab testing is right for you at this time.

If you've taken the Estrogen Dominance Quiz and it's likely you have either estrogen dominance or low progesterone, you may have all of the information you need right now to know the Foundation Protocol is the appropriate next step for you. Your answers to the quiz give you a handy way to identify your symptoms and notice how they are improving over the course of the protocol. If you implement the protocol and don't see the improvements you hoped for, consider testing to get a more specific sense of what's going on.

Order labs as a first step if you want to identify your baseline hormone levels before the start of the program. Do the labs again after the protocol to see what's changed. It can be very encouraging to have absolute proof in the numbers that you're moving in a positive direction and see the "before" and "after" in black and white. If this appeals to you, consider testing. I also recommend testing if you're suffering from many different symptoms, have a history of estrogenic cancer such as breast, ovarian, uterine, or thyroid, or you've tried many different ways to resolve your symptoms but are still struggling.

For the tests I suggest, please go to Recommended Lab Tests.

Hormones don't work in isolation. They work together and influence each other and other bodily systems, such as your gut, liver, and blood sugar regulation. For example, have you noticed stress makes your symptoms worse? That's because cortisol, the hormone your body releases to deal with stress, slows down our ability to get rid of excess estrogen, exacerbating estrogen dominance. Cortisol and each of the other hormones we'll cover in this chapter play a role in the symptoms you are experiencing—and in resolving them.

ORDER LABS IF YOU

- want a baseline, before and after doing the Foundation Protocol

- are suffering from many symptoms

- have a history of estrogenic cancers (breast, ovaries, uterus, thyroid)

- have tried to resolve your symptoms in many ways and are still struggling

Other Hormones and Their Role in Estrogen Dominance

Hormones are tiny chemical messengers that regulate nearly everything that happens in your body: growth, temperature, hunger, mood, sleep, libido, metabolism, and reproduction. Mainly produced by a network of endocrine glands, including the pituitary, pancreas, adrenals, thyroid, ovaries, and pineal gland, some hormones can be produced by excess or visceral fat cells. Hormones are released directly into the bloodstream then carried to the organs and tissues of the body to perform their functions. To enter a cell, each hormone must bind with a specific hormone receptor, like a key fitting a lock.

Key Hormone-Producing Glands

Thyroid Gland. Your body's gas pedal, the thyroid gland produces hormones that are responsible for your metabolism, conversion of fat to energy, body temperature, mental functions, and hair/skin quality. An underactive thyroid (hypothyroid) is frequently present in those with estrogen dominance. This is because most cases of hypothyroidism are the result of an autoimmune disease, when your body's immune system attacks the thyroid, such as Hashimoto's Thyroiditis. Excess estrogen is highly inflammatory and fires up the immune system's response.

Adrenal Glands. The adrenals are responsible for producing hormones that manage the stress response, regulate sugar levels, the immune system, water retention, and blood pressure. Cortisol is one of the main hormones produced by the adrenals.

Ovaries. Our prime reproductive glands, the ovaries produce eggs for fertilization and the reproductive hormones estrogen and progesterone. In menopausal women, the ovaries stop producing these hormones.

Steroid Hormones. Steroid hormones are made from cholesterol, a waxy, fat-like substance found in all cells of the body. Low HDL cholesterol can cause low steroid hormones in both women and men.

Pregnenolone. Produced in the adrenals, sex organs, brain, and spinal cord, pregnenolone is critically important as the source of several other steroid hormones: progesterone, cortisol, DHEA, testosterone, and estrogen.

Progesterone. As the name implies, progesterone is a "pro-gestation" hormone, which allows women to conceive and maintain a full-term pregnancy. It is essential in non-pregnant women, too, helping you to stay calm, clearheaded, fall asleep, and feel balanced. It is produced by the corpus luteum of the ovary during the menstrual cycle, and the adrenals when the ovaries are missing or have ceased production after menopause. Progesterone and estrogen are like two dance partners. A good balance between these two is vital. Low progesterone contributes to estrogen dominance.

Cortisol. Produced by the adrenals, this hormone influences many of the changes that occur in the body in response to emotional, physical, spiritual, or toxic stress. In times of high stress, the body will "steal" pregnenolone to make cortisol instead of progesterone. With less progesterone available, we end up with estrogen dominance. Cortisol can also block progesterone receptors and slow down our ability to get rid of excess estrogens.

DHEA. Produced by the adrenals, DHEA is converted by the body into testosterone and all three forms of estrogens. DHEA levels in the body begin to decrease after age 30 and decrease more quickly in women. DHEA is often touted as the "anti-aging" hormone because both testosterone and estrogen are critical hormones for women to feel physically strong and mentally sharp, in addition to having their joints and vaginas lubricated. Too much DHEA, especially when supplementing, can contribute to estrogen dominance and high testosterone.

Testosterone. The primary male sex hormone is also necessary, in smaller amounts, for women to feel and look good. Produced in the ovary and the adrenal glands, testosterone gets converted to all three estrogens, so adequate amounts of this hormone are necessary to maintain optimal estrogen levels. Women with high testosterone levels (and often PCOS – Polycystic Ovary Syndrome) can have estrogen dominance, too.

Estrogen. More accurately a group of steroid hormones as there are more than one type of estrogen, these are the primary female sex hormones. They are major players in our menstrual cycle and reproductive health as well as giving us breasts, a widened pelvis, and an increased amount of body fat, thighs, and hip region. But estrogen is responsible for so much more than sexual development and fertility. It plays an important role in bone health, helps protect against heart disease, and affects your mood. Estrogen impacts so many more areas of your health than you probably realize, which is why an estrogen imbalance causes a miserable cascade of symptoms.

If you are still cycling, your estrogen is primarily created by the ovaries and adrenals. It can also be produced by visceral fat, and in small amounts, by the liver and breasts. In menopausal and post-menopausal women, the ovaries stop

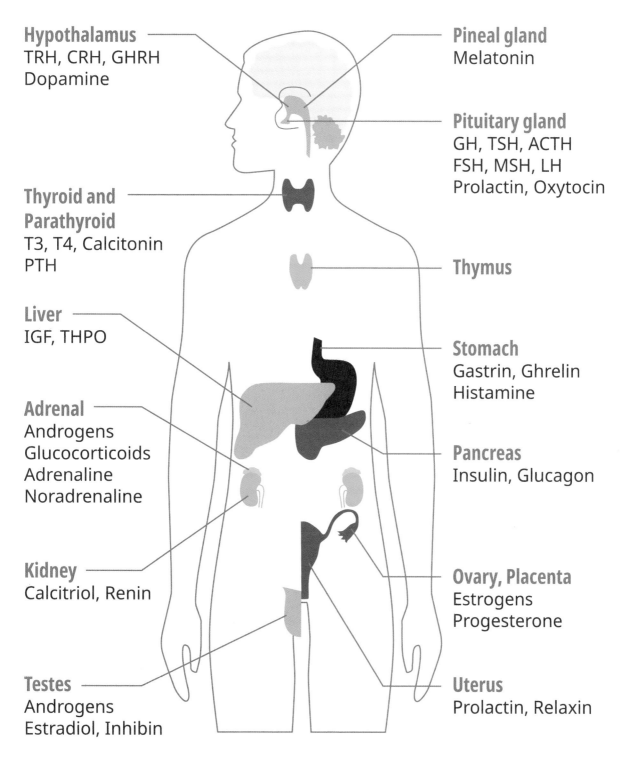

Hypothalamus
TRH, CRH, GHRH
Dopamine

Pineal gland
Melatonin

Pituitary gland
GH, TSH, ACTH
FSH, MSH, LH
Prolactin, Oxytocin

Thyroid and Parathyroid
T3, T4, Calcitonin
PTH

Thymus

Liver
IGF, THPO

Stomach
Gastrin, Ghrelin
Histamine

Adrenal
Androgens
Glucocorticoids
Adrenaline
Noradrenaline

Pancreas
Insulin, Glucagon

Kidney
Calcitriol, Renin

Ovary, Placenta
Estrogens
Progesterone

Testes
Androgens
Estradiol, Inhibin

Uterus
Prolactin, Relaxin

producing estrogen and modest amounts are produced by the adrenals, liver, breasts, and visceral fat.

There are three major forms of estrogen:

- Estrone (E1) is the "weaker" estrogen that is higher in pregnant and menopausal women.
- Estradiol (E2) is the strongest of the three estrogens and the predominant form in women of reproductive age who are not pregnant. It is responsible for maturing and maintaining the reproductive system and much of what happens during menstruation. An excess of estradiol causes estrogen dominance. Often called the "dirty" estrogen, it is also the leading cause of estrogenic breast, ovarian, uterine, thyroid, and lung (in nonsmokers) cancers.
- Estriol (E3) is the "protective" estrogen, released in large amounts by the placenta during pregnancy. It is very low in non-pregnant women, yet an important form of estrogen to have. Supplemental estriol has been shown to maintain healthy/youthful skin, keep the vagina moist/lubricated, and prevent hot flashes/night sweats. Estriol also plays an anti-carcinogenic role.

Because there are estrogen receptors throughout the body, low estrogen causes a wide-range of symptoms (think classic menopause), including forgetfulness, poor memory, depression, night sweats, hot flashes, leaky, overactive bladder, insomnia, and vaginal dryness. With high levels, you're prone to the many symptoms of estrogen dominance.

Nonsteroid Hormones

Nonsteroid hormones are made of amino acids. Here are a few of the most important ones that can have an indirect impact on estrogen dominance.

Thyroxine (T4) and Triiodothyronine (T3). The T4 produced by the thyroid can't be directly used by the body until it's converted, in the gut and liver, into the active T3 hormone. The amount of energy you have, your body fat, mental alertness, the quality of your hair, skin, and nails depend on the availability of the T3 hormone. Too much estrogen can stop the conversion of T4 into T3 and cause the liver to produce high levels of thyroid binding globulin (TBG), which as the name suggests, binds the thyroid hormone and decreases the amount of thyroid hormone that can be utilized by the body. Both scenarios result in the symptoms of hypothyroidism, including fatigue, sensitivity to cold, dry skin, and unexplained weight gain.

Insulin. A hormone made by the pancreas, insulin sweeps blood sugar (glucose) from the blood and delivers it to cells for energy. When a person eats a daily diet full of sugar and processed carbohydrates (such as flours, cereals, and packaged foods) the insulin receptors in the cells eventually shut down and won't accept insulin. This is called "insulin resistance" and 30% of the American population suffers from it. High levels of insulin cause the conversion of testosterone into excessive estradiol, promoting estrogen dominance. On the other hand, estrogen dominance makes the insulin receptors less susceptible to insulin.

Testing Methods

Urine/DUTCH. Urine is the gold standard for testing the steroid hormones progesterone, estrogen, DHEA, testosterone, and cortisol. The DUTCH (Dried Urine Test for Comprehensive Hormones) test, developed by Precision Analytical, provides a comprehensive assessment of these steroid hormones. It will tell you how your liver is breaking down estrogen so you'll know which metabolites you're producing, how you're converting testosterone to estrogen, give a very clear picture of your adrenal health, and so much more. The DUTCH tells a big story with a lot of detail (you'll need a doctor to help you interpret the results), providing insight into what is going on with your hormones.

Blood. Using blood to test the steroid hormones estrogen, progesterone, testosterone, DHEA, and cortisol is misleading and inaccurate. Urine gives a much more accurate and complete picture of these hormones. Blood testing doesn't allow you to see levels for more than a brief moment in time and not the ebb and flow through the day. It also only measures the total hormones in your bloodstream but not the "free" values that show how much is actually available for the body to use. Inflammation could be blocking the receptor so even though you have the hormone available, it can't be used. This is why a hormone panel from blood may look okay even though you are miserable with symptoms.

Blood testing is ideal for testing blood sugar levels (fasting glucose, insulin, and A1C), FSH, LH, thyroid hormones, and antibodies (such as in Hashimoto's).

Saliva. Saliva testing has gained in popularity as it's easy to collect a sample and noninvasive.

I appreciate saliva testing for its accurate reading of progesterone levels (something that urine won't show). Saliva tests are limited because they don't show the estrogen metabolites or the "dirty" estrogens. At the time of writing this book, there is no lab that combines the results on urine and saliva testing in one comprehensive hormone test.

How to Order Tests

You can order many labs yourself. You do not need to order them through a doctor unless you live in certain limiting states (at the time of writing this book NY, NJ, MD, and RI do not allow non-physicians to order lab tests). To get the most from your test results, especially the DUTCH test, I recommend working with a functional medical doctor. See Interpreting Your Results, below, for more.

Visit www.hormonesbalance.com/oed/testing to self-order DUTCH or saliva testing online.

Interpreting Your Results

Working with a professional to interpret your results will help you get the most out of them and craft the most beneficial healing plan. It is essential for reading a DUTCH test as it is complex and the results are meant to be interpreted by trained practitioners.

A note here on "normal" ranges. Conventional medical lab ranges vary from lab to lab and are based on the typical results found in the population the lab serves. These ranges may be "normal" for the testing population but aren't necessarily ideal for good health. Optimal ranges are functional medicine ranges that are associated with the lowest risk of disease and mortality.

Those are the ranges we want to be looking at and a functional medical practitioner will be able to read your results with those ranges in mind. Also, remember that what's "normal" for your female friend may not be best for you. Your body is unique. Listen to your symptoms to find the levels that are ideal for you.

Finding Balance

Optimal health means having hormones in balance, not too much or too little of any hormone. Now that you have a better sense of what estrogen dominance is and the major hormonal players that contribute to it, let's look at why these hormones can become imbalanced in the first place.

Optimal health means
having hormones in
balance, not too much or
too little of any hormone.

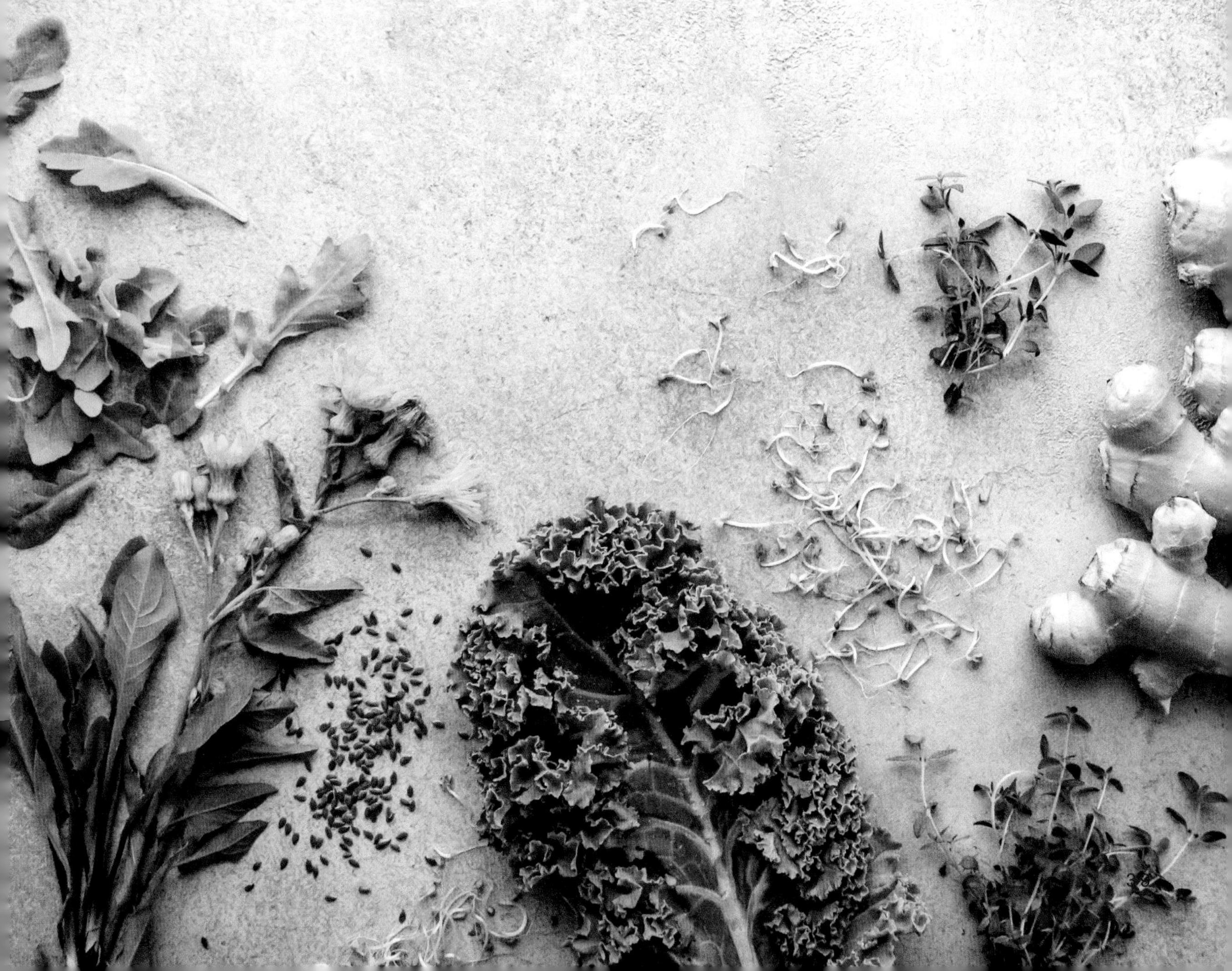

———————————————

Chapter 2

Why This is Happening

Causes of Estrogen Dominance

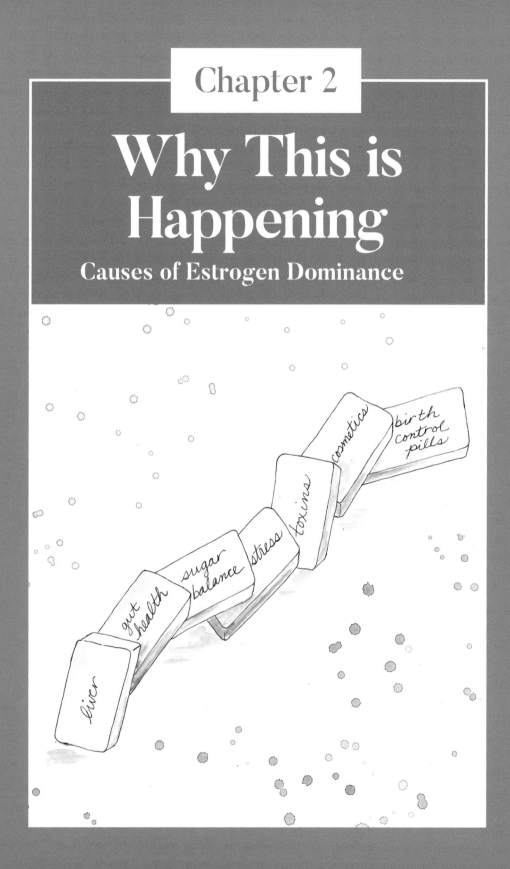

Estrogen dominance is a complex condition with several potential causes. Some are internal, meaning your physiology or your body's internal workings are contributing to your symptoms. Other factors are external, originating from outside of your body to cause hormonal imbalance. Most likely, a combination of internal and external factors are at work. Knowing where your estrogen dominance is coming from will help you reverse it and manage it for life. Let's take a look at some of the most common contributors to estrogen dominance to see what might be going on with you.

Internal Factors

Sluggish liver. Remember Scenario 2, the Ugly Breakup way to experience estrogen dominance? That's when the liver breaks down estradiol and estrone into too many potentially harmful "dirty" estrogens. When I was first diagnosed with estrogen dominance and my functional doctor asked about my liver, I was stunned that there was a connection. And yes, a sluggish liver is the main culprit, creating too many of the "dirty" estrogens, then struggling to bind them up and send them on their way to the gut for evacuation through your bowel movements. Your liver plays a critical role in estrogen detoxification and when it's not working optimally, either because of too many toxins or poor nutrition, your "dirty" estrogen levels will rise. This may also explain why estrogen dominance happens later in life (not always, but often)—when your liver gets taxed and becomes more toxic as we age. This explains why in your 20s you could down five tequilas, get up the following morning to go to class, and now you are hungover after two shots. The good news: There are a ton of things you can do. More on that, soon.

Poor gut microflora. A healthy gut needs a diverse assortment of bacterial microflora to properly support your immune system, absorb nutrients from food, and produce certain vitamins. A specific type of microflora called the estrobolome is in charge of metabolizing all of the various forms of estrogen. If your gut microflora is out of balance and there aren't enough beneficial estrobolome bacteria to break down estrogen so the body can dispose of it, too many "dirty" estrogens may end up back in your bloodstream, causing estrogen dominance.

Not enough fiber. We need to consume at least 20 to 30 grams of fiber each day, but most Americans only get about 15 grams per day, if that. More specifically, The U.S. Food and Nutrition Board of the Institute of Medicine recommends that women under 50 have a fiber intake of 25 grams per day and those over 50 consume 21 grams per day. The lack of fiber in our diets can lead to serious health consequences, including estrogen dominance.

Insoluble fiber, the kind found in most plant-based foods, including cruciferous vegetables, flax seed, oat bran, the hull of whole grains, beans, legumes, and sweet potatoes, does not dissolve in water. It stays intact throughout the digestive system and "sweeps" the colon, partly evacuating metabolized or "dirty" estrogens and preventing estrogen reabsorption. Eating enough insoluble fiber to have good, regular bowel movements is essential for maintaining estrogen balance.

Soluble fiber, the type of fiber that attracts and dissolves in water, turns into a gel-like substance in the colon. It helps to regulate the rate of digestion and prevents the reabsorption of estrogen, mitigating estrogen dominance. Soluble fiber is found in flax seed (yes, it has both kinds of fiber), apples, pears, asparagus, leeks, oats, and mushrooms.

In addition, all types of fiber feed the beneficial bacteria that maintain the mucosal layer lining the small intestine, which in turn decides which molecules enter into our bloodstream, and which stay out. When that barrier is compromised, chronic inflammation and a disruption of the gut microflora may occur. Both can lead to estrogen dominance.

Too much sugar. Sugar is linked to so many chronic conditions, from obesity to heart disease, diabetes, inflammation, and nonalcoholic fatty liver disease, it's no wonder it's called the White Death—and is a major cause of estrogen dominance. A diet high in sugar causes a cascade of troubles for your hormones. It elevates your blood sugar and insulin, paving the way for insulin resistance and estrogen dominance. Sugar is also a classic trigger for the release of cortisol. Too much cortisol not only promotes inflammation, it can also reduce the amount of progesterone available to balance out estrogen, contributing to Scenario 3, Unbalanced Partners. Your gut microflora takes a hit from too much sugar, taxing their ability to metabolize estrogen. And if that wasn't enough, all of this sugar turns to belly fat that further secretes estrogen. There's more, but what you need to know here is this: Sugar spells disaster for your hormones.

Belly fat. Belly fat, the visceral fat stored inside your abdomen and around your liver, stomach, and intestines, is often referred to as "active fat" because it produces hormones, such as estrogen, and specifically estradiol, the dominating and potentially harmful estrogen. The more belly fat you have, the more estrogen is being released by these cells and contributing to estrogen dominance. Belly fat also increases your risk for insulin resistance, another contributor to estrogen dominance.

Stress and trauma. Stress is a big one. It might sound cliché to say, "Oh, stress is a killer," but on a biochemical level, it is. When you're stressed out, you produce a high amount of cortisol to help you handle it. If you remain chronically stressed, your body will prioritize the conversion of pregnenolone into cortisol instead of progesterone and other sex hormones. This is called the "pregnenolone steal," and it means more cortisol and less progesterone available to offset estrogen. Many women who draw a health timeline notice that the majority of health problems started manifesting soon after a stressful or traumatic event. Women who experienced trauma are more likely to develop breast cancer (most breast cancers are estrogenic).

Too much testosterone is being converted to estrogen. All estrogens are created from testosterone in a process called aromatization. The enzyme aromatase is responsible for converting testosterone into estradiol. If too much testosterone is being converted, you could experience estrogen dominance because of an abundance of estradiol, the "bad guy" in Scenario 1, Too Much

The more belly fat you have, the more estrogen is being released by these cells and contributing to estrogen dominance.

of a Bad Guy. Insulin resistance increases the activity of aromatase and since aromatase lives in your fat cells, additional belly fat will contribute to the production of more estradiol.

No gallbladder or insufficient bile. We tend to overlook the gallbladder, but it's an important organ, especially for hormone balance. Sitting under the liver on the right side of the ribcage, the gallbladder stores bile, which is used to digest fats and help the liver excrete hormones including excess "dirty" estrogens. This explains why women who have their gallbladders removed often suffer from symptoms of estrogen dominance a few months after surgery. Most doctors won't mention this possible side effect. Even if you still have your gallbladder, you may not be making sufficient quantities of bile and can develop various seemingly unrelated health issues. Read more on bile and how to improve it in chapter 5.

Nutritional deficiencies. Your endocrine glands need raw ingredients in the form of vitamins and minerals in order to produce hormones. In the case of progesterone, we need vitamins A, B_6, C, and zinc to produce sufficient amounts, and oppose estrogen. As a society, we are collectively dealing with poor diets (many people don't even realize it), depleted soil that has lost the majority of its nutrients, and compromised digestion, which can result in poor absorption of nutrients.

Genetic predisposition. The expression of your genes can be turned on and off by your environment. Some genes can set the stage for developing estrogen dominance. But remember, the gene is like a loaded gun that you inherited— something has to pull the trigger. The field of epigenetics studies the influence of nutrients found in food and supplements, reduction of toxic lead, inflammation, and lifestyle choices on the expression of the genes. So, let me repeat:

Just because you have a genetic predisposition doesn't mean you will inevitably develop it, and I'm a perfect example of that. Even though I have a high genetic predisposition to estrogen-receptor positive (ER+) breast cancer, I have embraced lifestyle changes so cancer does not become my destiny (like it has in my family). The Estrogen Reset Foundation Protocol is designed to create the ideal environment for your body, cells, and genes so you can reset your estrogen pathways and support the beneficial breakdown of estrogen even if your genetics suggest differently.

These are some of the genes that can impact estrogen dominance and your symptoms:

COMT. The COMT gene provides instructions for making an enzyme that helps you break down neurotransmitters such as dopamine, epinephrine, and norepinephrine while ensuring estrogen is being processed through a protective pathway. As a side note, when you are stressed, your body will make more epinephrine and norepinephrine, which makes it harder for the slow COMT enzyme to break down these hormones. As you know, we need estrogen, but we don't want to hold on to excess estrogen nor do we want the unhealthy or cancer-promoting "dirty" estrogens. Unfortunately, my COMT gene codes for an enzyme that slowly breaks down my estrogens compared to the average woman. This is one of the reasons I experience chronically elevated estrogen levels. A lot of women who struggle with estrogen dominance have the slow COMT enzyme. Estrogen also acts on the COMT enzyme. So for those of you with the fast COMT enzyme and high estrogen levels, your body may behave as if you have a slow COMT enzyme.

MAOA. This gene helps to process several major neurotransmitters, including serotonin, dopamine, and norepinephrine. Women often have lower levels of serotonin, the "happy" calming hormone, with the gene that codes for the fast MAOA enzyme. When you break down your serotonin faster, you may be more prone to mood challenges, including mood swings and irritability. Like COMT, excess estrogen can also slow the MAOA enzyme, which can lead to increased anxiety and worry, even insomnia.

MTHFR. The MTHFR gene codes for an enzyme that creates a type of folate your cells can use. Folate plays an important role in a chemical process called methylation. It is essential for hundreds of functions in your body, including clearing toxins from the liver. Methylation is a process where your body adds methyl (CH3) to different nutrients, DNA, and estrogens. With folate, the addition of a methyl group takes folate from an inactive form to an active form. Folate and other B vitamins are critical for supporting detoxification. So if you don't provide the right nutrients to your body or your body cannot create the optimal version of the nutrient, your body is less efficient at this conversion and you may struggle to get rid of estrogen. Methyl groups are also very important for protecting your DNA. When your cells are copying DNA, the "copy enzyme" is designed to skip over areas with methyl groups and not copy that section of your DNA. Research suggests that having enough methyl groups in your body and on your DNA is important to help protect your body against cancer.

VDR. The VDR is a gene that codes for instructions for the vitamin D receptor protein. This protein joins together with calcitriol which is the active form of Vitamin D. Together this complex will signal other vitamin D genes to ensure you absorb your minerals such as calcium and phosphate. Poor absorption and low levels of vitamin D can compromise your immune system, make

you prone to mood issues, and weaken bones. Some studies suggest that vitamin D may also help maintain estrogen balance by reducing the amount of testosterone being converted into estrogen through aromatization and lowering estrogen's effects.

Other genes that work in the estrogen metabolism pathway. CYP1A1 encodes an enzyme that starts the estrogen breakdown process in the liver. Once estrogens have been converted by **COMT, SULT,** and **UGT** enzymes, estrogens get converted into the final form that can be put into the urine and removed from the body.

To order a genetic test to help you understand your ability to metabolize estrogen, please see Recommended Lab Tests on page 362.

External Factors

Xenoestrogens. You probably don't think twice about putting on makeup, applying lotion, cleaning your house with "nice-smelling" products, sipping hot coffee through a plastic lid, buying new furniture, or touching that receipt that the cashier just handed you. All these products have one thing in common: xenoestrogens, man-made chemicals that resemble estrogens without doing the work of true estrogens. They include BPA, phthalates, and parabens, which wreak havoc in your hormone balance. They create three problems (that we know of). First, they mimic estrogen, but unlike the real estrogen, they bind or block a receptor, preventing the cell from functioning properly. This is particularly detrimental to hormone sensitive organs like the uterus and the breast, the immune and neurological systems, as well as human development. Second, xenoestrogens cause DNA damage on the estrogen receptor, which has been linked to numerous cancers,

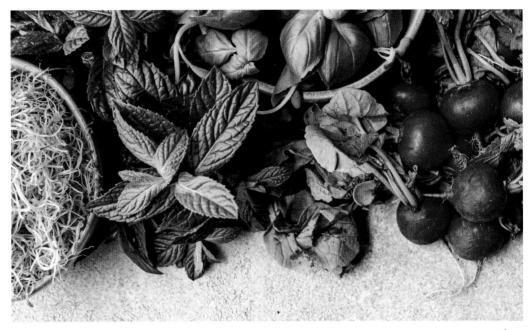

including breast cancer. Third, the body regulates the amount of estrogen it needs through intricate biochemical messaging pathways. When xenoestrogens enter the body, they increase the total amount of estrogen but the body isn't able to excrete them because the messaging pathways aren't functioning as they should. Xenoestrogens are not biodegradable, so they are stored in our fat cells. Buildup of xenoestrogens has been indicated in many conditions, including breast, prostate, and testicular cancer, obesity, infertility, endometriosis, early onset puberty, miscarriages, and diabetes.

Xenoestrogens are found everywhere nowadays: plastic bottles (the highest levels of xenoestrogens are found when heated up), mainstream makeup and skincare products (the leading culprits are the large multinational companies you see advertising on TV and in fashion magazines), household cleaning supplies, drinking water, new furniture, and cashier's receipts (the ink is very high in xenoestrogens). Avoiding these things is difficult, but it isn't impossible and later on I will share how I do it.

Phytoestrogens (the bad ones!). Phytoestrogens are foods containing a compound similar to the estrogen made by your body. Those found naturally in minimally processed plant foods, such as flax seeds, tempeh, edamame, soy sauce (fermented soy), and many other fruits and vegetables, are the good kind. It's the bad kind we want to avoid. Those are found in highly processed foods, like soy-made products and other imitation meats, conventionally raised meat, and dairy. These animals are usually fed a diet dominated by soy, and the phytoestrogens get passed along to us.

Birth Control Pills. Birth control pills are made with synthetic estrogen to disrupt your hormones and prevent ovulation and pregnancy. They work by keeping estrogen levels consistently high, essentially promoting estrogen dominance. In addition, your body doesn't recognize or break down synthetic hormones in the same way as the hormones it produces naturally or bioidentical versions, adding to the hormonal havoc. Women with the above mentioned genetic variants may be especially prone to experiencing symptoms of estrogen dominance when on birth control pills.

Synthetic Hormone Replacement Therapy (HRT). *Synthetic* hormone replacement therapy adds man-made hormones, most often estrogen and progesterone, to your body. These hormones have a slightly different chemical structure than natural hormones and your body metabolizes them differently. Piling on more of this kind of estrogen can lead to estrogen dominance and if you are already estrogen dominant, exacerbate your symptoms. Remember, you can be in menopause with low estrogen levels and still be estrogen dominant. (See the box on page 30.) Synthetic hormones are not the same as bioidentical ones. Bioidentical hormones are exact replicas of your body's natural hormones and are my preference. They are derived from soy or yams and modified in a lab to fit our cells perfectly. There is no research or evidence that bioidentical hormones cause cancers.

IF YOU ARE TAKING BIRTH CONTROL PILLS OR SYNTHETIC HRT

Birth control pills work by disrupting your hormones to suppress ovulation. They also harm your gut, rob you of essential nutrients, and mess with your thyroid hormones. Whether containing a combination of synthetic estrogen and progesterone (progestin) or only progestin, birth control pills contribute to estrogen dominance and you should be getting off of them. *Beyond the Pill* by Dr. Jolene Brighten is an excellent resource for transitioning off of the pill safely and with minimal side effects and finding contraception alternatives.

Did you start taking the birth control pill for a reason other than contraception, like to treat an irregular or incredibly long and heavy period or to relieve PMS? You're not alone. That's the story for most women. But here's the reality: The pill is just covering up your symptoms. Having a natural cycle is part of being a healthy woman and it doesn't have to be terrible and painful. If you've suffered in the past, it's likely due to estrogen dominance and the Foundation Protocol will help you address it.

Hormone Replacement Therapy (HRT) is a topic that often causes a lot of confusion. I'll explain the important differences between synthetic and bioidentical hormones (derived from yams or soy) in chapter 3. For now, I want you to know that I only recommend bioidentical hormones, if any at all. If you are taking any type of synthetic hormone, such as Climara, Provera, or Premarin, I encourage you to work with a functional medical doctor, naturopath, or nurse practitioner to discuss more natural alternatives. If you want to supplement with hormones, only use bioidenticals.

Bottom line: To address estrogen dominance and regain your health, you need to get off birth control pills, and synthetic HRT, as well as implement the Estrogen Reset Foundation Protocol.

Taking Control

It's no wonder so many women experience estrogen dominance given how many internal and external factors make us vulnerable. It can seem like a lot to take in but while several things could be going on to drive your estrogen dominance, there are only a few key areas—your gut, liver, and blood sugar—we need a fix to address all of them. And we can do so using natural solutions.

While several things could be going on to drive your estrogen dominance, there are only a few key areas—your gut, liver, and blood sugar—we need a fix to address all of them.

Chapter 3

What You Can Do About It

Natural Solutions for Estrogen Dominance

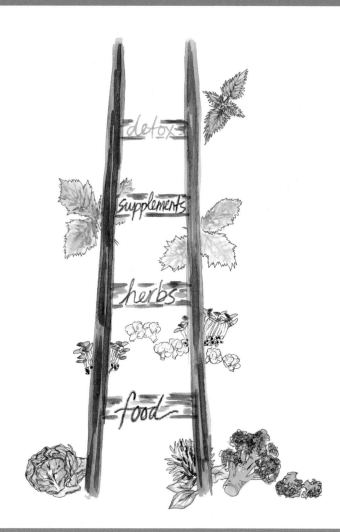

The great news is that estrogen dominance can be reversed naturally. And that's why I created the Estrogen Reset Foundation Protocol: to give you all of the tools you need and a clear, step-by-step plan to remove all of the obstacles for your body to heal and reset your estrogen. We're going to be using mostly food, herbs, and supplements to help you get there, freeing you from all of the symptoms. Most importantly, you will be future-proofing yourself so you never have to live in a state of fear, doubt, and confusion again.

The Tools: Follow the Healing Pyramid

This Healing Pyramid illustrates the tools we have in our toolbox for creating hormonal balance and healing. My motto is: Food is first and always. Herbs are often. Supplements sometimes. Medications only when needed.

Food

At the base of the pyramid is food. It is your foundation. It can move the needle on your health in a big way. I'm not saying that food is going to resolve all of your medical problems, but food is going to be fundamental on your healing journey. No amount of supplements will heal you if you don't adjust your diet.

Not long ago, I bought a beautiful house in Colorado in the Rocky Mountains just outside of Boulder. I fell in love with the views as soon as I walked inside, but the home is perched on the side of a mountain and that worried me. Before I purchased it, I made sure to have an engineer check to make sure the foundation was strong. What good is a beautiful home with a weak foundation? Your health is the same way. It needs a strong foundation of nutrient-dense, nourishing,

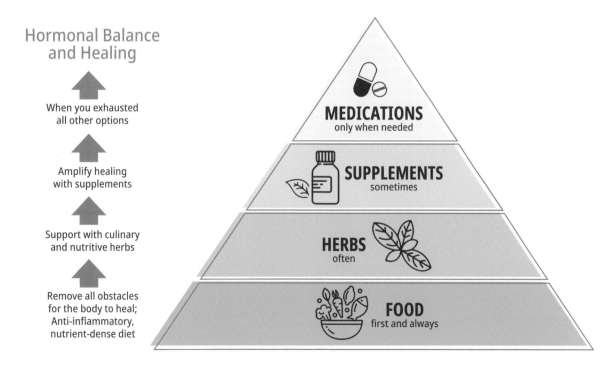

Hormonal Balance and Healing

When you exhausted all other options

Amplify healing with supplements

Support with culinary and nutritive herbs

Remove all obstacles for the body to heal; Anti-inflammatory, nutrient-dense diet

MEDICATIONS only when needed

SUPPLEMENTS sometimes

HERBS often

FOOD first and always

anti-inflammatory foods. In the Estrogen Reset Foundation Protocol and 28-Day Meal Plan we'll focus on:

- **Whole foods.** It's really simple. The next time you go grocery shopping, make sure 80% of your cart consists of fresh foods instead of packaged, processed items.
- **Organic, non-GMO foods, including meat.** If you think that organic food is just hype or a "hippie thing" to do, think again. "Conventionally" grown food contains a high amount of pesticides, fertilizers, growth hormones, and antibiotics that contribute to endocrine disruption in every way you can imagine.
- **Anti-inflammatory diet.** This way of eating cuts out the well-documented trigger foods: gluten, dairy, soy, eggs, corn, and nightshades; also limiting sugar. When you eat inflammatory foods, you add fuel to the fire of your hormonal imbalances. These foods compromise your small and large intestines, making the absorption of nutrients and supplements limited or sometimes outright harmful. In order to heal, it's best to avoid these foods. Give it a try and you will feel a difference. You may decide to add some of these foods back into your diet after the Foundation Protocol, but many women feel so amazing without them that they decide it's better to stay away.

Throughout the protocol, you'll discover an abundance of healthy, delicious, satisfying foods that will give your body all the resources it needs to heal while keeping you feeling full and nourished.

And don't worry. The protocol is designed to make eating this way effortless. There's nothing you need to figure out. All you have to do is follow the Estrogen Reset 28-Day Meal Plan. It is completely dialed-in for you, no guesswork required. Use the shopping lists and meal plan to build a strong food foundation with ease and confidence.

Herbs

Next are herbs. Culinary and nutritive herbs flood your cells with precious phytonutrients and can therefore help restore hormonal balance. Throughout the protocol, with the 28-Day Meal Plan, we'll be gifting and flooding the body with an abundance of herbs to restore balance and ease symptoms. Some of them may be familiar to you (ginger, rosemary, turmeric), while others may be new (chaste tree, raspberry leaf, milk thistle). I'll explain their benefits and share how they can be added to your daily diet or used to make simple salves, tinctures, and infusions.

As a certified herbalist, using herbs to heal the body is close to my heart. But I know they only really work well, amplifying and speeding up healing, when the food foundation is strong. That's why they're the next level up from food on the Healing Pyramid. Herbs build on a strong food foundation.

Supplements

Supplements are up next and like herbs, they work best atop a strong food foundation. Supplements are powerful tools for bridging the gaps in our nutrition and speeding up our healing.

The simple fact is, we can't always get all of the nutrients we need from food. Take magnesium. It's a key nutrient in hormone production and detoxification, yet a vast majority of women are severely deficient. Initially, some women need as much as 1,200 mg of magnesium per day to replenish. To get that much with food, they would need to eat 2.5 cups of raw cacao or 31 avocados per day. Per day! Vitamin D_3 is another good example—with 70% of Americans being deficient, this vitamin-cum-hormone is essential in keeping your immune system strong, protecting your bones, and mitigating cancer risks. It's practically impossible to get it from food alone. That's where a supplement steps in. Now, that's a major gap. Other times, the gaps are subtle and our symptoms are our guide. Supplements play a critical role in this case, too.

As part of the protocol, I recommend Foundational Supplements, a core list of supplements I've found most amplify healing, as well as additional ones for more targeted support to consider.

Getting Started with Supplements

I'm often asked "How should I start with supplements? Which supplements should I take first?" It's tough for me to reply because there is no one-size-fits-all answer. Each situation is different. These are the best practices I recommend:

Start with the Foundational Supplements covered in chapter 7. These are the supplements most women need and benefit from over the long-term.

Add additional supplements as needed. Pay attention to the potential benefits of the supplement and trust your intuition. Try it for a few weeks to see if your symptoms improve. If they do, great. If not, stop that supplement and try another.

Selecting High-Quality Supplements

The U.S. Food and Drug Administration (FDA) does not have authority to review dietary supplement products for safety and effectiveness before they are marketed. Companies have been caught putting low-quality ingredients in their products, not meeting label claims, and using materials with high levels of heavy metals. How can a consumer trust an unreviewed product? The answer is to research the company and evaluate them based on these five rules:

Rule #1: Identify Who Owns the Company and Check the Ingredient List Often

Know who currently owns the company and monitor the supplement ingredients frequently. I have found that independently owned supplement companies are a safe bet. Unfortunately, they often get bought out by larger companies that change the supplement formulas to be better for their bottom line but not for your health. For example, Nestlé, a company with a track record of putting profits ahead of consumer interests, is now the owner of Pure Encapsulations, Douglas Labs, and Garden of Life. The ownership changes aren't publicized, so the majority of consumers continue trusting the products. Large corporations' core responsibility is to create returns for their shareholders, and not improve your health. I therefore recommend to check the ingredients of your favorite brands regularly to ensure that they remain unchanged. In most cases, products bought by large conglomerates get reformulated, and not to consumers' health benefit.

Rule #2: Note Certifications

Look for a company with full transparency and traceability, uses all non-GMO ingredients, and has one or, even better, both of these certifications from the National Sanitation Foundation (NSF):

1. NSF/ANSI 173: This NSF/American National Standard Institute (ANSI) certification helps confirm what's on the label is in the product and that the product contains no unsafe levels of contaminants such as heavy metals, pesticides and herbicides.

2. Good Manufacturing Practices (GMP) Registration: This doesn't apply to individual products but rather confirms that a manufacturer's production facility is observing the good manufacturing practices established for their industry such as in record keeping, personnel qualifications, sanitation and cleanliness, and equipment maintenance.

SUPPLEMENT QUALITY CHECKLIST

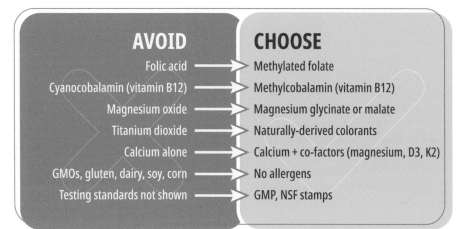

AVOID	CHOOSE
Folic acid →	Methylated folate
Cyanocobalamin (vitamin B12) →	Methylcobalamin (vitamin B12)
Magnesium oxide →	Magnesium glycinate or malate
Titanium dioxide →	Naturally-derived colorants
Calcium alone →	Calcium + co-factors (magnesium, D3, K2)
GMOs, gluten, dairy, soy, corn →	No allergens
Testing standards not shown →	GMP, NSF stamps

Rule #3: Know Which Ingredients the Product Does Not Contain

Pick supplements free of gluten, dairy, and GMOs. If intolerant or allergic, also avoid supplements containing soy, corn, peanuts, and yeast. Some of the dead giveaway ingredients you should never see in your supplements are: magnesium oxide (a cheap but ineffective and sometimes harmful form of magnesium), cyanocobalamin (a cheap but harmful form of vitamin B12), folic acid (a synthetic, poorly absorbable form of folate). Later on, I'll discuss what forms are safe and highly bioavailable for you to take. To avoid ingesting chemical solvents, such as the neurotoxin hexane, look for products processed through "supercritical extraction." Avoid titanium dioxide, a common colorant in supplements and cosmetics, recently classified as a possible carcinogen.

Rule #4: Make Sure the Product Does Not Contain Cheap Binders and Fillers

Choose "clean" products that have the nutrients in them you need to take and little to no low-cost fillers such as magnesium oxide or zinc oxide. These can dramatically reduce the bioavailability and absorption of supplements, while often causing gastrointestinal distress.

Rule #5: Pay Attention to Price Point

If a supplement from a reputable brand costs $30 and you just found a knock-off for $10, this should raise a red flag rather than create excitement. It's most likely the supplement is either made with inferior ingredients, is close to its expiration date, or is a fake (even if the label shows the reputable company logo). Fake supplements have become a problem, especially through online sales. This includes Amazon, which doesn't screen supplement sellers. Invest in yourself and quality supplements from reputable sources.

Medications/RX

Medications, at the very top of the pyramid, are used only when needed and when you have exhausted all other options. Certainly, there are times when you absolutely need medication and you should use them in coordination with your healthcare provider. And you know what? They will work better if you have a strong food foundation. That's absolutely true of the type of medication most relevant to this book and the kind I want to spend a little time on: supplemental hormones, more specifically, bioidentical hormones.

The difference between synthetic and bioidentical hormones. It's imperative for you to understand that all supplemental hormones are not the same. If you are interested in supplementing with hormones or your doctor has suggested you may benefit from supplemental hormones, you absolutely must pay attention to the kind of hormone on offer. Ask if it is synthetic or bioidentical. If you remember nothing else from this section, remember this: You want the answer to be *bioidentical.*

There is a big difference between synthetic hormones and bioidentical hormones. They are molecularly very different from each other and they cause very different results in women. Being unaware of the difference or how the difference impacts women's health is the source of so much of the fear and confusion around supplemental hormones. A lot of women hear hormones and they immediately think, *Oh, no. Not hormones. Those cause breast cancer!* And the reason they think this is because of one health study, the Women's Health Initiative (WHI).

The WHI was a randomized controlled government-funded trial designed to examine the long-term effects of hormone therapy—synthetic hormone therapy—on

ONLY CHOOSE BIOIDENTICAL, IF YOU DECIDE TO USE HORMONES

Bioidentical hormones, derived from yams or soy, have the same chemical structure as the hormones created by your body. Do *not* take synthetic hormones (Climara, Provera, Primarin, etc.), which do not have the same chemical structure as natural hormones and impact your body differently, leading to several potential health risks.

Some of the side effects of progestins (synthetic progesterone) include increased appetite, weight gain, fluid retention, irritability, depression, loss of energy, breast tenderness, and bloating. Progestins increase LDL (the "bad" cholesterol), decrease HDL (the "good" cholesterol), interfere with your body's own production of progesterone and don't help balance estrogen. Worse still, in numerous studies, progestins have been linked to breast cancers. None of these side effects have been identified in bioidentical progesterone.

over 27,000 postmenopausal women. In one clinical trial, women were given a combination of synthetic estrogen and progesterone (called progestin), while in another, synthetic estrogen alone. The combined trial was stopped early because of an increased risk of breast cancer, cardiovascular disease, and "more harm than benefit overall." The synthetic estrogen-only trial ended soon after because of an increased risk of stroke.

These are distressing findings and women are right to take them into account when thinking about hormone therapy. But, these studies were done with synthetic hormones, not bioidentical ones. Let me say it again: These negative outcomes are based on synthetic hormones, not bioidentical ones. If you are currently taking synthetic hormones, I encourage you to talk to your doctor about alternatives or switching to bioidenticals.

Here's the important difference between the two: Synthetic hormones mimic the natural hormones your body produces but have a slightly different chemical structure. Bioidentical hormones *have the same chemical structure as the hormones created by the human body*. They are not found in this form in nature but are made from yams and soy.

Now, you can't just eat soy or cook up a yam, eat it, and apply it to your skin while expecting results. Bioidentical hormones still have to be modified in a lab, but the significant point is that on the molecular level they are identical to our natural hormones and fit just as they do into our hormone receptors. If you want to supplement with hormones, only choose bioidentical ones.

The perfect candidate for supplementing with bioidentical hormones. Who should be supplementing? First and foremost, someone who has a strong food foundation, in addition to eating an anti-inflammatory and nutrient-dense diet. Then, you have:

- reduced your stress
- prioritized regular self-care and self-love
- tried supplements but are still symptomatic
- been going through a challenging time in life when extra support can help stabilize your symptoms
- had a hysterectomy (if one or both ovaries have been removed) and your body is adjusting to changing hormone levels

BIOIDENTICAL HORMONES

Progesterone, topically applied cream or oil

Estrogen (BiEst, TriEst)*

Androgens: DHEA and Testosterone*

A combination of any of the above*

* I recommend you only get these from a qualified healthcare practitioner who specializes in bioidentical hormones.

The bioidentical hormones available on the market. There are many bioidentical hormones available, but these are the ones I'm asked about most often: progesterone, estrogen, along with the androgens DHEA and testosterone. Except for topically applied progesterone and DHEA (available in creams, gels, and serums), I recommend you only get these bioidentical hormones from a qualified healthcare practitioner who specializes in bioidentical hormones. Only work with a practitioner who has experience with bioidenticals and a good reputation in the field.

Let's take a closer look at each bioidentical.

Progesterone, topically applied cream or oil. I feel progesterone, when applied to the skin, is a pretty benign hormone with extensive benefits for women with estrogen dominance, which is why it's included as one of the Foundational Supplements. For women in peri-menopause who are dealing with declining progesterone levels, supplementing with progesterone can be a saving grace, especially helping to regulate erratic periods and ease symptoms such as insomnia or mood swings. Progesterone can help:

- improve sleep
- promote a calmer, better mood
- increase libido
- regulate your cycle for more predictable periods
- eliminate mid-cycle spotting
- reduce fibrocystic breasts
- build stronger bones
- convert fat to energy
- lower the risk of developing estrogenic breast cancer
- reduce hot flashes
- lower high blood pressure
- lower systemic inflammation
- lower LDL ("bad" cholesterol)

The cream, gel, or oil delivers progesterone to your bloodstream through the fatty layer beneath your skin. You should always be cautious when incorporating a new supplement into your routine. Some women experience an immediate adverse reaction to it. In my experience, most women tolerate it well.

Some practitioners use oral progesterone. It works mainly in the GABA receptors, helping to calm nerves and promote sleep. Oral progesterone does not offer all the above mentioned benefits of topical progesterone.

For comprehensive FAQs on the use of progesterone, go to www.hormonesbalance.com/oed/downloads.

I advise consulting with a practitioner before using the following supplemental bioidentical hormones:

Estrogen. Bioidentical estrogen can come in different forms. Two of the most popular ways to take bioidentical estrogen are BiEst (bi-estrogen) and TriEst (tri-estrogen). BiEst is a combination of estriol and estradiol (often in an 80:20 ratio). TriEst includes all three estrogens: estriol, estradiol, and estrone in an 80:10:10 ratio.

JULVA

I personally love and use Julva, as do so many in the Hormones Balance community—and that's why I've decided to highlight it. Dr. Anna Cabeca formulated it to help women rejuvenate their vulva—to help with dryness and incontinence. Dr. Cabeca confirms that the DHEA found in the cream works only on the local tissue and does not increase your serum DHEA so you don't have the risk of converting it into more estrogen, which would cause more problems with estrogen dominance.

Who should consider it? This all-natural vaginal cream, available over the counter, supports vaginal health, moisturizing, lubricating, and improving skin elasticity and tissue resilience. If you're experiencing vaginal dryness, painful intercourse, or urine leaks—common symptoms of menopause—Julva could help you. It works on a deeper mucosal level as compared to estriol (E3), which is often prescribed to women for these symptoms.

How Julva can help:

- reduce incontinence
- relieve vaginal dryness and pain during sexual activity
- increase libido and arousal

I recommend working with a physician because you need a guide who is on top of your symptoms and measuring your hormones on a regular basis to see how you're doing. You know now that estrogen dominance can result from several different scenarios. Adding more estrogen through supplements may not directly exacerbate your estrogen dominance (though it could if you already have too much of the "bad guy," estradiol, as in Scenario 1), but if your liver and gut are breaking estrogen down into too many "dirty" estrogens, you will make things worse (Scenario 2). If you don't have enough progesterone to balance out all of the estrogen (Scenario 3), your symptoms could escalate as well.

Because of the chances of worsening your situation and the caution that needs to be taken if you have a history of estrogenic cancers, I recommend working with a physician.

Androgens: DHEA and testosterone. Symptoms of low androgens may show up as fatigue, lack of confidence, weakening of muscles, feeling unmotivated, forgetful, and/or having a belly fat that was never there before. Correcting your androgen levels may help support weight management, healthy blood sugar control, stress management, and can ease the symptoms of peri-menopause and menopause. However, taking androgens poses a few challenges when you're managing estrogen dominance. The reason is that DHEA gets converted into testosterone and all three types of estrogen (mainly estradiol), which exacerbates your symptoms. You therefore need to be cautious and ideally, work with a provider to watch how you are converting DHEA to testosterone and then from testosterone to estradiol. Also, DHEA is best avoided if you have a history of estrogen-receptor positive (ER+) breast cancer. Testosterone supplements, promoted to boost libido, strengthen bones and muscles, as well as improve mood pose similar challenges to DHEA:

It can be converted into estrogens in a negative way and contribute to estrogen dominance. It's best to monitor hormone levels carefully when taking testosterone.

Once you've built a strong food foundation and have tried nonhormonal supplements to resolve your symptoms, bioidentical hormones (never synthetic!) are a good option. I find that women working with a functional practitioner experienced with bioidentical hormones enjoy quicker and more lasting results when they first establish a good food foundation and nonhormonal supplement regimen.

The Plan: The Estrogen Reset Foundation Protocol

You now have many effective natural tools in your tool box to resolve your estrogen dominance—food, herbs, supplements, and bioidentical hormones. The Foundation Protocol makes it very practical and easy for you to apply them. Step-by-step, you'll use foods, herbs, and supplements to balance all three legs of your hormonal health:

Restore your gut. It's time to fall in love with your digestion! A healthy gut and good digestion are crucial when it comes to rebalancing your estrogen levels. You want a diverse, balanced microbiome to break down estrogen in a positive way and support your immune system. You'll learn how to restore your gut with healing anti-inflammatory foods and herbs, prebiotics and probiotics, as well as supplement support.

Detox your liver. Your liver works hard to help you detoxify estrogens and a sluggish liver is one of the main drivers of estrogen dominance. Let's show it some love. Now, you may see "detox" and

HELP FOR A
LOW-FUNCTIONING THYROID
OR THE SYMPTOMS OF ONE

Supporting your three-legged stool by restoring your gut, detoxing your liver, and balancing your blood sugar will help resolve your estrogen dominance and hypothyroidism or its symptoms. An inflamed digestive system causes immune system flare-ups that can worsen or cause an autoimmune thyroid disease, such as Hashimoto's. A poor gut or sluggish liver impairs the conversion of inactive T4 into active T3 so there won't be an adequate amount of thyroid hormone available for use. Those sugar spikes and crashes? They can damage the thyroid and curb thyroid hormone production. Help for your estrogen dominance is helpful for your thyroid, too.

think that you're going to starve yourself on a juice cleanse. That's absolutely not true. We're going to gently detox by eating liver-supporting foods, use bitters to stimulate bile to bind up estrogen, and get plenty of fiber.

Balance your blood sugar. I have not seen a woman with balanced hormones when her blood sugar levels were unstable, too high, or too low. Most of the time they're too high. By cutting back on sugar and amping up the protein, fat, and fiber at breakfast you'll curb your sugar cravings, steady your sugar levels, and reduce inflammation. Supplements with berberine and chromium can also really help rebalance your sugar levels, especially if you have insulin resistance.

Amplify with foundational supplements. With a strong food foundation, these baseline supplements will speed your healing and support long-term balance.

Add more healing practices. Now you're ready to move beyond food, herbs, and supplements to strengthen your three-legged stool even more. By reducing xenoestrogens in your home and personal care routine, getting hormone-supporting sleep, and incorporating healing practices

such as lymphatic massage, castor oil packs, sauna, or rebounding; you'll be well on your way to hormone balance.

Let's Get to It

It's your time to heal and thrive. With a strong food foundation and steady three-legged stool, you're removing all of the obstacles for your body to heal and creating the right environment to address any health issue. Turn the page and start learning how to restore your gut.

"JUST TELL ME WHAT I SHOULD EAT!"

Remember, you can always head directly to Part IV for the chapters covering the Foundation Protocol basics, including a quick-start overview chart of what foods/ products to add in and take out of your diet, along with the 28-day meal plan with recipes.

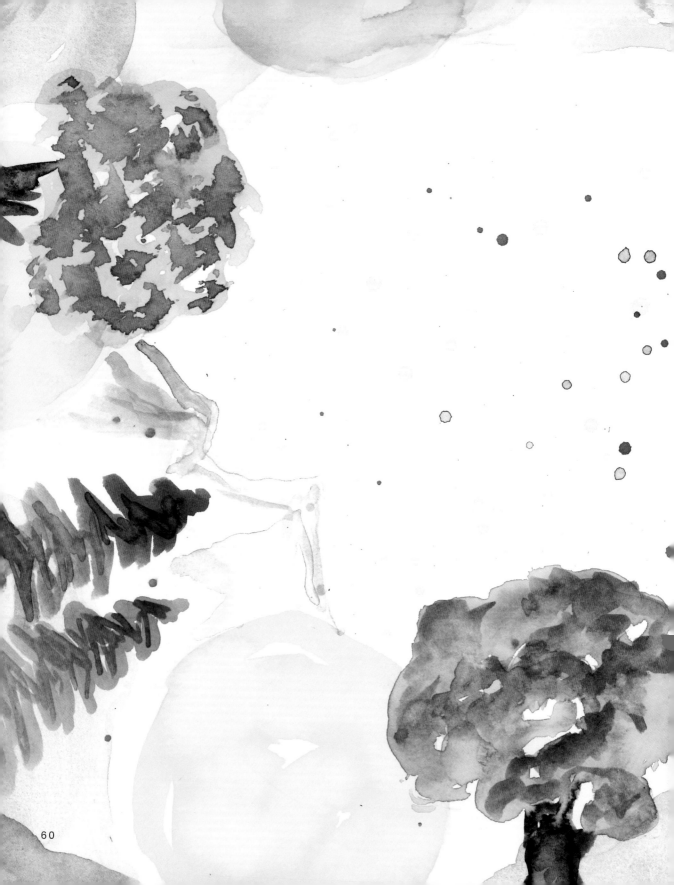

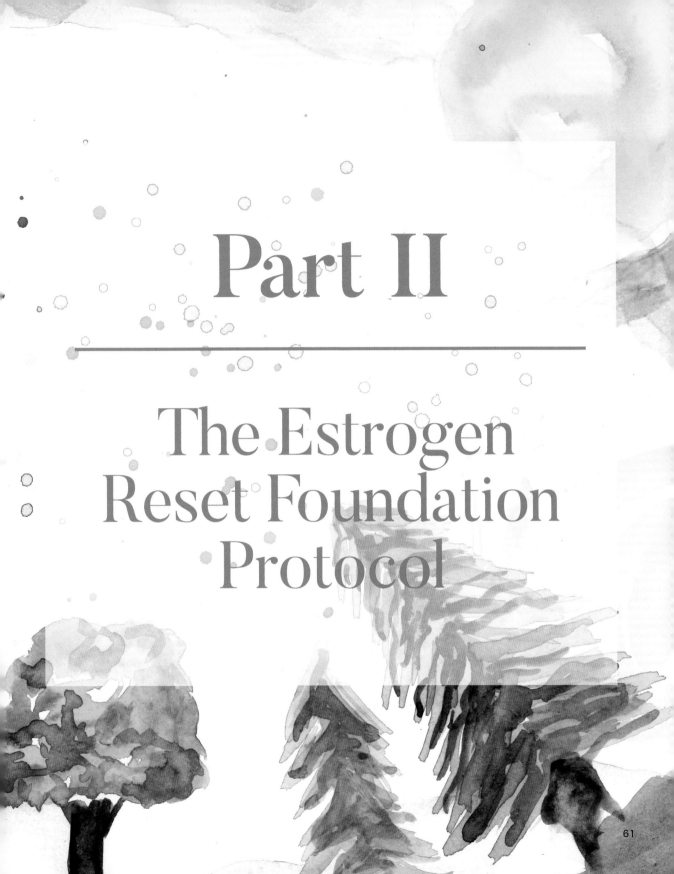

Part II

The Estrogen Reset Foundation Protocol

Restore Your Gut

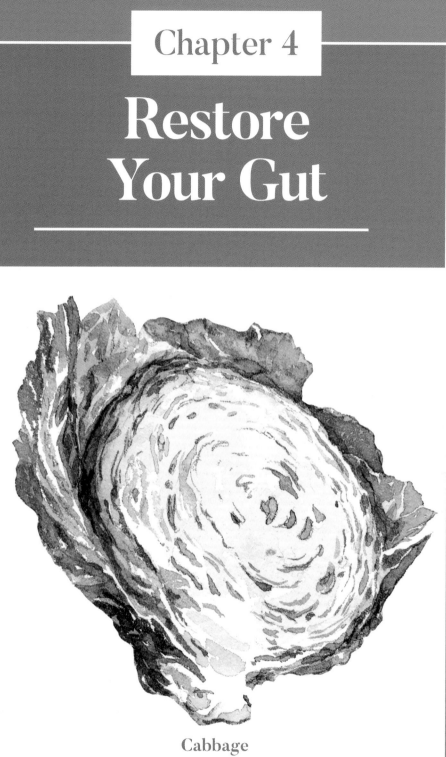

Cabbage

BRASSICA OLERACEA VAR. CAPITATA

HORMONAL BALANCE

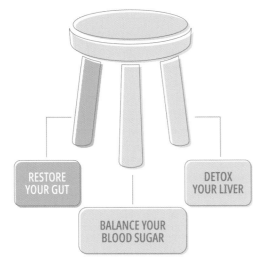

You may never have thought your gut was connected to your hormones, especially estrogen, but they are intimately linked. In this chapter, I will show you how critical your digestive health is, how restoring and maintaining a healthy gut is one of the most important steps you can take to resolve estrogen dominance, and restore hormone balance. If you follow my suggestions to heal your gut, chances are you're going to start feeling pretty amazing in the matter of days or weeks.

Tuning Into Your Body: Signs Your Digestion Needs TLC

Do you have to pop open a button or unzip your pants after a meal? Wake up and have acid reflux right off the bat? Only have a bowel movement once every other day? Burp after a meal? Many of us experience the signs of digestive distress so often that we've come to think of them as our normal. I want to assure you none of these symptoms are normal. They're signs your gut needs attention.

Here are digestive symptoms that should not be ignored:

- bloating
- constipation
- diarrhea or loose stool
- alternating between loose stool and constipation
- gas
- burping
- acid reflux
- autoimmune conditions such as Hashimoto's, Graves', multiple sclerosis
- bacterial infections such as SIBO and h.pylori
- fungal infections such as those caused by an overgrowth of the yeast Candida
- parasites or a history of parasites
- multiple food sensitivities

If you're experiencing any of these, it could be a sign your digestion needs some serious TLC. Rebalancing your gut will not only significantly reduce or resolve your digestive symptoms, it will help rebalance your hormones, and resolve the symptoms of estrogen dominance too.

How Poor Gut Health Impacts Your Hormones

Your digestive system, from your mouth, down through the esophagus, stomach, small intestine, large intestine, and out the rectum, is magnificently constructed to absorb nutrients, turn food into energy, and eliminate any waste. You probably knew that already. What you may not know is that it also makes and regulates hormones that impact nearly every bodily system, as well as has a direct impact on your estrogen levels. Most of the women I've known with estrogen dominance have weak digestive health. Poor gut health disrupts hormone balance in several ways by causing the below issues.

A lack of nutrient absorption, therefore, an inability to make the hormones you need. It may seem obvious, but it bears repeating: Breaking down food into smaller pieces that the body can use for energy, growth, and repair is a critical function of the digestive system. However, breaking down food is one thing; absorbing it so the nutrients can be used, is another. If the lining of the small intestine is compromised, nutrients won't be adequately absorbed and available for the body to use. You could be eating a diet rich in nutritious foods and taking top-notch supplements, but if you're not absorbing the nutrients, it'll do you—and your hormones—no good. Here are just a few examples:

- Proper thyroid function relies on sufficient vitamin B_{12}, selenium, and iron.
- Your adrenals depend vastly on your ability to provide them with vitamin C, magnesium, and quality fats.
- Your ability to make progesterone depends on the availability of zinc, vitamins C and E, vitamin B_6, and magnesium.

The new motto of functional nutrition has shifted from "You are what you eat" to "You are what you can absorb."

Elevated cortisol levels and chronic inflammation. Digestion issues (chronic constipation, bloating, stomach pain, or several food sensitivities) cause an inflammatory response in your body and trigger inflammation. It's a stress on the body, right? Cortisol levels rise and in order to keep up with demand, the body diverts pregnenolone away from progesterone production toward more cortisol production (the so-called pregnenolone steal). Now, you're low on progesterone and that's one of the reasons, Scenario 3, Unbalanced Partners, that you could be estrogen dominant.

Elevated cortisol levels also create systemic inflammation in the body and that inflammation causes hormone receptors to be less receptive to hormones. As a result, the progesterone you do have is blocked from getting into cells, making estrogen dominance even worse, and inhibiting all of your hormones from doing their work.

Compromised serotonin production and sleep. Most serotonin, known as the "happy hormone," is produced in your gut. Your gut and brain are directly linked and are in constant communication. Your gut is even known as the "second brain." It's why when you're nervous, you feel knots in your stomach, or you run to the bathroom (I do when I'm very stressed out or scared!). Well, the gut–brain connection works the other way, too. An unhealthy gut influences the brain. Low serotonin is associated with mood issues, such as anxiety and depression.

If you are low on serotonin, you are also low on melatonin, the hormone that signals your body it's time to sleep. Serotonin produced during the day is the precursor for melatonin. Without enough melatonin, you will struggle with insomnia or disrupted sleep, which fuel estrogen dominance.

A struggling liver. A healthy digestive system expels indigestible substances and other waste products of the digestive process, as well as toxins cleared through the liver, including "dirty" estrogens, as stool. Regular and efficient elimination prevents these toxins from getting reabsorbed. An unhealthy gut can't do its job properly so a lot of toxins and "dirty" estrogens get pumped back into the bloodstream, making the liver responsible, yet again, to clean them out. Working overtime and toxin reabsorption tax the liver in a huge way.

A compromised immune system. Your gut contains the majority of your immune system. Some, estimate up to 80% of it. A compromised gut means a compromised immune system and an increased vulnerability to infections, disease, and inflammation. The digestive tract also provides a natural defense barrier from bacteria, viruses, and parasites. Stomach acid, digestive enzymes, bile, and intestinal secretions can kill pathogens or prevent them from multiplying. A breach of this barrier will prompt an immune system response and if unresolved, keep it in overdrive.

An imbalanced gut microbiome unable to properly metabolize estrogen. A specialized subset of gut bacteria called the estrobolome processes estrogens and directly influences how much estrogen you have circulating in your system. An imbalance of these microflora contributes to estrogen dominance.

The Microbiome: Your New Best Friend

Your gut is home to a chemical factory of bacteria, yeast, and spores called the gut microbiome, which helps with digestion, regulates your immune system, protects you against other bacteria that cause diseases, produces vitamins, and processes hormones. The microbiome has such intricate and profound effects on human health that it is often referred to as the "hidden organ." One to be reckoned with, because it can alter your brain function, cancer risk, inflammation levels, sugar levels, immune system, and weight, as well as your hormonal balance.

A specific collection of bacteria that lives in our stomach and intestines is capable of metabolizing, or breaking down estrogens. They are called the estrobolome. If they become imbalanced, they can contribute to your estrogen dominance symptoms. On the other hand, a healthy and balanced estrobolome can relieve your symptoms.

Let's take a closer look at how estrogen travels through the body and makes its way to the estrobolome, where it can either be broken down into more "clean" estrogens and removed from the body (that's the goal) or returned to the bloodstream as "dirty" estrogens, which will drive estrogen dominance.

Estrogens produced by the ovaries, adrenal glands, and visceral fat are released into the bloodstream, where they are available for use by cells. Estrogen enters a cell through a receptor and once it has been used, it goes to the liver to be broken down, then bound up so it can be eliminated safely. The liver does this with the help of bile, which is why many women who have had their gallbladder removed struggle with estrogen dominance. Once the estrogens are prepared for elimination, the liver sends them to the large intestine for final elimination—your poop.

The bacteria of the estrobolome degrade the estrogens further. They do this with the help of an enzyme called beta-glucuronidase. It breaks down complex carbohydrates and detoxifies estrogen, thyroid hormone, and other environmental toxins. So we've got to have it. It helps expel "dirty" estrogens. But we don't want too little or too much of beta-glucuronidase. Too much can cause "dirty" estrogens to reenter the bloodstream and make your estrogen dominance symptoms worse.

Why does B-glucuronidase become too high? An imbalance in the bacteria of the estrobolome typically caused by a diet high in processed foods, conventionally raised meat, alcohol, and antibiotics. Having a history of intestinal bacterial or fungal overgrowths, such as Candida and SIBO is also a sign the estrobolome is unhealthy.

The Link Between the Microbiome and Estrogen-Driven Breast Cancer and Other Estrogenic-Conditions

Researchers have found links between an imbalanced microbiome and several estrogenic conditions, including estrogen positive (ER+) breast cancer, PCOS, and endometriosis. This is likely because of the increase in circulating estrogens caused when beta-glucuronidase gets too high. Do we have all of the answers when it comes to the connection between the estrobolome and these conditions? Absolutely not. But we're beginning to see a significant correlation that shouldn't be ignored.

Estrogen-driven breast cancer. Several studies suggest a connection between a lack of gut bacteria diversity and breast cancer. In one, postmenopausal women with breast cancer were found to have a less diverse gut microbiome compared to the control group. A less diverse microbiome means an estrobolome with high levels of beta-glucuronidase and excess free estrogen. Those excess free estrogens may promote estrogen-sensitive cells to proliferate, causing cancer. Claudia S. Plottel, MD, a leading scientist on the estrobolome and a professor at New York University, confirms that "states of estrogen excess are associated with an increased risk of developing estrogen-related cancers."

As a woman who is at high risk for estrogen-related problems, including breast cancer, this research is close to my heart. Here's what I take away from it: A healthy gut with a diverse microbiome is important for clearing estrogens and reducing the risk of these types of cancers.

Endometriosis. Studies have also linked an altered gut microbiome and endometriosis. The estrobolome of women with endometriosis may have larger numbers of beta-glucuronidase-producing bacteria, leading to increased levels of circulating estrogen, which drives endometriosis.

PCOS. A low-diversity gut microbiome and disrupted estrobolome have also been implicated in PCOS, a condition with symptoms including

THE IMPORTANCE OF MICROBIOME HEALTH FOR MENOPAUSAL AND POST-MENOPAUSAL WOMEN

Estrogen is critical for heart/bone health and helps to regulate metabolism, along with body weight. In menopause and postmenopause, estrogen naturally declines, increasing your risk of cardiovascular disease (the leading cause of death in menopausal women), osteoporosis, declining mental health, and stubborn weight gain, especially around the belly. Guess what can drive your estrogen levels even lower and amp up the likelihood of these issues? Low beta-glucuronidase. In fact, breast cancer patients, along with obese and overweight patients show poor microbiome health, especially in postmenopausal and menopausal women. Now more than ever, it's time to repair your microbiome and balance beta-glucuronidase.

ovarian cysts, high DHEA, high testosterone levels, high blood sugar levels, insulin resistance, stubborn belly fat, frontal baldness, irregular periods, infertility, and irritability. In this case, women with PCOS have low beta-glucuronidase activity and low estrogen levels, but it all links back to the gut.

More studies are needed. The hope is that eventually characteristics of the gut microbiome could be used to determine if you have a risk for estrogenic cancers or conditions then identify the best ways to prevent and treat them.

What You Can Do to Restore Your Gut

Perhaps everything you have read sounds complicated. Don't worry, because you have a lot of control over your microbiome and digestion. And it is not complicated; I've made the recipes and meal plans in this book easy for anyone to follow and meet the objectives of enriching your microbiome. Here's how to improve microbiome diversity, balance beta-glucuronidase, support your estrobolome, and help your estrogen dominance.

- eliminate inflammatory foods (by doing the Elimination Diet)
- ensure sufficient stomach acid
- get the digestive bitters and/or digestive enzymes going
- ensure a daily bowel movement
- get plenty of prebiotics and probiotics

All five ways to restore your gut are built into the Foundation Protocol and 28-Day Meal Plan in Part IV. You don't even have to think about it!

Eliminate inflammatory foods

This might be the most profound step in the program, since it reduces or completely eliminates a host of health issues you've been experiencing for decades, hormonal and otherwise. The foods listed here are the main inflammation-causing culprits, so it's key to cut them out during the four-week Foundation Protocol. Do not pick and choose foods from this list. Commit to doing the complete Elimination Diet by removing them all. You will be cutting out:

- gluten (wheat, barley, rye, farro, and products containing processed gluten-containing grain flours such as breads, pastas, cookies, and muffins)
- dairy (cheese, butter, milk, yogurt, including lactose-free)
- eggs (both the yolk and whites)
- corn (in all forms, including taco shells)
- soy (in all forms, including soy sauce and tempeh)
- nightshades (tomatoes, white potatoes, eggplant, peppers, chiles, goji berries)
- processed or packaged foods, including protein powders (you'll be eating only whole foods)
- limit conventionally grown vegetables, grains, meat, and fish (aim to eat as much organic, non-GMO, and pasture-raised food as possible)
- limited (or none at all) coffee and caffeine
- limited sugar and no artificial sweeteners

Instead, you're going to fill up on healing, nutrient-dense, and anti-inflammatory foods that taste amazing!

If you feel a little overwhelmed and sad that I'm asking you to cut out some of your favorite foods (many women feel they can't live without cheese,

> This might be the most profound step in the program, since it reduces or completely eliminates a host of health issues you've been experiencing for decades

eggs, and coffee), the good news is that you will be eliminating these foods for only 28 days. You can start reintroducing gluten, dairy, etc., after that. Many people continue avoiding these foods beyond the 28 days because they feel so good without them.

When you reintroduce these foods, you will gain clarity on which ones cause digestive problems (and many other symptoms). Many women who have followed this protocol are surprised at how many of their health issues were caused by foods such as eggs and coffee. But maybe that won't be the case for you! The important thing is to identify the foods that inflame your body and don't agree with you. Then as much as possible, cut them out of your diet. There is a possibility you would be able to eat some of them again (such as eggs), once your gut is fully healed. I've found that people who struggle with numerous food sensitivities have a highly compromised gut. Heal

your digestion and gain the freedom to eat some of these foods. So, please, please, do not skip this step.

How to Reintroduce Foods After the Elimination Diet?

Once you complete the Elimination Diet, you may want to reintroduce the potential culprit foods to see how they affect you. Use your Food Mood Poop Journal (see box page 91) to track your emotional and physical reactions. When you reintroduce a suspect food, do it during each meal on that day. It is best to start off with a food that you suspect is not a problem for you. Reintroduce commonly problematic foods such as dairy and gluten only at the end.

Let's say you start by reintroducing eggs on Monday. The process is simple: Eat eggs (or foods that contain eggs) for breakfast and perhaps lunch or dinner. Tune into your body right away. There are two possible outcomes: You start feeling some changes (digestive issues, brain fog, fatigue, headaches, anxiety, skin rash, mood swings, just feeling "off") within 30 minutes to two days later, or you get no reaction at all.

If you develop no symptoms on the first day, continue eating the food you are testing on the second day as well. Sometimes the food reaction manifests after the first day. Even if no symptoms occur immediately on the second day, stop eating these foods and wait two more days and observe whether you get any reactions. The reactions you are looking for vary from physical (GI issues such as constipation, diarrhea, gas, bloating, acid reflux or pain, low energy, skin issues, itching, headaches, food cravings), mental (anxiety, depression, brain fog), to emotional (anger, crying, feeling "blah"). If you do not react, it is a sign you have no problem with that food. It's best not to reintroduce foods around your period or major life events (like weddings or house moves) because you may not know what is causing these symptoms. "Am I bloated because of my period or the eggs I've just reintroduced?"

Weight gain can be a common sign of food intolerance as well. Measure your weight toward the end of the Elimination Diet, first thing in the morning. Let's say you are ready to reintroduce gluten on a Monday. Jot down your weight on Monday morning before you start eating gluten. Weigh yourself on Tuesday morning; if your weight shoots up by more than two pounds in one day, there is a high likelihood this food is a suspect.

A Note on Reintroducing Dairy

Even though I advise eliminating all dairy products from your diet, I know that it can be difficult to do and for some people, it's okay to have it once in a while. Therefore, when reintroducing dairy, test each as if it was its own food category:

A. cow's milk and cheese
B. cow's yogurt, kefir, or cottage cheese
C. goat or sheep cheese
D. goat or sheep yogurt

You may find it easier to digest fermented dairy products or dairy from a goat or sheep.

Even if you find you can tolerate some dairy (such as goat cheese or fermented dairy like yogurt), I advise you treat dairy as an occasional indulgence and not an everyday food.

Long-Term Food Game Plan

After reintroducing all of the foods you have eliminated, you will know your food intolerances. Remove these foods from your diet to heal your digestion and reduce inflammation, which is essential for regaining hormonal balance and overall well-being. I have also found that once you heal your digestion, you may be able to have some of your problem foods with no reactions. For example, I can have an occasional good-quality cheese (such as Parmigiano-Reggiano) and get no reactions. If I eat it often, it triggers my Hashimoto's disease and IBS, as well as brings on other food sensitivities. And, yes, I'm not perfect and it has happened a couple of times, especially after trips to Italy!

Alternatives to the Elimination Diet

In case the Elimination Diet does not produce concrete results, you can also try IgG testing, the heart rate method, or kinesiology (also known as "muscle testing").

Ensure Sufficient Stomach Acid

Stomach acid is a really good thing. It is essential for good digestion, enabling the stomach to extract nutrients from the food you eat and stimulating the release of digestive enzymes. It aids the absorption of vitamin B_{12}, iron, zinc, folate, calcium, and magnesium, essential nutrients for hormone health. And, it helps you maintain a healthy microbiome by killing pathogens that threaten to disrupt it.

Unfortunately, many of us don't have enough stomach acid, especially as we age. Head's up all of you with acid reflux! Acid reflux is *not* caused by too much stomach acid; the issue is that you do not have enough of it.

Symptoms of low stomach acid include:

- bloating or belching immediately following a meal
- a sense of fullness after eating, like a rock sitting in your stomach
- feeling like food sits in the stomach forever
- gas after eating
- iron and B_{12} deficiency; anemia (even if you're supplementing)
- undigested food in stool (See kale leaves or pieces of carrot?)
- weak, peeling, or cracked fingernails
- being prone to parasite infections, especially if they return soon after treatment
- chronic intestinal infections such as h.pylori
- a history of multiple food allergies and intolerances

You can find out if you have low stomach acid by doing the HCL Pill Test (see below) at home. If you're low, you can increase stomach acid with food or by continuing to use the Betaine HCL supplement.

To increase stomach acid with food:

Drink 2 tablespoons of apple cider vinegar, lemon, lime, or sauerkraut juice in six to eight ounces of room temperature water, 15 minutes before eating. Start by having it first thing in the morning and if after a few days you're still experiencing symptoms of low stomach acid, drink it before every meal. This mixture won't interfere with thyroid medication.

If you can't tolerate any of the above, try drinking 1/2 teaspoon of sea salt in six to eight ounces of room temperature water before meals. Do not take this with thyroid medications as it will interfere with absorption.

You'll know you're doing enough to increase your stomach acid when you get a burning sensation in your stomach. You should start to feel better and see no food in your poop.

To increase stomach acid with supplements:

Use Betaine HCL. To determine the proper dose, take the HCL Pill Test. All you need are Betaine HCL with pepsin pills, which help increase the level of hydrochloric acid in your stomach. Prepare a high-protein meal of at least six ounces of meat. Take one pill with or after the meal.

TOOLS FOR SUCCESS: FOOD-MOOD-POOP (FMP) JOURNAL

This is a super helpful tool for helping you keep track of what you're eating, how it makes you feel, and how it makes you poop (an indicator of exactly what's going on in your gut). It's good to start an FMP while you're on the Foundation Protocol so you get used to keeping it and tuning into your body. The Meal Plan removes a lot of the foods that tend to cause people problems but you may find, for example, that coconut or grains don't sit well with you, and your tummy feels heavy or your thinking is foggy.

The FMP Journal is invaluable if you decide to try adding foods back in after the 28-day Foundation Protocol. It'll help you to notice patterns. If cheese makes you feel bloated and gassy or causes constipation, it clearly is the problem food for you and it should be cut out for now.

You can download a digital version of the FMP journal at: www.hormonesbalance.com/oed/downloads

Hormones
&BALANCE

MY FOOD – MOOD – POOP JOURNAL (SAMPLE)

DATE: May 10

TIME:	FOOD/DRINK CONSUMED:	HOW I FEEL: Mood, stomach/digestion, energy level, quality of sleep, skin, aches & pains, etc.	POOP: Refer to the Bristol Stool Chart to give it a number (#) and describe color
8 AM Breakfast	I bowl whole grain cereal with low fat milk		Constipation, Type #1. Brown. Feels like there is more left.
9:30 AM		Feel tired and moody, slight headache, already hungry again	
11:30 AM Lunch	Water, turkey sandwich on whole wheat bread, potato chips, apple		
12 PM		Feel slightly better: less moody, headache gone, still tired	
3 PM Snack	Small bag of trail mix		Got diarrhea
6:30 PM Dinner	Roast chicken, I bowl of vegetable soup, salad (lettuce, cucumber, tomato, carrot, Italian dressing)		
7 PM	I bowl whole grain cereal with low fat milk	Feel much better after dinner	
9 PM Snack	Bowl of chocolate chip ice cream with a banana		
9:20 PM	Water	Feel exhausted and bloated, just want to go to sleep	

If you feel stomach distress, such as heaviness, burning, or hotness, you have sufficient stomach acid. If you don't feel any discomfort, then you are low in stomach acid and you'll add pills to each meal until you feel stomach distress: heaviness, burning, or hotness. Once you experience a reaction, you'll need to take one pill less at each meal to have sufficient stomach acid and well-functioning digestion. For example, if you need four HCL pills to feel discomfort, you'll take three pills at each meal. Do not take more than eight capsules with a meal. Here's what your first few days could look like as you try to find the number of pills you need.

Be sure to take HCL pills with a meal that contains at least six ounces of protein.

Day 1:

- 1 pill with dinner

Day 2:

- 1 pill with lunch
- 1 pill with dinner

Day 3:

- 1 pill with breakfast
- 1 pill with lunch
- 1 pill with dinner

Day 4:

- 1 pill with breakfast
- 1 pill with lunch
- 2 pills with dinner

Day 5:

- 1 pill with breakfast
- 2 pills with lunch
- 2 pills with dinner

Day 6:

- 2 pills with breakfast
- 2 pills with lunch
- 2 pills with dinner

And so on, going up, up, up until you feel a burning sensation in your stomach or a lot of discomfort. Then you stop and continue with the last dose before the burn.

If your stomach acid stays consistently low despite your changes, consider trying digestive enzymes instead. Also, ask your doctor to test for H. pylori with the Gastrointestinal Microbial Assay Plus (GI-MAP) test. It tests for gastrointestinal microbiota from a single stool sample. I've found it to be much more accurate than blood tests and other stool tests. A lot of other tests failed to register my H. pylori infection; this is the one that finally showed it.

Get the Digestive Enzymes Going

Digestive enzymes break down food into smaller molecules—and only in the broken-down form can they be digested and absorbed by the body. They are made in the mouth, stomach, pancreas, and small intestine. Without enough digestive enzymes, your body can't access the nutrients it needs and all that undigested food causes all sorts of digestive distress.

To promote excretion of digestive enzymes with food (my recommended way #1):

Eat bitter greens. Dandelion leaves, mustard greens, radishes, parsley, arugula, and cilantro are all considered bitter foods that are really great at creating all of the digestive juices.

To promote digestive enzymes with herbs (my recommended way #2):

Make digestive bitters a daily routine. Bitter taste is a lost and underappreciated taste in our culture. We have developed a taste for sweet, salty, and some of us, sour. Most frown at bitters. I agree, it's an acquired taste, but once you embrace it, your body will crave it. The bitter flavor sends a cascade of not only digestive but also neurological signals, including activating the parasympathetic nervous system, which will calm you down and aid digestion.

To me, digestive bitters are magical and that's part of the reason why I formulated my own. I love them for the array of benefits they offer, namely:

- increase digestive enzyme excretion and stomach acid production
- ease constipation and encourage regular bowel movements
- promote bile production and flow (key for fat digestion and estrogen binding)
- aid in protecting gut tissue and encourage healing through supporting the innate self-repair mechanism of the gut cells
- help with acid reflux by improving esophageal sphincter tone
- regulate bacterial environment
- regulate the body pH (for most people, to a more alkaline state)
- detoxify the liver and help clear "dirty" estrogens
- lower blood sugar levels

Almost every culinary culture has a bitter element to it. In ancient Egypt, wines were infused with bitter herbs to aid digestion. In South Indian cooking, a meal is often accompanied by a delightfully bitter green mango chutney. What are you offered after a rich Indian meal? A teaspoon of fennel and cumin seeds—slightly bitter seeds that will aid and calm digestion. Orange bitters, popularized by the British before the 19th century, have found varied renditions in digestifs found in most European cultures—a Campari in Northern Italy, Gammel Dansk in Denmark, Jägermeister in Germany, and the list goes on.

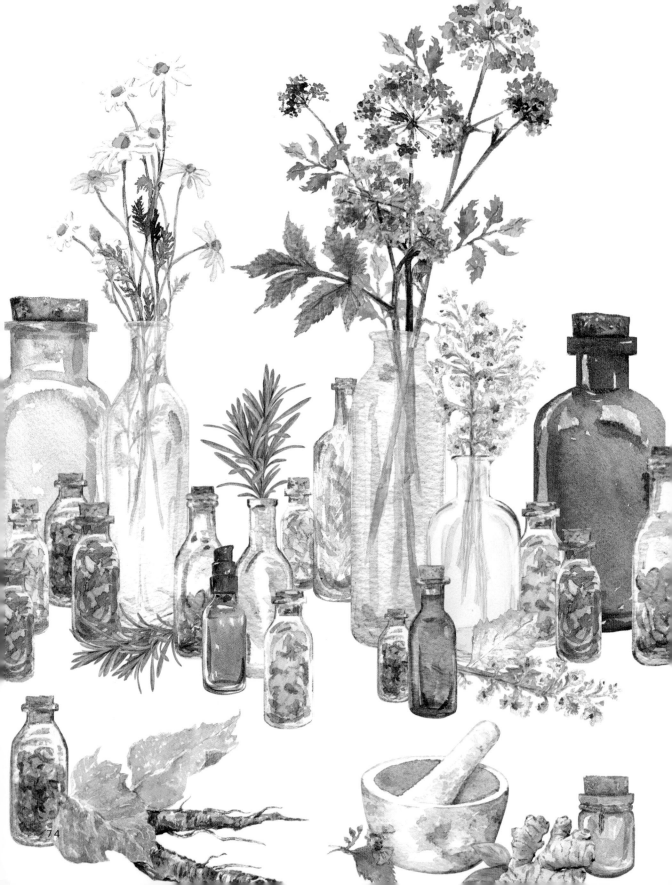

You may think of them as libations, but they were first marketed as tonics and digestive medicines.

Now, we can take our supplemental bitters in a more healthful way, *before* and *after* we eat. Digestive bitters are plants, roots, leaves, and stems with a bitter flavor, usually extracted in alcohol. The classical bitters contain dandelion root, burdock root, yellow dock, fennel, gentian, or orange peel.

(Note: The most effective bitters are still alcohol-based. If alcohol isn't an option for you, supplement with digestive enzymes instead.)

I have a personal affinity for digestive bitters because my body craves them and my digestion behaves better when I take them. I've developed the Before Digestive Bitter and After Digestive Bitters to create a special experience for you. The Before Meal bitters warm up your digestion, preparing it for receiving food and extracting maximum nutrition from it. It contains bitter and warming herbs such as gentian, schisandra, angelica, ginger, rosemary, meadowsweet, and cloves. Creating heat in the digestion is essential and this is why patients of Traditional Chinese Medicine are always told not to drink iced drinks with a meal—you are shutting down your digestion.

The After Digestive Bitters were developed to feel like having a tiny dessert. It's slightly sweet, licorice-y, and calming to the digestive system. This formula contains burdock root, chamomile, angelica, anise, andrographis, catnip, and fennel.

The digestive bitters you have tried might have been so intense (from the alcohol

In the latest discovery, taste receptors have been found to appear in the form of thirty receptors that aren't just located in the mouth. Turns out, we have bitter receptors in the whole upper gastrointestinal tract, as well as lungs and kidneys. They can even be found in the bile ducts and even though their role isn't fully understood yet, my bet is: Bring on the bitters for better bile flow and digestion!

and the bitter herbs) that you may not want to try them again. We spent months formulating our Before and After Digestive Bitters by including some glycerin, making them delicious, very rounded in taste, and a pleasure to sip before and after every meal. You may fall in love with them even more after experiencing less stomach pain, bloating, heartburn, have more regular bowel movements, fewer food sensitivities, lower inflammation, and more energy.

I hope you try them and make them a part of your daily meal ritual.

If alcohol-based bitters are not right for you, try supplementing with digestive enzymes.

Encourage a Daily Bowel Movement

I'm often asked, "What's the big deal about constipation?" So many women are chronically constipated that they assume it's the norm. The big deal is regular elimination is how the body removes harmful toxins, including "dirty" estrogens, from the body. If these toxins aren't removed, they go right back into your bloodstream, increasing your body's toxic load, taxing your liver, and exacerbating your estrogen dominance. Constipation promotes pathogenic organism growth in the colon too.

You want a good bowel movement that:

- occurs at least once daily
- leaves you feeling emptied
- is brown, never yellow or green
- is shaped like a banana and well formed
- is #3 or #4 on the Bristol Stool Chart (see next page)
- does not have visible food particles
- takes 12 to 24 hours to move through your digestive system

If you struggle with constipation, here are a few suggestions to help get things moving:

- A fiber deficiency is a common cause of constipation. Get more fiber by taking 2 tablespoons of whole flax seed (not ground) before bed or consider a fiber supplement. A highly efficacious source of fiber is acacia gum (from the acacia tree).
- Drink enough water. How much in ounces equals half of your body weight (in pounds). If you weigh 140 pounds, you should drink 70 ounces of water each day.
- Encourage healthy gut microflora by getting plenty of prebiotics and probiotics. More on those on page 78.
- Address food intolerances by eliminating problematic foods. Dairy is often an issue when it comes to constipation.
- Address a magnesium deficiency by taking magnesium citrate or baths with Epsom salts.
- Improve stomach acid by using the suggestions previously mentioned in this chapter.
- Try digestive bitters before meals. So many women report eliminating constipation by using bitters.
- Assess your current prescription medications with your doctor as they are a common cause of constipation.

Eat enough fiber

A fiber deficiency is a common cause of constipation, a contributor to hormone imbalance, and estrogen dominance. When you are constipated, metabolized or "used up" hormones reenter the body instead of being evacuated. A lack of fiber also compromises the health of your gut and microbiome. We need to consume at least 20 to 30 grams of fiber each day, but most Americans only get about 15 grams per day. More specifically, the U.S. Food and Nutrition Board of the Institute of Medicine recommends women under 50 have a fiber intake of 25 g per day and those over 50, have 21 g per day. If you choose to supplement with fiber, I highly recommend the formula contains acacia.

Eat plenty of fermented foods

Fermented foods have a place in every culinary history—for good reason. Making sure you have enough of each fermented foods supports a balanced microbiome and estrobolome.

Lacto-fermented foods (see Note), those made using lactic-acid bacteria to break down the sugars in food and not vinegar, are rich in probiotics. Probiotic-rich foods include:

- sauerkraut, lacto-fermented (find it in the refrigerated section of your supermarket or health store; avoid shelf-stabilized sauerkraut in vinegar—they are not fermented)
- dill pickles, lacto-fermented (found in the refrigerated section; avoid shelf-stabilized pickles in vinegar—they are not fermented)
- cultured olives, lacto-fermented
- preserved lemon, lacto-fermented
- beet kvass, lacto-fermented
- kimchi, lacto-fermented (chili found in kimchi is a nightshade, so only eat if after

WHAT DOES
HEALTHY POOP
LOOK LIKE?

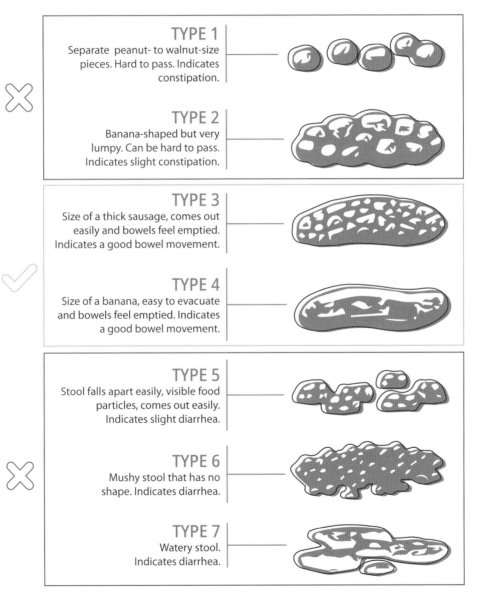

TYPE 1
Separate peanut- to walnut-size pieces. Hard to pass. Indicates constipation.

TYPE 2
Banana-shaped but very lumpy. Can be hard to pass. Indicates slight constipation.

TYPE 3
Size of a thick sausage, comes out easily and bowels feel emptied. Indicates a good bowel movement.

TYPE 4
Size of a banana, easy to evacuate and bowels feel emptied. Indicates a good bowel movement.

TYPE 5
Stool falls apart easily, visible food particles, comes out easily. Indicates slight diarrhea.

TYPE 6
Mushy stool that has no shape. Indicates diarrhea.

TYPE 7
Watery stool. Indicates diarrhea.

the 28-Day Foundation Protocol if you decide to reintroduce nightshades to your diet and tolerate them well)

- miso, the soy-free type (if it contains soy, only eat it if after the 28-Day Foundation Protocol if you decide to reintroduce soy to your diet and tolerate it well)
- Kombucha, with caution (I'm not a fan because it is full of yeast and many women struggle with Candida, a yeast overgrowth; I'd avoid it while on the 28-Day Foundation Protocol and drink sparingly, if at all)

Add Prebiotics and Probiotics

Resistant starch is a pretty awesome type of prebiotic because it is not digested in the stomach or the small intestine and serves as a fuel for the bacteria in your intestines. It contributes to insulin sensitivity, satiation, weight loss, and colon health (see Note).

Prebiotic foods high in resistant starch include:

- seeds
- cashews
- unprocessed whole grains
- legumes
- cooled (cold from fridge) cooked rice and white potatoes
- raw green bananas, most often found in the form of flour

> **Note:** if you are sensitive to FODMAPS or have SIBO, you may react adversely to many of the foods on this list so proceed with care. Prebiotic-rich foods high in resistant starch won't cause digestive distress.

Prebiotic foods high in soluble fiber provide fuel for the bacteria in your colon. These include:

- Jerusalem artichokes
- onions
- whole grains
- bananas
- garlic
- onions
- shallots
- leeks
- cabbage
- root vegetables, such as beets, dandelion, and chicory
- apples
- beans
- legumes
- asparagus
- nuts and seeds, such as flax seeds

Check out the Supplement Guide (page 361) if you want an out-of-the-box RS Fiber.

Probiotics supplements contain live "good" microorganisms that support a healthy gut microbiome and the integrity of the intestinal lining, promoting estrogen detoxification, a healthy immune system, and good digestion. Probiotics and other friendly bacteria feed on prebiotics, a type of fiber the body can't digest.

When choosing a supplement, quality is key. There are several challenges with probiotics, the main ones being: the quality of the supplement (strain diversity and amount, how it's made, how fresh it is, the preservation technique used, how it bypasses the stomach to get into your intestines) and the current bacterial diversity of your microbiome. It's key not to overpopulate with just a few strains and rather focus on the biodiversity of your microbiome. An interesting factoid: people who were not breastfed tend to be low in bifidobacteria.

Every manufacturer will make promising claims about their products. In reality, the efficacy of the product will depend on your current bacterial microflora and what you need in order to improve your health. Some people see no improvements from one probiotic but feel improvements with another. It might be a tedious and expensive process to test various probiotics but probably one worth it. Include these various forms of probiotics:

- lactobacillus and bifidobacterium strains
- spores
- soil-based bacteria
- for dosage, follow manufacturer's instructions.

Add collagen, the tissue glue

Collagen is very rich in various amino acids which are the building blocks for proteins. Your body is largely made up of protein; skin, hair, and your gut included. Collagen rebuilds your gut mucosal lining, strengthens bones, supports joints, promotes strong hair, skin, and nails, as well as minimizes wrinkles. It's rich in glycine, necessary for phase 2 liver detoxification and a precursor to glutathione, a master detoxifier. The best form of collagen is made of the skin, bones, and the connective tissue of an animal. Studies show this form of collagen improves bone density, helps with cartilage recovery (such as after surgeries), and skin elasticity (includes gut mucosa and wrinkles). Marine collagen, which is getting a lot of medical attention these days, is also worth exploring if you are a vegetarian or vegan; look out for sourcing and low toxicity levels due to ocean pollution. One scoop per day containing 11 grams of protein is a suggested dose unless otherwise determined by your practitioner.

Back on Track

The first leg of your three-legged stool for hormone balance is a healthy gut with a balanced microbiome and estrobolome. If this leg is shaky, not only will you experience digestive troubles, a compromised immune system, and mood issues, but estrogens won't be broken down and eliminated from your body properly. To heal your estrogen dominance, heal your gut with the suggestions included in this chapter and found in the Foundation Protocol and 28-Day Meal Plan in Part IV. Everything you need to do from eliminating inflammatory foods to getting enough probiotics and prebiotics is built right in.

COULD HISTAMINE BE A PROBLEM FOR YOU?

If eating fermented foods causes you to sneeze, tear up, break out in hives, feel congested, or itch, you may have a histamine intolerance. Histamines are chemicals made by your immune system to get rid of an allergen or other threat. We take antihistamines to reduce the uncomfortable reactions we experience as they work to remove the invader. When histamine levels get too high, we can develop histamine intolerance. High levels are caused by systemic inflammation and a barrage of debilitating symptoms. Excess estrogen (like in estrogen dominance) can also trigger the release of histamines. With time, restoring gut health, lowering overall body inflammation, and rebalancing estrogen levels will improve your tolerance to histamine. Progesterone is a histamine antagonist and regulator. If you are low on progesterone and correct it, your histamine intolerance might improve as well.

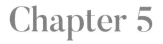

Chapter 5

Detox Your Liver

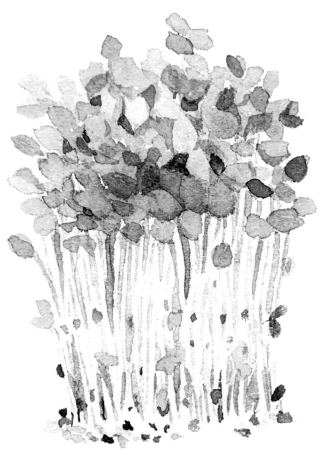

Broccoli Sprouts

BRASSICA OLERACEA ITALICA

HORMONAL BALANCE

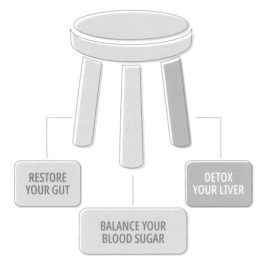

RESTORE YOUR GUT

DETOX YOUR LIVER

BALANCE YOUR BLOOD SUGAR

A healthy liver is the second leg of your three-legged stool for hormone balance. The liver is often overlooked when it comes to women's hormonal struggles, but it shouldn't be. In this chapter, I'll show you what a large role the liver plays in regulating our hormones, especially estrogen. The liver is instrumental in breaking down used estrogens and metabolizing them so they can be safely excreted. If the liver is overburdened, it may not be able to detoxify as quickly and efficiently, allowing "dirty" estrogens back into the bloodstream and contributing to estrogen dominance. By following my suggestions to support your liver, you'll feel better than ever and relieve the symptoms you're suffering from right now.

Tuning Into Your Body: Signs Your Liver Needs TLC

Your liver performs about 200 functions, most of which are vital for overall good health and hormone balance. Because it influences so many systems, a sluggish liver impacts almost every aspect of how you feel, physically and emotionally. It's tough to know from one specific symptom if the culprit is a less-than-optimal liver, but the below signs are a good indication that it needs some attention:

Hormonal Imbalances

- intolerance/adverse reactions to hormone replacement therapy (HRT)
- severe menopausal symptoms
- PMS
- estrogen dominance
- mood swings

Blood Sugar Problems

- sugar cravings
- hypoglycemia (low blood sugar)
- type 2 diabetes
- energy slumps
- waking in the night

Immune System Dysfunction

- allergies (seasonal and to many environmental triggers)
- chemical sensitivities (for example, unable to stand fumes from cleaning products or perfumes)
- chronic fatigue/fibromyalgia
- frequent illness

Digestive Issues

- no hunger in the morning
- gallstones
- inability to digest fatty foods
- sensitivity to alcohol and/or caffeine
- acid reflux
- bloating or constipation

Abnormal Metabolism of Fats (Lipids)

- abnormal level of fats in the blood, such as high LDL ("bad cholesterol") and reduced HDL ("good cholesterol")
- elevated triglycerides
- blocked arteries, raising your risk of hypertension, heart attacks, and strokes
- fatty liver (indicated by the ALT and AST enzymes blood tests)
- obesity

Mood and Other Nervous System–Related Issues

- anger and irritability
- foggy brain
- overheating
- frequent headaches

External Signs

- skin rashes
- furry tongue
- bad breath
- acne and rosacea
- yellow, red, or itchy eyes
- easy bruising
- brown spot on hands, back, and face

How many of these symptoms do you experience? If there are several, take it as a sign your liver needs some support. The truth is, the modern world is very hard on the liver and all of us could stand to give it some extra attention.

How a Sluggish Liver Impacts Your Hormones

Your liver does so much more than you ever imagined, much more than just detoxing. Think of your liver as a sieve. Everything you breathe, ingest, or apply on your skin gets into your digestive system and bloodstream, which eventually passes through the liver. It's the largest organ in the body, weighing about three pounds, and it's the only organ that can regenerate itself (isn't it fascinating?!). It purifies your blood at an astounding rate of 50 ounces or 1.4 liters per minute!

Do you know where your liver is located? Sit or stand up straight. Put your hand over your right rib cage, under your right breast. Your hand is now over your liver. Most of the liver is protected under the rib cage, but a little bit sticks out, about where the tips of your fingers rest. Tucked underneath the liver is a little pouch, your gallbladder, where bile is stored (bile is produced in the liver).

Your liver plays numerous roles in your body, just about all of which influence hormone balance. A sluggish liver disrupts your hormones by causing:

Blood sugar problems. One of the main functions of the liver is to maintain stable blood sugar levels. If blood sugar increases, the liver starts storing excess sugar in the form of glycogen. When blood sugar runs low, the liver breaks down glycogen and releases sugar into the blood. Erratic blood sugar fluctuations caused by a sluggish liver can

In Chinese medicine, the liver is called the "anger organ." Smiling into your liver, sending positive energy into it, can dissolve anger and resentment. Take a moment now to put your hand over your liver, close your eyes, take a deep breath, and smile into your liver.

lead to a host of serious conditions, including insulin resistance and type 2 diabetes.

Poor storage of minerals and fat-soluble vitamins. In addition to storing sugar (in the form of glycogen), the liver also stores fat-soluble vitamins (A, D, E, and K) and minerals (iron and copper), and releases them into the blood when needed. Nutrient deficiencies hurt hormone production.

Abnormal metabolism of fats. The liver is responsible for maintaining a healthy level of fats in the bloodstream. For an average person, approximately 80% of their cholesterol is generated by the liver—and that's a good thing! We need cholesterol; it's a primary building block for our cells and the precursor for all of our steroid hormones, which include progesterone, estrogen, DHEA, testosterone, and cortisol. Liver cells also break down fats to generate energy and produce bile, an important liquid for the digestion and absorption of fats in the small intestine. A sluggish liver produces less bile, slowing this process while causing many digestion and hormonal problems.

A weakened immune system. The liver is a member of the immune system and helps to fight against infections. A sluggish liver won't be able to adequately respond to a threat, including parasites .

Inadequate detoxification, toxic overload. Detoxification is the liver's most recognized function. The liver makes fat-soluble toxins, such as pesticides, preservatives, food additives, heavy metals, pollutants, plastics, and other environmental chemicals, less harmful to the body then removes them from the bloodstream. If the liver is unable to do its job and toxins remain in the body, inflammation skyrockets, jeopardizing hormone balance and causing a variety of symptoms. Skin irritation or skin allergies is one of the first signs of liver damage.

Estrogen dominance. The liver is responsible for processing metabolized, or "used up" hormones and removing them from circulation, including estrogens. A sluggish liver will prioritize the toxins and take care of the more harmful toxins, such as heavy metals or PCBs first, leaving metabolized hormones out—this can be a big contributor to hormone imbalance and estrogen dominance by allowing a build-up of harmful "dirty" estrogens.

Let's take a closer look at the liver's detoxification process and how it removes toxins and estrogen from circulation.

Liver Detoxification 101

The liver's detoxification happens in two phases.

Phase 1 is known as oxidation. Most toxins are fat-soluble and can't be cleared without the liver's help. In phase 1, the liver uses oxygen and enzymes to break down these toxins, making them water-soluble so they can be more easily excreted from the body through urine, bile, and stool. This is also the phase when used up estradiol and estrone can either be broken down into the antagonistic "dirty" estrogens 4-OH and 16-OH or the "good" estrogen 2-OH. We want to support a balanced breakdown and not tip too much toward 4-OH and 16-OH.

In order to complete this phase the liver needs key nutrients including: B vitamins (B_2, B_3, B_6, B_{12}), folate, glutathione, flavonoids, sulforaphane, and diindolylmethane (DIM).

Phase 2 is known as conjugation. In this phase the broken down toxins and estrogens from phase 1 (more toxic now than they were before) are coupled with another compound that will safely evacuate them via several different detoxification pathways. The companion that will evacuate them could be a methyl group, along the methylation pathway or sulfur, along the sulfation pathway.

If phase 2 is not working effectively, then the highly toxic chemicals formed in phase 1 cannot be happily paired off and successfully sent down a pathway. This can cause a lot of toxicity issues in the body and allow excess hormones, like "dirty" estrogens, to circulate through the bloodstream instead of being excreted. The result is hormonal imbalances, including a flair of estrogen dominance symptoms. I have

never met a person with a sluggish liver who is hormonally balanced.

In order to complete this phase, the liver needs key nutrients including: Methionine, cysteine, magnesium, glutathione, B vitamins (B_5, B_{12}), vitamin C, glycine, taurine, glutamine, folate, choline, and sulforaphane.

If more science is not your thing, skip ahead to the next section, What You Can Do to Detox Your Liver, where I make it crystal clear which foods you should eat to support phase 1 and phase 2 detoxification.

But if you want to dig a little deeper into phase 2, take a look at the following table. It provides a snapshot of four major pathways, items each pathway is responsible for conjugating

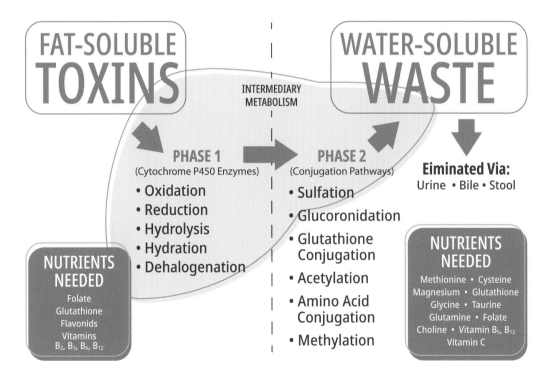

OVERCOMING ESTROGEN DOMINANCE

or carrying off to be evacuated and detoxed, what can inhibit this action, along with what can activate it.

Taking the methylation pathway as an example, you'll see estrogens are one of the hormones cleared through this pathway. Oral contraceptives, proton pump inhibitors (PPIs) for GERD, antibiotics, and Ibuprofen inhibit this pathway so you want to cut them out as much as possible. The activators, the foods and nutrients that kickoff this process, are high in choline and vitamin Bs, beets, and SAMe (a supplement).

See chart on the next page.

There you have it: Your liver needs a lot of nutrient support to make sure both phase 1 and phase 2 detoxification happens smoothly as well as ensuring toxins, used up hormones, and "dirty" estrogens are removed safely. The next section covers the superfood allies that will help you provide the needed support.

What You Can Do to Detox Your Liver

I hope you are excited to show your liver some love! Not only will your hormones rebalance, but so much of your total health is going to improve as well. You'll sleep better, your LDL cholesterol will probably drop, and overall, you'll feel like a million bucks. It's not complicated. It boils down to one easy action: eating liver-supporting foods.

> Everything you need to detox your liver gently and consistently is built into the Foundation Protocol and 28-Day Meal Plan in Part IV. Just follow those guidelines and you'll be all set.

Eat liver-supporting foods. Food has to be first. After all, it's the biggest part of what you are putting in your body. Bring more of these anti-inflammatory and liver-supporting foods into your diet. Don't be intimidated by this long list. All of these foods are part of the Foundation Protocol recipes and meal plans. Just follow those and you'll be eating to encourage phase 1 and phase 2 detoxification.

Visit
www.hormonesbalance.com/oed/downloads
to get the Superfoods Printable Poster.

PATHWAY	RESPONSIBLE FOR CONJUGATION OF:	INHIBITORS	ACTIVATORS
METHYLATION	• Estrogen • Dopamine • Histamine • Heavy Metals	• Oral contraceptives • proton pump inhibitors • antibiotics • ibuprofen	• Choline: eggs, non-GMO soy lecithin and avocado (less) • Vit Bs • Beets • SAMe
GLUTATHIONATION	• Pesticides • Paracetamol (painkiller) • Heavy Metals; mercury, lead, cadmium, etc • Penicillin • Tetracycline (antibiotics) • Petroleum distillates • Alcohol • Bacteria	• Low iron • zinc • Vit Bs • selenium • fluoride • aspirin	• Glycine, glutamine, & cysteine • Methionine (from meat, fish and dairy) • Fish oil • Limonene (lemon rind) • DIM/Cruciferous vegetable • Vitamins B_2, B_6, C • Selenium • Milk Thistle • Glutathione (NAC) • SAMe • To up glutathione levels; whey protein, Vit C and NAC
SULPHATION	• Progesterone • Thyroid • DHEA • Melatonin • Histamine • Dopamine • Adrenalin • Noradrenalin	• NSAIDs	• Sulphur-rich food: garlic, onions, cabbage • Cruciferous vegetables • MSM • Sulphur-containing amino acids: methionine, cysteine, taurine
GLUCURONIDATION	• Sex Hormones: estrogens, cortisol androgens • Paracetamol • Pollutants, food, additives • NSAIDs (aspirin, Tylenol, etc) • Benzodiazepines (ant-depressants)		• Calcium d-glucarate • Zinc • Vitamin B complex • Essential Fatty Acids

DIRTY DOZEN AND CLEAN 15

Each year the Environmental Working Group (EWG.org) analyzes test data from the Department of Agriculture to determine the amount of pesticides on produce then ranks fruits and vegetables in order to help shoppers make educated decisions. I advocate always buying organic, but if you have to make financial choices, always go organic when it comes to the Dirty Dozen.

Dirty Dozen

These fruits and vegetables are infamously high in toxic chemicals from pesticide residues. You definitely want to choose organic.

1. strawberries	7. peaches
2. spinach	8. cherries
3. kale	9. pears
4. nectarines	10. tomatoes
5. apples	11. celery
6. grapes	12. potatoes

Clean 15

These were found to have the lowest amounts of residues. If you don't have the budget for organic, you can feel more comfortable buying non-organic versions.

1. avocado	9. kiwi
2. sweet corn	10. cabbage
3. pineapple	11. cauliflower
4. sweet peas, frozen	12. cantaloupe
5. onion	13. broccoli
6. papaya	14. mushrooms
7. eggplant	15. honeydew melons
8. asparagus	

Cruciferous vegetables. Put away the lettuce. Crucifers are so much more nutritionally dense.

They are rich in diindolylmethane (DIM), which helps the detoxification pathways and clears "dirty" estrogens, high in fiber, anti-inflammatory, and packed with nutrients. They are also safe for the thyroid. (See the box for more.)

- cabbage
- cauliflower
- kale
- broccoli
- broccoli sprouts
- Brussels sprouts
- collard greens
- mustard greens
- watercress
- arugula
- bok choy
- radishes
- rapini
- romanesco broccoli
- kohlrabi
- rutabaga
- horseradish
- daikon

Broccoli sprouts. These are a cruciferous vegetable, but are so amazingly nutrient-dense they deserve a category all their own. They contain the highest levels of sulforaphane—a magical compound we now know can help phase 1 and phase 2 liver detoxification and clear out "dirty" estrogens. Sulforaphane is anticarcinogenic and

kills cancer stem cells! Broccoli sprouts are safe for the thyroid. (See the box for more.)

What you can do with them:

- Add them to salads, smoothies, and soups.
- Treatment dose (for someone going through or having recently undergone treatment for thyroid cancer or breast cancer): 1 cup per day
- Maintenance dose: 1/4 to 1/2 cup per day

Flax seed. A powerful ally when it comes to dealing with estrogen dominance. It binds up "dirty" estrogens and evacuates them, blocks "dirty" estrogens from getting into estrogen receptors, and lowers beta-glucuronidase, the enzyme in our estrobolome that promotes "dirty" estrogens when it gets too high. Studies have also shown that flax seed helps reduce thyroid cancer, alleviates PMS, and improves fertility. Plus, it's a great source of both soluble and insoluble fiber. And flax seed is safe for the thyroid.

What you can do with them: add to salads, smoothies, soups or a glass of water.

How to use it:

- Always use freshly ground. It keeps for a maximum of five days in an airtight container.
- Do not buy "flax seed meal" because it's old and likely oxidized.
- Do not cook. The flax seed that you put into muffins doesn't count. For liver-supporting benefits, the flax seed must be raw.
- Consume 2 tablespoons per day.

Fiber-rich foods. These aid the liver in moving toxins out.

- seeds and nuts, such as flax seed, sesame seeds, sunflower seeds, and pumpkin seeds
- vegetables, such as artichoke, sweet potato, carrots, beets
- fruit, such as avocado, pear, apple, berries
- lentils, including chickpeas
- beans
- whole grains, such as oats, brown rice, buckwheat

THE FEAR OF FLAX SEED (IT'S "ESTROGENIC" AND "WILL SLOW MY THYROID")

Many women fear flax seed because it contains phytoestrogens (naturally-occurring estrogens), and is "goitrogenic" and may therefore interfere with the thyroid. This information got popularized by well-meaning bloggers who unfortunately don't fact check and lack deeper context. Naturally-occurring estrogens don't cause estrogen dominance, I explained what does in chapter 1. Flax seed contains low amounts of glucosinolates (that get broken down to goitrin, the disliked compound). Research has shown the risk for hypothyroidism increases only when consumed in large quantities and accompanied by iodine deficiency. It's also worth noting that 90% of patients with hypothyroidism suffer from Hashimoto's, which is an autoimmune condition and most don't have iodine deficiency. Treatment requires addressing the immune system and removing "goitrogenic" foods won't help. This would explain why I've never met a woman who has given up flax seed (or other "goitrogenic" foods such as the cruciferous vegetables) and healed her hypothyroidism or Hashimoto's. Instead, this is a food that will help with estrogen dominance and improve the conversion of T4 to T3 thyroid hormone.

Dandelion (leaf and root). The leaf detoxes the kidneys while the root works on the liver. The whole root will help a lot because it's bitter and we know bitter greens and tinctures are great for our digestion. They are also liver-supporting, promoting bile excretion to help expel toxins and "dirty" estrogens. Dandelion is a stand-out superfood.

What you can do with them:

- Sauté the leaves or add them raw to salads. Dress with orange and/or lemon juice to balance out the flavors.
- Use the root to make tea.
- Use tinctures containing dandelion root.

Iodine-rich foods. Iodine detoxifies our "dirty" estrogens while playing a key role in breast and brain health. We have iodine receptors in our breasts, thyroid, brain, adrenals, and ovaries. An iodine deficiency compromises energy levels, cognition, immune function, and factors into breast lumps as well as breast cancer. I cannot tell you how many women regain energy and mental sharpness after eating more kelp (they put it into a bone broth). This is why you will find a few of our recipes containing seaweed. Many people in the United States are iodine deficient. Choose clean, toxin-free products, harvested in the United States. Do not buy seaweed from China.

Seaweed is a fantastic source of iodine and can be found in:

- kelp (kombu), has the highest amount of iodine
- hijiki
- wakame
- nori, low in iodine

What you can do with them:

- Add dried kelp, hijiki, or wakame to bone broths or soups.
- Use them to make salads. Beware of bright green seaweed salad. This color is fake. Natural seaweed is a dirty green color.

Caution: Do not consume iodine in high amounts if you have Hashimoto's and elevated TPO antibodies.

Sulfur-rich foods. Sulfur is a compound needed by the liver in phase 2 detoxification to "marry" estrogens and some of the toxins in order to evacuate them. Rich in sulfur, these foods support liver detoxification and clear "dirty" estrogens. They are also anti-inflammatory and antibacterial.

- onions, especially red onions because they contain the flavonoid quercetin, are a powerful antioxidant and anti-inflammatory
- garlic
- leeks
- chives
- scallions

Collagen-rich foods. Collagen has phenomenal health benefits. It rebuilds your gut mucosal lining, strengthens your bones, supports your joints, promotes strong hair, skin, and nails, as well as minimizes wrinkles. It's rich in glycine, necessary for phase 2 liver detoxification, and a precursor to glutathione, a master detoxifier.

Eat chicken, beef, or lamb bone broth made with a variety of collagen sources: joint tissue, cartilage, skin, feet, and knuckles. Note: marrow bones do not contain collagen. (See recipe on page 260.)

Additional notes:

If you do not have access to good-quality bones, use a collagen supplement instead.

Pomegranates. My absolute favorite fruit, pomegranate is a liver-supporting powerhouse, rich in antioxidants, vitamins C and E, a good source of folate, potassium, and vitamin K. It's also high in selective estrogen receptor modulators (SERMs). SERMs attach to an estrogen receptor and block "dirty" estrogens from entering the cell. Isn't that just absolutely phenomenal? With its high content of phytoestrogens, it is no surprise that in India and Iran pomegranates are prescribed for fertility and PMS as much as for menopausal symptoms.

What you can do with them:

- Add to salads and smoothies.
- Eat them as a snack with some nut butter.
- Juice them, but don't buy ready-made juices. They are pasteurized, get oxidized, and lose their potency.

Turmeric (curcumin). Makes you feel healthy just looking at that rich yellow color, doesn't it?

TOOLS FOR SUCCESS: HOW TO REMOVE POMEGRANATE SEEDS

People shy away from trying pomegranates because of the time and effort it takes to get the seeds out. No more! Check out a quick video at www.hormonesbalance.com/oed/downloads and learn how to remove those precious seeds quickly and easily.

The active ingredient in turmeric, curcumin, helps detox the liver and is anti-inflammatory. It also supports digestive, heart, and brain health, and boots your immune system. If you can't buy it fresh, consider a supplement with high bioavailability.

What you can do with it:

- Add to any dish or drink.
- Juice it. I add a little ginger and an orange or lime.
- Consume 1/2 to 1 teaspoon per day.
- Add black pepper to help with absorption but only a tiny bit. Too much pepper can damage the gut lining.

Wild Salmon. A high-quality protein, wild salmon is high in selenium, which helps break down toxins, a potent anti-inflammatory, high in omega-3s and B vitamins. Selenium is also good for women with thyroid issues.

Words of advice:

- Buy only wild caught, never farmed. Farmed salmon is filled with antibiotics, growth hormones, and colorants (to make the flesh look pink).
- Meat should be tight and muscular, not flabby, and a dark, rich color.
- Frozen is okay.

Culinary tip: Try baking for 20 minutes at 300°F so you don't overcook it.

Beets (root and leaves). The roots *and* leaves are amazing for the liver. They are a blood cleanser and liver detoxifier while full of fiber, folate, and vitamin C. Beets are also highly anti-inflammatory and support digestive, brain, heart, and immune system health.

- Can be consumed raw or cooked.
- Don't chuck the leaves! I like to sauté them.

Berries. Berries are packed with powerful nutrients and antioxidants that help protect the liver from damage and prevent cardiovascular disease, cancers, diabetes, and some metabolic diseases. They are low on the glycemic index so they won't elevate your blood sugar levels, a good source of fiber, and highly anti-inflammatory. Berries can also combat microbial infections.

- blueberries
- blackberries
- raspberries
- gooseberries
- strawberries (higher in sugar than other berries)

Cacao. High in magnesium and containing 20 times more antioxidants than blueberries, cacao is a good source of protein, calcium, carotene, thiamin (B_1), and riboflavin (B_2).

What you can do with it:

- Add to smoothies
- Make low-sugar truffles.

Additional notes:

- Only choose chocolate above 70% cacao with no dairy and little sugar.
- Choose organic cacao.

Citrus zest (lemon, lime, and orange). The peel is high in a potent liver detoxifier, d-limonene, plus it stimulates stomach acid production.

Zest only the surface, not the pith (the white part).

What you can do with it:

- Add to dressings, salads, and smoothies.

Sardines. I know sardines aren't everyone's favorite, but if you haven't given them a try, do so. Sardines are much lower in toxins than other fish, such as tuna. They are highly anti-inflammatory due to high Omega 3 content—a key benefit for a healthy liver. Sardines are also a great source of clean protein, as well as calcium, and magnesium from the bones. This is why it's best to buy sardines with bones (not boneless), and if buying canned, I recommend brands such as Crown Prince or Wild Planet.

What you can do with them:

- Mash on toast with avocado and sauerkraut (I like using the Polish Sourdough Buckwheat Bread on page 254.)
- Add to salads, mashed

Thyme. Thyme is packed with vitamin C and is also a good source of vitamin A. It is full of antioxidants, phytoestrogens, and is highly anti-inflammatory. Thyme is also great for people with histamine intolerance as it helps block histamine and its release. You can use dried or fresh, which is very easy to grow indoors.

What you can do with it:

- Add to salads or sprinkle on top of meals. Many of our recipes in this book contain thyme.

NAC and glutathione. NAC (N-Acetyl-L-Cysteine) is the darling of the detoxification world because it gets converted to glutathione, the master detoxifier capable of preventing damage to important cellular components caused by reactive oxygen species, such as free radicals, peroxides, lipid peroxides, and heavy metals. NAC also helps protect the liver. Studies show that NAC can help estrogen metabolism (by producing more of the "clean" estrogens) and protect the cells from estrogenic cancer growth. Glutathione supplements vary in quality and are infamously unstable in its delivery. I therefore recommend taking NAC, an inexpensive and easy-to-convert to glutathione supplement.

Liver herbs. Herbs are incredible liver allies, in nuanced ways. There are those that can "move" the liver, meaning they regenerate and protect the liver. Here are a few of my favorites.

- Mild liver herbs: burdock root, St. John's Wort, calendula
- Liver stimulants: dandelion root, chicory root, andrographis, Oregon grape root
- Liver protectors: turmeric, schisandra, milk thistle, licorice

For recipes, see the Liver Tea (Decoction) on page 345.

Our Before Meal and After Meal Digestive Bitters contain many bitter herbs (such as gentian, burdock, and andrographis) that stimulate bile production in the liver—essential action in enabling digestion of fats (which many of your hormones are made of) and binding up "dirty" estrogens. Other liver allies in these bitters are schisandra (this is my personal favorite), angelica archangel, ginger, and rosemary.

Your Gallbladder: What You May Not Know

Your gallbladder is a sachet tucked under the liver. It stores the bile the liver produces and releases it when you eat fat-containing foods.

Bile also helps the liver to excrete excess hormones and "dirty" estrogens. There are 250,000 surgeries performed in the United States to remove the gallbladder just because we technically can live without it. It's true that we can, but with what quality of life? Removal causes a host of issues that you probably haven't heard about. Sadly, doctors don't share this, therefore many women don't connect the two events—gallbladder removal and the subsequent onset of estrogen dominance along with a host of other health issues.

First, how can you tell if you have gallbladder problems? Symptoms include:

- gallstones
- pain or tenderness on the right of the abdomen
- pain in the right shoulder blade
- trouble digesting fatty foods
- food sits in the stomach
- light or chalky stool
- fatty stool
- constipation
- nausea, vomiting
- hormonal problems

Next, while we can live without a gallbladder, it's not uncommon to experience these issues:

Trouble digesting and absorbing fats, causing diarrhea and gas. Some women have embarrassing toilet episodes.

Vitamin and mineral deficiencies. When you don't have fat available as a raw material, then vitamins D, A, and K won't get absorbed very efficiently (unless you take supplements that use oil as a delivery method).

REMEMBER TO AVOID THESE INFLAMMATORY FOODS DURING THE 28-DAY FOUNDATION PROTOCOL. YOUR GUT AND LIVER WILL BE VERY GRATEFUL.

- gluten (wheat, barley, rye, farro, and products containing processed gluten-containing grain flours like breads, pastas, cookies, and muffins)

- dairy (cheese, butter, milk and yogurt, even lactose-free)

- eggs (both the yolk and whites)

- corn

- soy (in all forms, including soy sauce and tempeh)

- nightshades (tomatoes, white potatoes, eggplants, peppers, chili, goji berries)

- processed or packaged foods, including protein powders (you'll be eating whole foods only)

- conventionally grown vegetables, grains, meat, and fish (eat organic, non-GMO, and pasture-raised meat as much as you can)

- coffee and caffeine

- sugar, in limited quantities only

Bone and muscle problems. Lack of bile avail-ability leads to low testosterone and estrogen, building blocks for muscles and bones.

Hormonal imbalance. Losing a gallbladder means losing access to bile on demand. One of bile's functions is to bind up the "dirty" estrogens that are causing problems. This is why women who have their gallbladders removed often start having estrogen dominance issues. It doesn't happen right away, maybe three to six months after surgery. Most of the time they don't realize the connection. Loss of bile can also lead to low DHEA, testosterone, progesterone, and estrogen.

Here's what to do if you're suffering with gallblad-der issues right now.

- Follow the 28-Day Foundational Protocol Meal Plans to avoid dairy, eggs, gluten, and other problematic foods.
- Make sure fresh vegetables comprise 70% of your plate.
- Add bitter greens, such as dandelion leaves and arugula.
- Do not avoid all fats unless close to an attack; extra virgin olive oil and fish oils are great.
- Eat fresh or juiced beets and cucumbers.
- Add digestive bitters before and after meals.

If you feel like your gallbladder isn't working at its optimal level, start taking our Before Meal and After Meal Digestive Bitters—they contain herbs that stimulate bile production.

Consider ox bile. If your gallbladder has been removed, add an ox bile supplement. It will help you digest and absorb fats as well as proteins, aid in the absorption of vitamins A, D, E, and K, while also assisting in the support of healthy bones and muscles. Bile supports binding of "dirty" estrogens, helping to evacuate them through stool. In those who lost their gallbladder, extra bile supplemen-tation will help metabolize the fats, which are the precursor for all your steroid hormones includ-ing estrogen, progesterone, cortisol, DHEA, and testosterone. Try 125 mg of ox bile, standardized to 45% cholic acid, with meals, once per day.

Why I'm Not a Fan of One-Off Detoxes

How often do you tidy up and clean your house? Probably daily (tidying up) and weekly or so (cleaning)? Once a year you may do some deep spring cleaning, right? Imagine now that you never tidied up or cleaned your house through-out the year, but you waited to do that once-a-year spring cleaning. What would your house feel and look like? Your liver is the same way. It needs daily care to function properly and keep your hormones in check. I'm not opposed to you doing a deep detox once a year (just the way you would do spring cleaning), but please remember to use every meal as an opportunity to support your liver, too. It is not difficult because our 28-day meal plan features recipes that will give your liver the TLC it so deserves. I hope you enjoy the recipes we created here for you and make some of them a part of your daily cooking repertoire.

Let the Healing Continue

I hope you have a new appreciation for your liver and its powers beyond detoxification. A well-functioning liver, capable of getting rid of "dirty" estrogens along with other toxins, is essential for hormone balance and the second leg of your hormone balance stool. In healing a sluggish liver, you'll look and feel better than before, have more energy, experience better moods, while significantly reducing or resolving estrogen dominance. Detox your liver with the suggestions included in this chapter and found in the Foundation Protocol and 28-Day Meal Plan in Part IV. All of the liver-supporting foods are in the recipes and meal plans so just follow those and you'll be giving your liver all of the love it needs.

Chapter 6

Balance Your Blood Sugar

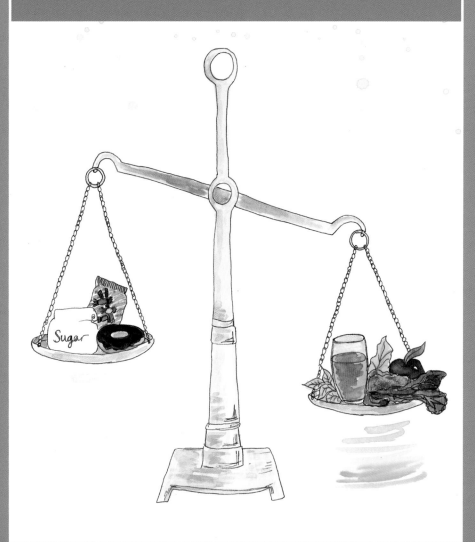

HORMONAL BALANCE

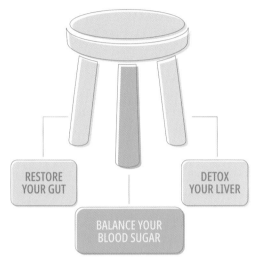

RESTORE YOUR GUT

DETOX YOUR LIVER

BALANCE YOUR BLOOD SUGAR

Balanced blood sugar is the third leg of your three-legged stool for hormone balance. Your hormones depend on stable blood sugar just as much as a healthy gut and liver. Blood sugar that fluctuates wildly throughout the day or is consistently too high or too low can really mess with your hormones and exacerbate your estrogen dominance. Many of the women I work with feel controlled by sugar; struggling with sugar cravings and sugar addiction. It's no wonder given how much our food is loaded with sugar. The numbers are shocking. According to the Diabetes Council, the average American eats 126 pounds of sugar each year. That's 156 grams or 39 teaspoons (1 teaspoon = approximately 4 grams) of sugar each day.

1 teaspoon = 4 grams of sugar

One of the big surprises I experienced when I first moved to the United States was how sweet everything tasted. Another thing that surprised me was people didn't feel the food and drinks were too sweet—an indication of how desensitized they were to sugar. Sugar is everywhere, from savory foods like soups, salad dressings, bread, kielbasa, and condiments to snacks, energy drinks, and granola bars. The foods you may think of as "healthy" are often packed with sugar. Many of us simply don't realize how much sugar we eat each day.

Here's an example of how easy it is to overdo it: You start out the day with a bowl of Kashi Go Crunch Honey Almond Flax cereal, 12 grams of sugar (3 teaspoons). On the way to work you grab a venti Java Chip Frappuccino blended coffee, about 88 grams of sugar (22 teaspoons). For lunch, you have a mixed salad with dried cranberries and dressing, 4 grams of sugar (1 teaspoon). But lunch came with a free Snapple lemon tea, setting you back with 36 grams of sugar (9 teaspoons). By late afternoon, you need a pick-me-up and reach for an Almond Butter Chocolate Chip Larabar, 16 grams of sugar (4 teaspoons). Dinner is a piece of roasted chicken and a sweet potato, 4 grams (1 teaspoon). But hey, it's been a long day and you feel like you deserve a bit of a treat. One serving of Ben and Jerry's Cherry Garcia will set you back 31 grams of sugar (nearly 8 teaspoons). The grand total? 191 grams of sugar—48 teaspoons or 1 cup! If you skipped that sugar-bomb Frappuccino, it's still 26 teaspoons of sugar.

That's even more than the average American. And these foods aren't what you think of when you think of "junk" foods, right? In this example, I've tried to show you how incredibly easy it is to consume way more sugar than you think.

Play sugar detective yourself for a few days. Read the nutritional label of foods you eat on a regular basis and add them up by the end of the day.

I guarantee you will be surprised at the quantity of sugar they contain.

Bottom line: It's too easy to fall into the sugar trap. To balance your hormones and estrogen dominance, you need to be much more conscientious about the amount of sugar and the kinds of sugar you eat.

Signs Your Blood Sugar Balance Needs TLC

If you recognize any of the following symptoms of hypoglycemia (low blood sugar) and hyperglycemia (high blood sugar), you have some work to do to balance your blood sugar levels. We tend to start with low blood sugar causing us to feel shaky, anxious, and unfocused—and desperate for sugar to make us feel better. If you need a soda, coffee, chocolate, or granola bar at 4:00 p.m. to make it through the rest of your day, you know what I mean. We eat those sugar-filled treats and then our blood sugar spikes making us feel better for a short while until we crash again, perpetuating the vicious sugar roller-coaster cycle and setting us up for an unhealthy relationship with sugar.

Symptoms of Sugar Imbalance

Hypoglycemia (Low blood sugar)

- Having to eat every few hours to avoid crashing
- Needing sugar to "bring sugar levels up" two hours after eating

- When hungry, feeling:
    - shaky, nervous, or anxious
    - moody and unfocused
    - sweating, experiencing chills, and clamminess
    - irritable or impatient
    - confused, even delirious
    - rapid or fast heartbeat
    - light-headed or dizzy

Hyperglycemia (High blood sugar)

- blurry vision
- difficulty concentrating
- frequent urination
- constant thirst
- constant hunger (even after a large meal)
- fatigue after eating
- stubborn belly fat
- blood glucose level greater than 90 mg/dL—even though labs/doctors say 99 mg/dL is acceptable (see Note)
- HA1c greater than 5.4 (even though labs/doctors say 5.6 is acceptable)
- insulin greater than 15 IU/mL (even though labs/doctors say 24.9 IU/mL is acceptable)

Note: Use functional medicine ranges that are more stringent than lab ranges (what you see on your results). Functional ranges are for optimal health whereas lab ranges are only averages of patient results and should not be used to manage your health.

Let's take a closer look at what happens in your body when you eat sugar to better understand this cycle of spikes and crashes, as well as what you can do to find a better balance.

What Happens When You Eat Sugar

When we talk about sugar, we're talking about carbohydrates. Sugar is just a general term for sweet, short-chain, soluble carbohydrates. When you eat carbohydrates, whether a plate of pasta, slice of bread, or sweet potato, your body converts them into glucose, a type of sugar your cells use for energy. The glucose circulating in your bloodstream is called your blood sugar. High levels of glucose in your blood triggers the pancreas to release insulin, a hormone that "sweeps up" glucose from the blood and carries it into cells. Excess glucose is stored by the liver as glycogen for future use. When those stores are filled, glucose is turned into fat for storage in cells throughout the body. This is how eating too many carbs packs on the pounds: extra sugar is converted to fat.

Paying attention to the amount of carbohydrates you eat matters but so does the type of carbohydrate you consume. Not all carbs are created equal. Choose carbohydrates carefully because different types affect you in different ways.

Processed carbs are sugars and grains that have been refined or altered in some way to remove their fiber, vitamins, and other nutrients. Processed carbs only have one or two sugar atoms, so they are sometimes called "simple carbs." These include table sugar, all kinds of flour, and refined grains (even if they are gluten free), and all of the foods made with these ingredients such as white bread, cereals, rice crackers, quinoa puffs, doughnuts, cookies, protein shakes and powders (yes, most are of full of sugar), and additives and preservatives. Because the fiber in them has been

largely or completely removed, these foods are digested quickly, causing a rush of glucose into your bloodstream and a huge spike in insulin.

In contrast, foods in a whole form, such as quinoa, buckwheat, or brown rice are complex carbs. It takes your body longer to digest these because they still contain plenty of fiber. Fiber helps to slow down the metabolism of sugar. This is a good thing, helping to maintain blood sugar balance, preventing the sugar rush, and insulin spike of processed carbs. The sugars in the fiber are not completely broken down until they reach your large intestine, keeping you full for longer and providing longer-lasting energy.

These two charts illustrate the difference in blood sugar and insulin levels after eating a complex, slowly digested carb versus a processed, easily digested carb.

TESTS TO CHECK YOUR BLOOD SUGAR LEVELS (IN FUNCTIONAL RANGES—FOR TRULY HEALTHY PEOPLE!)

Order these three tests to check your blood sugar levels and measure against these functional medicine ranges for acceptable levels:

1. Blood glucose (70 to 90 mg/dL)

2. Insulin (0 to 15 IU/ml)

3. HA1c (4.8 to 5.4%)

Chart 1 shows the result of eating a slowly digestible carbohydrate on a person with healthy blood sugar levels. As you can see, their blood sugar and insulin go up following the meal and as insulin moves glucose into the cells, both steadily fall, taking about four to five hours to digest. Their blood sugar never dips below baseline.

Chart 2 shows the result of either eating a super sweet smoothie, cereal, or muffin, or drinking a cup of coffee with sugar in it. Their blood sugar and insulin levels go up quickly and then crash below baseline within three hours. Now they're experiencing signs of hypoglycemia: bad mood, disorientation, brain fog, even physical shakiness. Some people crash in as little as two hours and this is when they reach for another muffin, cup of coffee, or energy bar "to bring up their sugar levels."

Being caught up in a cycle of sugar dependency is not a good place to be. After all, there are good reasons why sugar is called the White Death.

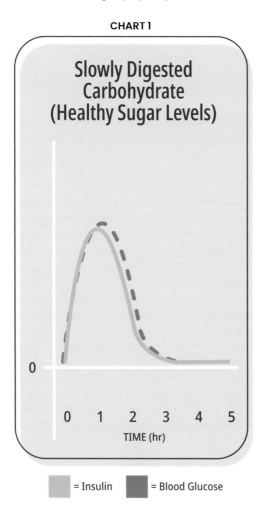

CHART 1

Slowly Digested Carbohydrate (Healthy Sugar Levels)

0

0 1 2 3 4 5

TIME (hr)

= Insulin   = Blood Glucose

How Sugar Impacts Your Hormones

Sugar sabotages your hormonal health in the following ways:

Amplification of **your current symptoms.** Sugar makes *everything* worse. It will amplify every one of your symptoms, from body aches and pains to autoimmune conditions, insomnia, terrible PMS, or the growth of fibroids and breast lumps.

Taxing of **the endocrine system, resulting in a host of hormone imbalances.**

High blood sugar raises testosterone. High blood sugar levels are the leading cause of high testosterone in women. High blood sugar levels suppress the Sex Hormone Binding Globulin (SHBG), a hormone responsible for, as the name implies, binding and regulating excess sex hormones such as testosterone. A lack of SHBG means more available testosterone. This can lead to the development of polycystic ovarian syndrome (PCOS) and estrogen dominance as testosterone gets converted to estrogen, contributing to high estrogen levels.

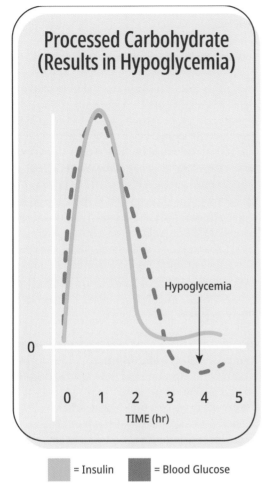

CHART 2

Processed Carbohydrate (Results in Hypoglycemia)

Hypoglycemia

0

0 1 2 3 4 5

TIME (hr)

= Insulin   = Blood Glucose

High blood sugar raises estrogen. Estrogen is made from testosterone, so as testosterone levels rise because of high blood sugar so does the likelihood of estrogen dominance.

High blood sugar raises insulin and cortisol. Chronically high blood sugar levels lead to high insulin levels. In turn, high insulin levels trigger the release of cortisol by the adrenals to try to bring insulin levels back to baseline. This not only taxes your adrenals but high levels of cortisol disrupt your body in a variety of ways. They are associated with an increased risk of many health problems including digestive issues, sleep problems, anxiety, depression, and heart disease.

Low blood sugar stresses your adrenals. That sugar crash does more than ruin your mood; it zaps your adrenals too. Sugar dips put stress on the body, signaling the adrenals to release cortisol and rebalance our sugar levels. Many women already suffer from compromised adrenals and these sugar lows weaken them even further. Compromised adrenals have been linked to premature aging, dry skin, fatigue, coffee addiction (another skin-aging factor), weight gain, moodiness, frequent sickness, feeling depleted and unmotivated.

Blood sugar fluctuations worsen hot flashes. The mechanism isn't fully understood but we know dropping blood sugar levels can bring on or worsen hot flashes. I once polled our online community, asking what had helped them reduce or stop hot flashes and night sweats. The answers were overwhelmingly unanimous; changed my breakfast to PFF (Protein, Fat, Fiber), reduced or stopped coffee, dropped desserts and alcohol before bedtime, added a supplement like chromium or berberine. Guess what? All these point to one thing: improved blood sugar levels, which helped with hot flashes and night sweats.

Depletes vitamins and minerals. Sugar is not just empty calories, a food with no nutrients. It's worse; it robs us of key vitamins and minerals. Sugar depletes us of magnesium, calcium, zinc, chromium, potassium, copper, and B vitamins. Without these nutrients, we're more likely to experience leg cramps, low blood pressure, hair loss, gray hair, wrinkles, ADD, ADHD, depression, asthma, osteoporosis, and of course hormonal imbalances.

No surprise as our endocrine system needs these raw materials to make hormones. And our liver relies on B vitamins to detoxify us from estrogens.

Triggers systemic inflammation. Chronic inflammation can shut down hormone receptors, making them unresponsive to hormones trying to enter cells to do their job. For example, inflammation can block progesterone from entering cells, widening the gap between estrogen and progesterone, therefore promoting the estrogen dominance caused by these "unbalanced partners."

FRANCIS'S HOT FLASHES IN THE EMERGENCY ROOM

Dr. Francis is an emergency physician who used to experience debilitating hot flashes at exactly 11:00 a.m. each morning. The problem was they would strike in the middle of her shift when she was often saving lives. Something had to change. After initial reluctance, she sent me her food journal, which said her 8:00 a.m. breakfast consisted of cereal, topped with fruit and yogurt. She had also noted that if she had a handful of walnuts (full of protein, fat, and fiber!) around 10:45 a.m., she wouldn't get a hot flash. This was a great observation and one that proved her dropping blood sugar level around 11:00 a.m. was the cause of her hot flashes. She wasn't always able to snack to prevent a hot flash. I wanted to focus on the bigger picture and prevent her blood sugar levels from dropping in the first place. We changed her breakfast to a PFF (Protein, Fat, Fiber) kind of breakfast and her hot flashes immediately stopped. This is why most of the breakfast recipes in this book are based on the PFF principal.

Sugar is a major contributor of inflammation in the body.

Lowers the immune system. The vitamin and mineral depletion caused by sugar weakens the immune system. Ever gotten sick after a couple of big nights out? Alcohol is sugar so it's not surprising after a major overdose your immune system can't fend off illness.

Feeds Candida, a yeast overgrowth. Candida disrupts the microbiome, which we know is terrible for our hormones, estrogen dominance, and is a leading cause of sugar cravings. Candida loves to gobble up sugar, which helps it thrive and multiply. It uses sugars to strengthen its cell walls and give it the energy to fight off your body's natural defenses. Regular sinus, yeast, or vaginal infections, bloating, and a white coating on the tongue, are all typical signs of Candida.

Changes the body's pH, making it more acidic and promoting inflammation. Sugar lowers stomach acid production and pulls our body's pH into a more acidic state.

Messes with neurotransmitters including serotonin, dopamine, and beta-endorphins. When you eat sugar, your brain rewards you by releasing mood-enhancing neurotransmitters such as serotonin (a mood balancer), dopamine (a feel-good neurotransmitter associated with reward and pleasure), and beta-endorphins (natural pain killers), resulting in a short-lived high. It is no surprise then that many former drug, gambling, sex addicts, and alcoholics recover from their addictions only to become sugar addicts. A diet high in sugar has been linked to poor mental health, including an increased risk of depression, worsened anxiety symptoms, poor memory, and mood swings.

Causes insulin resistance. Insulin resistance happens when the insulin receptors on a cell won't open and allow glucose entry. It's as if the key—insulin—no longer fits the lock—the insulin receptor. The cell has become "resistant" to the influence of insulin. This can happen because of a diet overloaded with sugar, processed carbohydrates, and systemic body inflammation. Cells become starved of the glucose they need for energy, yet blood sugar and insulin levels remain high. The result is symptoms including fatigue, trouble losing weight, belly fat, depression, prediabetes, and type 2 diabetes. One in three Americans—including half of those age 60 and older—is insulin resistant.

Drives fatty liver disease. Fatty liver disease is when too much fat gets deposited in the liver. Where did all of the fat come from in the first place? Sugar. Remember, the liver can only store so much leftover sugar as glycogen and when that space gets filled up, the liver converts it to fat. And you know from chapter 5 a healthy liver is key in balancing your hormones.

Creates sugar addiction. The more sugar you eat, the more your body will crave it. It takes higher and higher amounts of sugar to achieve the high.

Sugar is bad for your health and hormones, but it's a problem with a solution. There are some very practical steps you can take to kick the sugar habit and balance your sugar levels.

What You Can Do to Balance Your Blood Sugar

I hope you are inspired to break your sugar addiction. The good news is once you do that, your taste buds will recalibrate and you will find sugary things taste disgustingly sweet. When I was in private practice, my clients would report their favorite cocktails would taste awful. Afterwards, their smoothie would need juice from vegetables such as celery, cucumber, or fennel bulb to feel nourishing. Their cravings had vanished. You won't spend time searching for a sugar "pick me up" to beat a 3:00 p.m. slump.

Here's how to beat sugar for good:

- become more aware of how much sugar you consume
- limit the amount of sugar you consume
- be smart about the kinds of sugars you eat
- eat according to the PFF (Protein, Fats, Fiber) principle, especially breakfast
- support with supplements

Become more aware of how much sugar you consume. (You will be so surprised!) One of the biggest steps you can take toward self-healing is to become more aware of the amount of sugar you consume daily. I'm not into micromanagement (such as counting calories) because it's an unsustainable way of living. I will ask you to do this exercise for only a few days, or until you feel you get into a habit of reading product labels before putting a product into your shopping cart. Start by examining the sugar content of every product you buy. Take stock of the foods you have in your refrigerator and pantry. Look at the back of

> Everything you need to balance your blood sugar is built into the Foundation Protocol and 28-Day Meal Plan in Part IV. The Meal Plans are designed to be low in sugar and help you to maintain stable blood sugar levels throughout the day. Follow those and feel the results..

the packaging for the amount of "Total Sugars" listed in the nutritional information and not the often empty promises on the front of the package. Divide the number of grams by four to get the approximate number of teaspoons of sugar the product contains.

Watch out for the serving size. Oftentimes, a product we typically consume in one sitting reads "2 servings" and it creates an illusion of a lower sugar content. For example, a bottle of kombucha states one serving contains 8 grams (that's 2 teaspoons) and there are two servings per bottle. "Not bad," you think. If you drink it in one sitting like most people, you will actually drink 16 grams or 4 teaspoons of sugar.

When you do buy packaged foods, check the label to catch sugars masquerading under other names including: dextrose, fructose, glucose, high fructose corn syrup, malt, golden syrup, honey, maple syrup, maltose, lactose, brown sugar, caster sugar, palm sugar, raw sugar and sucrose, while some newer varieties include agave syrup and rice malt syrup.

This may feel like micromanaging your diet, which is not what I would ever want to promote in the long term. This is just a temporary measure for you to develop your sugar detective muscle. In no time, you will learn which products to stay away from. Or when evaluating new products, your first intuition will be to turn the product around and read the ingredients list, including sugar content. This new habit will be instrumental in balancing your sugar levels and hormones.

Limit the amount of sugar you consume.

Eat no more than 5 teaspoons or 20 grams per day. The Estrogen Reset Meal Plans only contain 20 grams of sugar each day (or less) so you don't even have to think about counting grams if you follow those. If you have Candida or are doing a Candida cleanse, you'll want to eat almost no sugar at all.

To put this number in context, the Dietary Guidelines for Americans from the U.S. Department of Agriculture is 32 grams of sugar = 8 teaspoons per day. This covers *all* sugar, the "good" kind which naturally occurs in whole foods such as fruits, vegetables, and unrefined grains, as well as the "bad" kind, found in processed foods, added to packaged foods with salt or additives to increase sweetness and addictiveness. It's important to look at the total sugar content (not just what has been added) because your body doesn't know the difference and has to process everything you put into it.

Be smart about the sugars you eat. I'm often asked what the best and worst sugars are. Some sugars are better than others. I rank them based on three factors:

1. The amount of fructose they contain (the less the better). Fructose is a form of sugar found naturally in many fruits, vegetables, and sweeteners such as agave, honey, and brown rice syrup. Because fructose is sweeter than glucose

ALCOHOL IS SUGAR, TOO

If you must drink, limit it to two to three drinks per week, always with or after food. Avoid drinking late at night as it may disturb your sleep and tax your liver. Avoid drink mixers as they contain high fructose corn syrup.

and acts as a preservative, it is very popular with processed food manufacturers. It is often added to packaged foods and beverages (soda or fruit-flavored drinks). Only the liver can metabolize fructose so it won't raise your blood sugar levels and insulin but breaking down a lot of it, taxes the liver. When you have estrogen dominance, you want to show the liver some love and ease its burden, not overload it.

Does this mean you should stop eating all fruit to avoid fructose? No. Cut out processed forms of fructose (this is where it's most concentrated) and pay attention to how much fruit you consume as well as how it makes you feel.

2. The glycemic index (how quickly a serving elevates your blood sugar levels) and glycemic load (a number that takes into account the amount of carbohydrates in a serving of food along with how quickly it raises blood sugar). The glycemic index of a food is a value assigned to it based on how slowly or quickly it raises glucose levels in your bloodstream. Index values range from 0 to 100, with 100 being pure glucose. High-value foods cause blood sugar to rise most rapidly and are generally the most processed. The glycemic load factors in the actual amount of carbohydrates present in one serving of the food. For example, a food can be high on the glycemic index but have so few carbs actually present in one serving that its glycemic load is low. Take cantaloupe. It has a high glycemic index (65) but a low glycemic load (4). A glycemic load of 10 or less is considered low, 11 to 19 medium, and greater than 20 high. To maintain good blood sugar balance, you want to stick with foods low on the glycemic index and with a low glycemic load.

3. The degree of processing it took to make it. We want the least amount of processing as possible.

The "Best to Consume" sweeteners in the Sugar Chart contain less than 40% fructose and their glycemic index is below 60 and glycemic load is below 20 (which is medium range).

Some may be new to you. Here are a few things to keep in mind:

Artificial sweeteners. Stay far away from artificial sweeteners. Seriously, do not consume these. They've been linked to breast cancer, glucose intolerance (an umbrella term for conditions resulting in high blood sugar), gut microbiome imbalance (contributing to obesity and weight gain), and hypertension. Artificial sweeteners to avoid at all cost are:

- acesulfame potassium, used in Sunett, Sweet One
- aspartame, brand names are NutraSweet, Equal, Neotame
- saccharin, brand names are Sweet 'N Low, Sweet Twin, Sugar Twin
- sucralose, brand name is Splenda

Sugar alcohols. These are a new form of sugars that have entered the market under names such as xylitol, sorbitol, mannitol, and erythritol. On the plus side, they're naturally derived, very low in calories, and do not increase your blood sugar levels. On the negative, they are highly processed and can cause gut issues in some people. They can also be terrible with IBS or SIBO patients. I have found erythritol is the best tolerated. If you want to try them, I suggest starting with erythritol and seeing how you respond.

Natural sweeteners that are not sugars. These include monk fruit and stevia. Monk fruit, also known as luo han guo or Buddha fruit, is a small round fruit grown in the South of China. It's been used for centuries in traditional Chinese medicine and approved by the Food and Drug Administration (FDA) as a sweetener in 2010. Buy with caution as monk fruit is often mixed with sugar alcohols such as erythritol. Stevia might be a good option; it's easy to obtain nowadays, has no bad side effects (if you don't consume excessive amounts), and don't mind the taste (I personally don't like it). I don't recommend brands such as Truvia and Sun Crystals; even though they use stevia, they are highly processed.

Which sugars do I use? (sporadically, no more than 1 tablespoon per day) I like several (check out my favorite brands in Resources):

- coconut nectar (my absolute favorite, low in fructose, fairly low on GI/GL index and minimally processed)

- raw, unfiltered, local honey
- maple syrup
- monk fruit (if you don't like the taste of pure monk fruit in the dish you're making, try adding a bit of honey to mask it and add sweetness)

Eat a PFF (Protein, Fats, Fiber) Breakfast

Protein, fats, and fiber slow down sugar ingestion, prevent sugar spikes and crashes. The way to stabilize your blood sugar levels is to surround yourself with foods high in protein, good fats, soluble, and insoluble fiber, or the PFF Principle, for short. Set yourself up for success by starting your day with a good PFF breakfast, and little to no sugar or fried foods. Follow the Chinese proverb that says, "Let your breakfast be your best friend, lunch your acquaintance, and dinner your enemy," meaning eat a big breakfast, a light lunch, and a smallish dinner. Instead of crashing, crashing, crashing throughout the day after a breakfast of fruit, flavored yogurt, grains, cereals, bars, and oatmeal you'll be stable with no dips at 11:00 a.m. and 4:00 p.m. You'll sleep better at night too. A member of our online community once posted, "In order to change my nights, I had to change my breakfast." By changing her breakfast and stabilizing her blood sugar levels throughout the day, she improved the quality of her sleep, so much so eventually she didn't need sleeping pills anymore.

What does a PFF breakfast look like? The sources of proteins in your breakfast could come from fish, beef, chicken, bison, lamb, tempeh (if you can tolerate soy), and coconut butter, but also from moderate amounts of presoaked nuts and seeds, if tolerated. I know, these probably don't sound like traditional breakfast foods to you, but people around the globe have savory,

BEST TO CONSUME	JUST OK	BEST TO AVOID	NEVER CONSUME
Coconut nectar Dates (whole) Yakon syrup Fruit juice (real, fresh) Honey (raw, unfilered) Maple syrup (gradeB) Blackstrap molasses, molasses Stevia (dry, green leaf or extract)*	Brown sugar Cane juice and sugar Date sugar and syrup Turbinado Raw sugar	Agave and agave nectar Barley malt Beet sugar Brown rice syrup Caramel Carob syrup Corn syrup Dextran and dextrose Ethyl maitol Fructose Fruit juice concentrate Glucose Golden sugar/syrup Grape syrup High fructose corn syrup Lactose Malt syrup Maltodextrin Maltose Manninol Sorbitol Sorghum syrup Sucrose Table or white sugar Xylitol	Acesulfame K (Sweet One) Aspartame (Equal, Nutra-Sweet) Saccharin (Sweet'N Low) Stevia white/bleached (Truvia, Sun Crystals) Sucralose (Splenda) Tagato

low-sugar breakfasts. For example: The Turks eat plenty of salami and cheese, the Moroccans sip on a bean soup, while the Japanese eat miso soup and fish for breakfast.

All of the breakfasts in the meal plans are nutrient-rich PFF breakfasts. Give them a try over the next four weeks. People who follow the PFF breakfast recommendations report massive improvements. Many of them start losing weight, feel more energetic, focused, and grounded. Their sugar addiction ends or lessens, their skin clears of acne, eczema, dryness, and they sleep better, while many report less PMS and fewer hot flashes.

Coffee and Blood Sugar Levels

This isn't going to be very popular with the coffee lovers here, but you need to know this: coffee jacks up your blood sugar levels. According to research, the spike happens two to four hours after consumption. One way to mitigate it, if you must drink coffee, is to have it after a meal and not before. Decaf doesn't raise blood sugar levels.

Support with supplements

If you've been struggling with blood sugar balance, you may benefit from some extra support from these supplements. I encourage you to fix your food first because doing so will make the supplements more effective. You'll feel better faster when you do both. Supplements such as berberine and chromium picolinate can be helpful.

Berberine. Many studies show that berberine can improve insulin sensitivity, significantly reducing blood sugar levels in individuals with type 2 diabetes. In fact, it has been shown to be as effective as metformin, a popular diabetes drug (Glucophage) without the side effects. The recommended dosage is 500 mg per day.

Chromium picolinate. Several studies have shown that this trace element improves insulin sensitivity and lowers glucose levels. The recommended dosage is 300 to 500 mcg.

Inositol. This nutrient can help balance blood sugar and regulate polycystic ovarian syndrome (PCOS)-related issues such as insulin resistance and elevated testosterone. Look for the form D-chiro-inositol, a good regulator of insulin metabolism. It's best when inositol comes in two forms: myo-inositol and D-chiro-inositol. Myo-inositol has been shown to be more involved with the health of the ovaries and overall reproductive and hormonal function, while D-chiro-inositol is a good regulator of insulin metabolism. The recommended dosage is 3.2 g per day.

In Control

I hope you are inspired to take control of your blood sugar levels and add a strong third leg to your hormonal balance stool. By becoming more aware of the hidden sugars in your food and knowing what to look for on nutrition labels, you'll start to lower your intake, break your addiction, and balance your hormones. But, of course, the easiest fix is to start following the meal plans and recipes in the Foundation Protocol in Part IV. All of the recipes support blood sugar balance. By following the meal plans, you'll support stable blood sugar levels while rebuilding your digestion and detoxifying your liver naturally. It's incredible how quickly your symptoms will start going away by taking care of your gut, liver, and blood sugar levels.

In the previous three chapters, I've covered many ways to do so, primarily with food. In the next chapter, I'll share the Foundational Supplements you can use to amplify your healing.

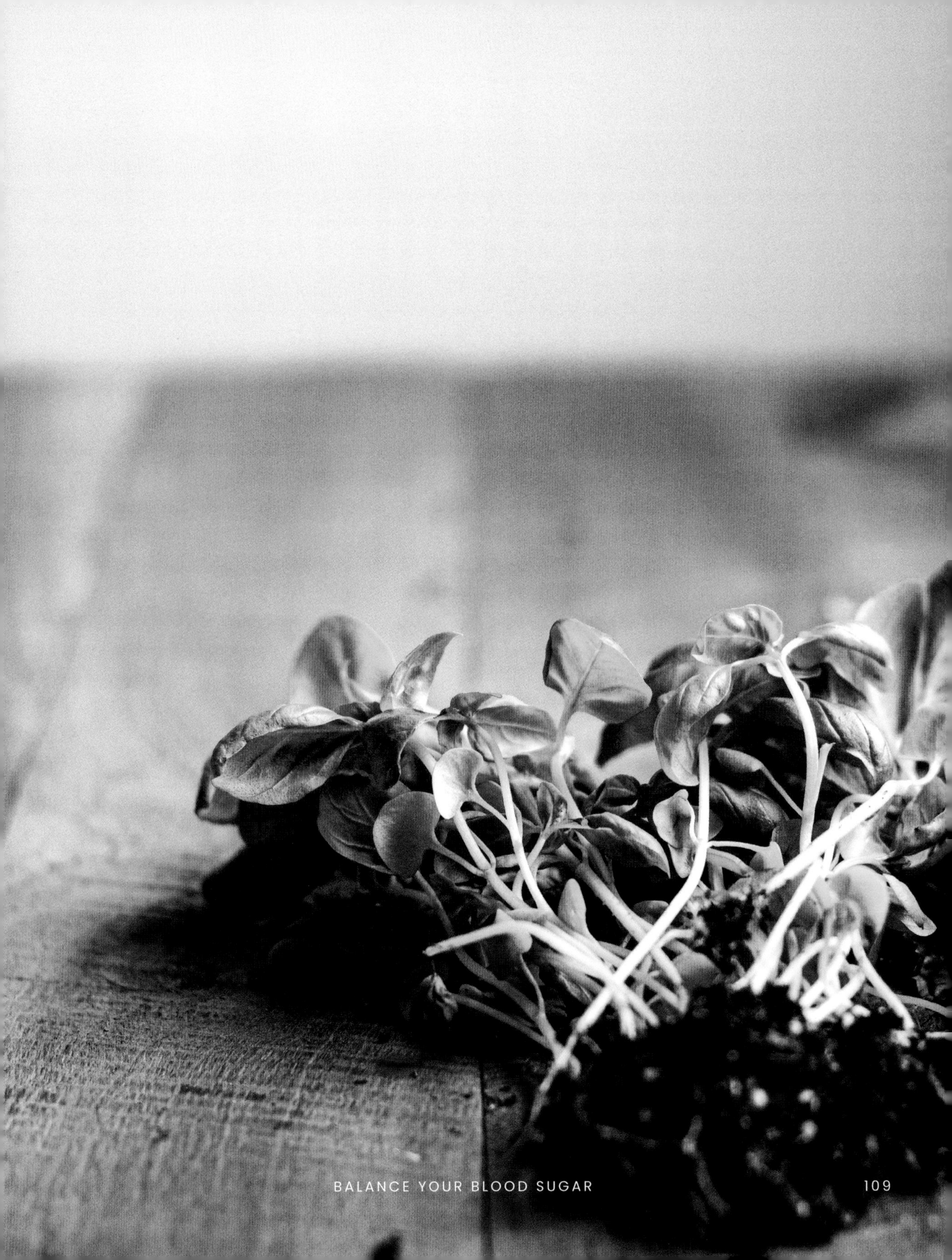

Chapter 7

Foundational Supplements

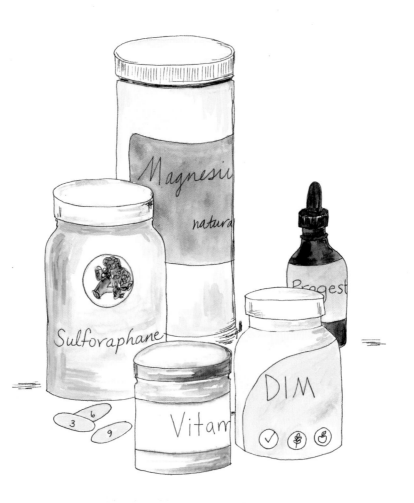

While food is always first, supplements are powerful allies for bridging the gaps in our nutrition and speeding up our healing. Most women are deficient in several essential nutrients, for example magnesium. Those of us with estrogen dominance can benefit from a few key supplements aimed at addressing the root causes driving our symptoms, such as by helping us clear "dirty" estrogens as well as improving our estrogen to progesterone ratio.

Used atop a strong food foundation, the following Foundational Supplements will amplify your healing. Add these as part of your Foundation Protocol. For the brands I personally use and recommend, see Resources, page 361. If you choose to use your personal favorite brand of supplements, please read "Getting Started with Supplements" in chapter 3, page 52, for how to evaluate the quality of your supplements. It is an unregulated industry and therefore the quality of supplements can vary from highly efficacious and clean to harmful junk.

Foundational Supplements for Estrogen Dominance

- Magnesium
- Vitamin C
- Vitamin B Complex
- Zinc
- Vitamin D$_3$
- DIM
- Sulforaphane
- Calcium D-glucarate
- Omega 3 Fatty Acids
- Vitamin B$_6$
- Bioidentical Progesterone (Topical)

What About Food?

Food is not only foundational, but nonnegotiable if you want to fix your hormones and overall health. When I first started practicing, I was convinced food could fix everything. In fact, I used to bash supplements, partly because my private clients would come with a bag of supplements which cost them $500 per month and provided no results. Why? Because my clients barely made any diet changes or the supplements were of very poor quality. Over the years, I've come to a solemn conclusion that food alone (organic included) may not be enough to correct many nutritional deficiencies. The fact is our food isn't as nutrient-rich as it once was. Modern farming practices, including organic, don't adequately restore important minerals to the soil. As a result, produce is lower in nutrients, including magnesium, calcium, selenium, and zinc.

As much as I would love for food to be the only source of nutrients, it may not be enough for most of us unless you have access to food grown on biodynamic farms. This is why supplements can be a great help and I have certainly seen them help my own health and the health of our Hormones Balance community.

Magnesium

If you want to achieve balanced hormones and optimal health, you need adequate levels of magnesium. A widely used mineral, magnesium has many important roles in the body and is involved in multiple processes, including energy production, musculoskeletal support, digestive regulation, detoxification, nervous system function, mental health, cellular homeostasis, and hormonal balance. Yet most of us aren't getting enough. In fact, researchers have estimated up to 75% of Americans may be deficient in magnesium. Magnesium is needed for over 300 hundred enzyme reactions in the body, helps clear estrogen, lowers inflammation, promotes good sleep, and regular bowel movements. It supports:

- calm, relaxation, and sleep
- blood sugar balance
- breast health (lumpy breasts)
- bone health
- digestion and regular elimination
- cardiovascular health
- kidney health

- thyroid function
- the relief of body pains, muscle aches, twitches, or cramps at night
- the relief of weak, tired muscles

Magnesium and Hormone Balance

Magnesium, as part of the three-legged stool analogy, plays a supportive role in the body's digestive health, sugar balance, and liver detoxification pathways, as well as helps neutralize toxin and heavy metal exposure. Sufficient magnesium levels in the body can naturally and effectively help balance a majority of our most important hormones. Magnesium directly affects our hormonal health by supporting:

Digestion and elimination. A magnesium deficiency is a common cause of chronic constipation, which prevents the "dirty" estrogens from being expelled from the body.

Sugar balance and insulin sensitivity. Current research has shown there is an inverse relationship between the intake of magnesium and the risk for developing type 2 diabetes. Further studies have shown supplementing with magnesium may positively affect glucose regulation in patients with type 2 diabetes and even improve insulin sensitivity in healthy individuals.

Lower cortisol. Magnesium moderates the way cortisol is produced in the body during times of stress, may influence a person's anxiety level, and how she or he responds to stress. Another study confirmed supplementation with magnesium helps to significantly decrease serum cortisol levels.

Thyroid function. Magnesium, when taken by those with low thyroid function, is highly beneficial.

There are two forms of thyroid hormone: T3 (the active one) and T4 (the less active one). People with hypothyroidism either have issues with the production of T4 or the conversion of T4 to T3 hormones. Magnesium facilitates the conversion. This explains why women with hypothyroidism feel energized when taking magnesium.

Sex hormone production. Magnesium plays a role in the proper production of estrogen, progesterone, and testosterone.

Estrogen and liver detoxification. Magnesium is needed not only in estrogen production, but it is also a co-factor in breaking estrogens into "clean" and "dirty" estrogens. Magnesium shifts the balance in the "clean" direction. "Dirty" estrogens are produced mainly due to poor phase II liver detoxification. If magnesium is not available in sufficient quantities, the detoxification process may be inefficient and affect the clearance of "dirty" estrogen metabolites from the body. Women suffering from estrogen dominance benefit greatly from adding high-quality magnesium to their daily supplement regimen.

Recommended Dosage

The RDA for magnesium is around 320 milligrams per day. If levels drop below this, the ramifications can quickly be seen. Many women need a higher magnesium intake than the RDA suggests, particularly if they are being robbed of magnesium by genetic issues, conditions such as thyroid autoimmune disease, or stress.

To know if you need a higher dose, try the "bowel tolerance test" described below. This means you go up in doses every two days until your stool becomes loose. Some women are so depleted (stress and sugar are common magnesium robbers) that they need as much 1,200 mg per day to replenish their reserves. Once you get a loose stool, back off to a lower dose.

Here is an example:

- Day 1: 300 mg per day; regular stool or constipation
- Day 2: 300 mg per day; regular stool or constipation
- Day 3: 600 mg per day (300 mg in the morning and 300 mg at night); regular stool or constipation
- Day 4: 600 mg per day (300 mg in the morning and 300 mg at night); regular stool or constipation
- Day 5: 900 mg per day (600 mg in the morning and 300 mg at night); regular stool or constipation
- Day 5: 900 mg per day (600 mg in the morning and 300 mg at night); loose stool
- Day 6: Back off to 600 mg per day (300 mg in the morning and 300 mg at night) to go back to regular stool

Continue taking 600 mg per day until you develop loose stool, then back off again. If not, stay on this dose. Magnesium is one nutrient I recommend taking long-term. In times of stress, you may need to up the dose.

To settle on the best dose of magnesium, you need to listen to what feels right for your body. If you overdo it, you will experience loose stool or intestinal rumbling and then you will know to reduce your daily intake.

Recommended Form

There are various forms of magnesium; not all of them are recommended and their uses vary. I recommend these forms:

Magnesium glycinate

- Highest bioavailability, non-laxative effect; best used to replenish low magnesium levels quickly.

Magnesium malate

- High bioavailability, non-laxative effect; can be energizing for some; good to replenish low magnesium levels quickly.

Magnesium citrate

- Good absorption but can create a laxative effect in many. Hard to replenish low levels because of that. Great for women with constipation or those who travel and get constipated.

Magnesium chloride

- Used topically, it's a great way to increase magnesium levels and bypass the gut, especially helpful for people with leaky gut, digestive issues, or those who don't want to take pills.

Worst: Magnesium oxide

- Only has 4% bioavailability and can cause negative reactions. Companies that use it tend to add other low-quality ingredients. I do not recommend using it at all.

Magnesium Rotation Method

The magnesium rotation method is a quick and easy way to optimize your magnesium levels by capitalizing on the unique benefits of each form of magnesium throughout the day. Here's how it works:

Breakfast (6:00 to 8:00 a.m.)

Magnesium Malate (1 capsule providing 180 to 200 mg magnesium). This form of magnesium will help promote sustained energy levels and mental vitality throughout the day along with healthy cardiovascular function. Take 1 capsule with or immediately following breakfast.

Dinner (5:00 to 7:00 p.m.)

Magnesium Glycinate (1 to 2 capsules providing 150 to 300 mg magnesium). This form of magnesium will help promote sleep, easy bowel movements, and relaxation in general. Take 1 or 2 capsules (depending on magnesium status and/or goals) with or immediately following dinner.

Magnesium Citrate (1 teaspoon provides 300 mg magnesium). Take this form at night if you tend to get constipated. It will help you to have a healthy and complete bowel movement in the morning.

Bedtime (9:00 to 10:00 p.m.)

Magnesium Chloride (¼ teaspoon applied to arms and legs provides 150 mg magnesium). This form of magnesium will help relax your muscles to avoid cramps and pain, reduce hot flashes, as well as promote good, uninterrupted sleep. If you find the magnesium is tingling, wash it off after 20 minutes that's all the time needed for absorption.

As needed: for constipation or travel

Magnesium Citrate (1 teaspoon provides 300 mg magnesium). This form of magnesium helps promote bowel regularity and soft stools. It also helps calm the nervous system for relaxed travel.

Start with 1 teaspoon and titrate up until you get a bowel movement or loose stool. You can add it to a mug of warm water, which can additionally ease constipation, or mix with your choice of juice. If you're taking it before bedtime, you might want to add it to some tart cherry juice, which can additionally help with sleep and pain.

For travel, add a good amount to a small ziplock bag along with a 1 teaspoon measuring spoon. Keep it in your carry-on bag to easily add to hot water or even green tea during your flight.

For brand recommendations, see Supplement Guide on page 361.

Precautions

Magnesium intake may influence the absorption of certain medications therefore caution should be taken in patients with kidney and heart problems. Specifically, avoid taking magnesium with drugs that reduce urinary output, such as glucagons, calcitonin, and potassium-sparing diuretics, which may all increase magnesium levels in your blood.

Magnesium may also influence the absorption of the following drugs: aminoglycosides, bisphosphonates, calcium channel blockers, fluoroquinolones, skeletal muscle relaxants, and tetracyclines. In these cases, always talk to your doctor first before supplementing with magnesium.

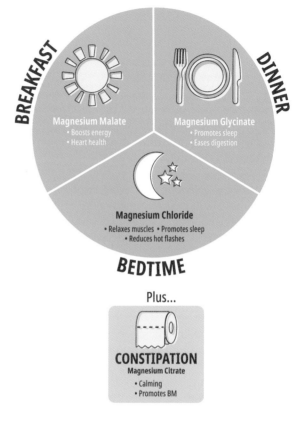

MAGNESIUM ROTATION METHOD
The Fastest Way to Replenish Magnesium Levels

BREAKFAST

Magnesium Malate
• Boosts energy
• Heart health

DINNER

Magnesium Glycinate
• Promotes sleep
• Eases digestion

Magnesium Chloride
• Relaxes muscles • Promotes sleep
• Reduces hot flashes

BEDTIME

Plus...

CONSTIPATION
Magnesium Citrate
• Calming
• Promotes BM

Vitamin C

The first thing that comes to mind when you think of vitamin C is immune health. Many people take vitamin C when coming down with a cold or when already feeling bad to shorten the duration of a virus. In addition to immune support, vitamin C is a cofactor for enzymes involved in the synthesis of important neurotransmitters like serotonin and norepinephrine. These neurotransmitters help maintain a positive mental outlook and deal with stress.

Vitamin C also has a crucial role in making some of the hormones necessary for maintaining your adrenal glands and these glands also contain one of the highest concentrations of vitamin C in the body.

Collagen synthesis requires vitamin C. Collagen is a primary structural protein in connective tissues such as bones, tendons and ligaments, as well as in hair, skin, and nails. Vitamin C helps maintain blood vessel health which is why inadequate amounts of C can result in easy bruising or bleeding.

Another very researched and talked about role for vitamin C is its antioxidant function. Vitamin C is a potent neutralizer of free radicals, helping to recycle other antioxidants, including vitamin E and glutathione.

Vitamin C and Hormone Balance

It has also consistently shown improved levels of endogenously produced progesterone. This is because the corpus luteum has some of the highest concentrations of vitamin C in the body. I have come to appreciate vitamin C a whole lot more when taking higher doses during the COVID-19 pandemic (1,200 to 1,800 mg per day). My period cycle, which originally shortened to 21 days, suddenly returned to a full 28-day cycle with very little PMS. It's typical of women with dropping progesterone levels to experience shorter cycles and once progesterone comes back up, the cycle gets more regular.

In the same fashion, raising your progesterone naturally will mitigate all your symptoms of estrogen dominance.

In the Nurses' Health Study, pre-menopausal women with a family history of breast cancer who consumed an average of 205 mg per day of vitamin C from food had a 63% lower risk of breast cancer than those who consumed an average of 70 mg per day. In the Swedish Mammography Cohort, overweight women who consumed an average of 110 mg per day of vitamin C had a 39% lower risk of breast cancer compared to overweight women who consumed an average of 31 mg per day.

Recommended Dosage

The RDA for vitamin C is 70 milligrams per day for women. Most RDAs state minimal values for a person to live and survive, not thrive in optimal health. You may therefore consider higher doses, with 2,000 mg per day being the upper limit.

To know what dose of vitamin C you need, try the "bowel tolerance test" described below. This means you go up in doses every two days until your stool becomes loose. Some women are so depleted that they need as much 4,000 mg per day to replenish their reserves. Once you get a loose stool, back off to a lower dose.

Here is an example:

- Day 1: 600 mg per day; regular stool or constipation
- Day 2: 600 mg per day; regular stool or constipation
- Day 3: 1,200 mg per day (600 mg in the morning and 600 mg at night); regular stool or constipation
- Day 4: 1,200 mg per day (600 mg in the morning and 600 mg at night); regular stool or constipation
- Day 5: 1,800 mg per day (1200 mg in the morning and 600 mg at night); regular stool or constipation

- Day 5: 1,800 mg per day (1,200 mg in the morning and 600 mg at night); loose stool
- Day 6: Back off to 1,200 mg per day (600 mg in the morning and 600 mg at night) to go back to regular stool

Typically, when you replenish your levels of vitamin C, you will start getting loose stool even with 1,200mg per day; lower the dose then to 600mg or even less until your stool returns to normal.

Recommended Form

Many natural supplement makers proclaim the best form of vitamin C comes from berries, such as unripe acerola, amla, or camu camu. Yes, these berries contain a very high content of vitamin C, but the amount of the vitamin C in them varies (which is normal, nature isn't "standardized") and doesn't contain more than 25% ascorbic acid, the active compound. What's often shown on these labels is the grams of the berries but not the actual vitamin C content, which can be misleading to a consumer. I therefore recommend using a supplement that uses a combination of natural sources and ascorbic acid.

For brand recommendations, see Supplement Guide on page 361.

Precautions

Before taking vitamin C, consult your physician if you suffer from blood disorders such thalassemia, G6PD deficiency, sickle cell disease, and hemochromatosis. Avoid taking vitamin C immediately before or following angioplasty.

Vitamin B Complex

Have you ever wondered why B Complex is such an in-demand supplement and why so many people need it? For starters, it consists of eight different B vitamins combined together into one super formula. It contains the always popular B_{12}, usually known for helping with energy and weight loss (although, in reality, it does so much more), along with seven other B vitamins that are essential for overall health and hormonal balance. Below are the eight vitamins that are usually contained in a B Complex supplement and their main functions in the body.

- Thiamine (B_1): energy production, detoxification, glucose metabolism
- Riboflavin (B_2): thyroid function, fatty acid metabolism, detoxification
- Niacin (B_3): nervous system function, estrogen metabolism, detoxification, cholesterol management, blood sugar regulation, mood enhancement, adrenal health, circulation, healthy skin
- Pantothenic Acid (B_5): production of sex hormones, detoxification, adrenal function, brain health, inflammation
- Pyridoxine (B_6): mood, hormonal balance, liver health, and much more
- Biotin (B_7): adrenal function, nervous system support, metabolism of fats and carbohydrates, healthy hair, skin, and nails, inflammation, blood sugar support, cholesterol management
- Folate (B_9): brain health, mood, proper fetus development (Caution: Avoid the form called "folic acid," as it's a synthetic form of the vitamin that does more harm than good)
- Cobalamin (B_{12}): energy production, detoxification, brain function, sleep, nervous system maintenance, cardiovascular health

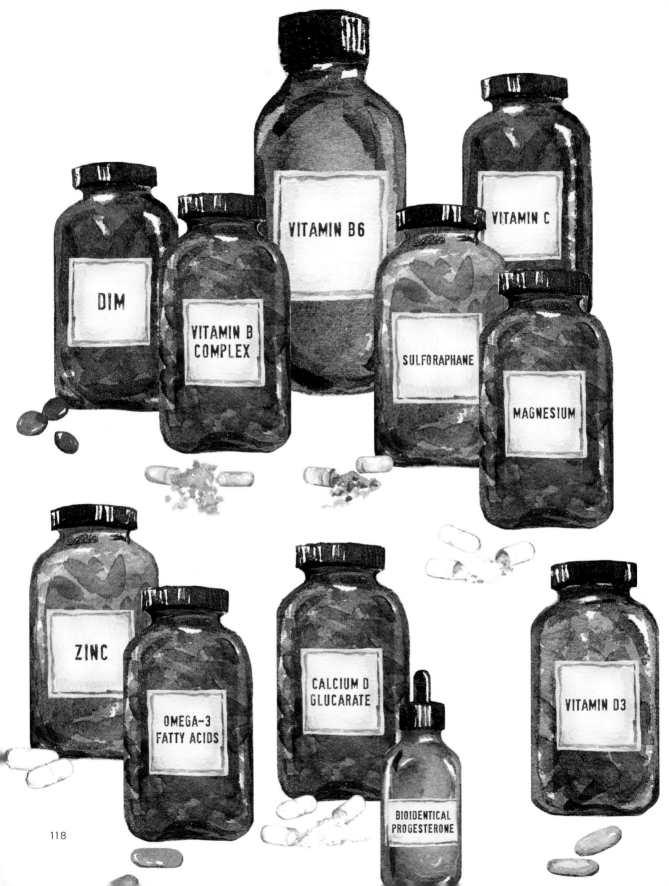

These eight very important vitamins have many benefits for the body, especially when combined into one formula. As a group of water-soluble vitamins, they play key roles in a majority of our bodily systems and processes; they are often synergistic in their actions. A deficiency compromises the function of every cell in the body.

Vitamin B-Complex and Hormone Balance

When it comes to hormonal health, B vitamins are integral to the proper production and balance of a majority of our hormones.

- Sex hormones: B vitamins are crucial to balancing the sex hormones estrogen and progesterone, especially in the case of estrogen dominance, as well as for overall support of the female cycle from menarche through menopause.
- Progesterone production: Vitamin B_6 is essential for the development of the corpus luteum. This gland is produced in the ovary after the egg has been released and it is what makes progesterone.
- Cortisol and DHEA: B vitamins support our adrenal glands, which produce two key stress hormones, cortisol and DHEA. The proper production and balance of these hormones is imperative to overall health.
- Thyroid: Another important aspect of hormonal wellness is the function of the thyroid gland and how it produces the thyroid hormones. One study concluded almost half of all the hypothyroid patients in the study were deficient in vitamin B_{12} and replacement with a B_{12} supplement led to improvement of symptoms. Vitamin B_{12} is essential in converting the inactive T4 to the active T3.
- Blood sugar balance: Lastly, insulin, which is involved in proper regulation of blood sugar, is under the influence of multiple B vitamins.

Recommended Dosage

Optimal daily doses:

- Thiamine (B_1): 25 to 50 mg
- Riboflavin (B_2): 25 to 50 mg
- Niacin (B_3): 25 to 50 mg
- Pantothenic Acid (B_5): 25 to 50 mg
- Pyridoxine (B_6): 25 to 50 mg, not to exceed 100 mg per day
- Biotin (B_7): 30 to 100 mcg
- Folate (B_9): 400 to 800 mcg
- Cobalamin (B_{12}): in its most effective form, methylcobalamin: 50 to 100 mcg

Recommended Form

Look for a supplement with B vitamins in their active or methylated form. The body can use them right away, without having to convert them through the methylation process. A methylated supplement is especially beneficial if you have the MTHFR SNP and your body's methylation is compromised. In its methylated form, B_{12} is called methylcobalamin and B_6 is pyridoxal-5-phosphate. Poor-quality supplements would present B_{12} in the form of cyanocobalamin. Folate in its methylated form is 5-methyltetrahydrofolate, not folic acid, which can be inflammatory and harmful. These are some of the factors you can check to assess the quality of your supplement brand.

For brand recommendations, see Supplement Guide on page 361.

Precautions

People with certain conditions should be cautious when taking niacin in high doses: jaundice, heart conditions, digestive issues, kidney failure, and gout. Vitamin B_6 should not be taken with the drug levodopa. Women who are nursing should not take more than 50 mg per day in order to maintain proper lactation. Folate should always be avoided by anyone taking the drug methotrexate.

I recommend taking B vitamins in the morning; they can be too energizing for some when taken in the evening.

Zinc

Zinc might be one of the more underappreciated nutrients, known by many but understood by few. As an essential trace element, it is utilized by multiple bodily systems and processes. Unfortunately, we are not able to produce it on our own and it therefore needs to be obtained from outside sources, either from food or supplements.

There are many benefits from supplementing with zinc:

- immune system function and support (It helps the body fight off bacterial and viral infections. This is especially important during critical periods of immune system development or challenge such as early childhood, pregnancy, and later life.)
- helps with autoimmune disorders (By supporting the immune system, zinc is important for women with autoimmune conditions such as Hashimoto's, especially when combined with selenium.)
- aids in DNA creation and repair in our cells by supporting protein synthesis
- promotes wound healing
- supports growth and development, starting as early as pregnanc, through infancy, and childhood
- promotes hormone production and balance, especially progesterone

- supports your senses: smell, taste, and vision
- provides overall metabolic support, including enzyme production and blood sugar stabilization.
- encourages better muscle recovery after exercise
- gives healthy blood pressure maintenance
- may improve fertility

A zinc deficiency compromises many bodily systems—and hormone balance.

Zinc and Hormone Balance

Zinc is essential for proper hormone balance, when it comes to both production and maintenance of many of our hormones. Zinc has a direct effect on:

- Estrogen and progesterone: These sex hormones, involved in all aspects of a woman's cycle from menstruation and fertility to menopause, are greatly influenced by the presence of zinc in the body, which is involved in their metabolism. Zinc also plays a part in stimulating the production of the follicle-stimulating hormone (FSH) and luteinizing hormone (LH), which in turn support the production of estrogen and progesterone.
- Testosterone: Zinc has a very important job when it comes to testosterone levels, especially when they are elevated, as is the case with PCOS. Zinc inhibits an enzyme that converts testosterone into its less-desirable form, dihydrotestosterone (DHT), thereby preventing unwanted facial hair growth and head balding, two common problems for women suffering from PCOS.
- Thyroid hormones: Both free T3 and free T4, as well as TSH, are negatively affected

in a zinc-deficient state. Furthermore, zinc is needed to convert the less active T4 to the more active T3 hormone. A study on hypothyroid women showed 30 mg of zinc supplementation helped reduce TSH (a good thing) and increase free T3 (also a good thing).

- Immune function: Zinc supports the immune system, which is vital in women who suffer from Hashimoto's thyroiditis.
- Cortisol: Zinc has the ability to inhibit cortisol secretion acutely and temporarily, which comes in handy during "fight or flight"–type of stress reactions. Further studies have supported zinc's role in the adrenal gland response. It is also interesting to point out the relationship goes both ways and high levels of cortisol can inhibit zinc metabolism.
- Growth hormone: Growth hormone (GH), secreted by the anterior pituitary, regulates multiple processes, including growth and metabolism. Research has shown both GH levels and growth rate in children increased with zinc supplementation. Not only is zinc responsible for an increase in GH levels in times of need, but zinc plays a pivotal role in GH storage, transport, and normal secretion. Growth hormone helps with cell regeneration and is therefore called the "anti-aging" hormone.

Recommended Dosage

A healthy adult needs 30 to 40 mg of zinc daily from both food and supplement sources.

Recommended Form

The best, most bioavailable forms are zinc picolinate and bisglycinate, which is well tolerated and is a readily-absorbed form of zinc. One precaution to consider is taking too much zinc accidentally, which can cause mild symptoms of nausea, vomiting, abdominal cramping, poor appetite, and headaches.

For brand recommendations, see Supplement Guide on page 361.

Precautions

A few interactions to keep in mind:

- Excess zinc inhibits copper absorption and can lead to a deficiency.
- Excess zinc inhibits iron uptake and can lead to a deficiency.
- Copper inhibits zinc absorption and can lead to a deficiency.
- Iron interferes with the absorption of copper and zinc, so take them separately if using both.

Vitamin D$_3$

Vitamin D$_3$, probably the most well-known and talked about of any vitamin, is crucial for nearly every aspect of our health. It plays a role in multiple metabolic processes and organ systems. It can also help prevent and recover from breast cancer. Several studies, including one from The Stanford University School of Medicine, have found vitamin D$_3$ inhibits the growth of breast cancer cells and stimulates apoptosis, the death of cancer cells.

The best source of vitamin D is the sun, so during summer aim for 15 to 20 minutes of unprotected sun exposure (without sunblock) between 10:00 a.m. and 12:00 p.m. Various factors play a role on how much vitamin D you can be absorbed, including the month of the year, your skin color, altitude, and percentage of body exposure. If you have a smartphone, I recommend using D Minder, an app that will help you calculate the values. Whatever you do, do not get fried in the sun.

Unjust fear of common-sense sun exposure along with the deceitful conclusion that any form of sun exposure causes skin cancer is erroneous and outright harmful. This propaganda (and marketing play by many skincare companies) has caused 70% of people in Western countries to be severely deficient in vitamin D. This deficiency has now been linked to autoimmunity, fatigue, depression, hormonal troubles, and several cancers, among other conditions. Interestingly, most people with melanoma are vitamin D deficient.

In the winter months, prevent deficiency or maintain a good level in your body by taking a high-quality vitamin D supplement.

Vitamin D is more than just a vitamin because it acts as a steroid hormone in our bodies. It "influences the bones, intestines, immune and cardio-vascular systems, pancreas, muscles, brain, and the control of cell cycles," which covers pretty much the whole body head to toe.

Here are some everyday benefits of vitamin D:

- bone development and protection, including osteoporosis prevention
- muscular support
- skin integrity
- immune system support
- cardiovascular protection
- mood enhancement
- brain function and nervous system support
- hormone production and balance (specifically thyroid, adrenal, and sex hormones)

Vitamin D and Hormone Balance

This mighty vitamin is a building block for many of the hormonal pathways in the body, such as:

- Blood sugar balance: Vitamin D_3 helps make insulin receptors more sensitive, hence balance blood sugar levels.
- Thyroid hormones: New research finds an association between vitamin D deficiency and autoimmune thyroid conditions, Hashimoto's thyroiditis and Graves' disease. Furthermore, there have been reports that impairment of the vitamin D signaling pathway has been observed in thyroid cancers, but more research still needs to be conducted. TSH, a critical hormone in the regulation of thyroid function, has been shown to have an inverse correlation with vitamin D, meaning the lower the vitamin D level in the body, the higher the TSH will be, which is usually the first step in developing hypothyroidism. It is important to note more research needs to be done to determine if vitamin D is a cause or consequence of hypothyroidism.
- Adrenal hormones: Over the last few years, some research has come to light demonstrating the role of vitamin D in endocrine diseases in particular, adrenal-related issues. A recent study researched the effect of vitamin D supplementation on cardiovascular disease risk factors, including elevated stress hormone cortisol. Results showed generally healthy adults who supplemented regularly with vitamin D had lower levels of cortisol in their urine when compared to the placebo group. Furthermore, vitamin D helps fight daily and chronic fatigue, whether it is or isn't the result of decline in adrenal function.

- Sex hormones: Vitamin D is a key nutrient involved in the production and regulation of many hormones in the body, including the sex hormones, such as estrogen and testosterone. It specifically plays a role in estrogen biosynthesis via calcium regulation. A recent study found a level of 25(OH)D greater than 32 ng/mL in the blood was associated with "significant reductions in bioavailable estradiol, free and bioavailable testosterone, compared to women whose circulating 25(OH)D remained below 32 ng/mL." This is important for women who suffer from estrogen dominance and excessive testosterone production. Perhaps most important, it can play a positive role for women with estrogen-receptor positive (ER+) breast cancer.

Recommended Dosage

If your blood lab result shows a deficiency, 5,000 IU to 10,000 IU is necessary to replenish the vitamin D in your body. It typically takes three months to get the levels up. Retest your levels, once satisfactory (and in the functional range), switch to a maintenance dose of 2,000 IU per day.

Always read supplement labels; you may think your multivitamin has enough vitamin D_3, but the truth is most multivitamins rarely have vitamin D_3 in sufficient doses even for maintenance.

Recommended Form

There are two forms of vitamin D available: D_2 and D_3, with the latter being far more effective in raising blood levels and usually of better quality. Vitamin D_3 is sourced from animal and marine sources, while vitamin D_2 is sourced from plants, but it is also often synthetically-derived.

Vitamin D needs the help of other nutrients (vitamins and minerals) to be able to do its work. They include vitamins A, C, E, B_6, B_{12}, and folate, as well as minerals such as zinc, magnesium, copper, and selenium. Vitamin D_3 works well with vitamin K_2 and is needed for optimal bone health; as well as for calcium, magnesium, phosphorus, and K_2 to get into the bones.

For brand recommendations, see Supplement Guide on page 361.

Precautions

It's possible to overdose on vitamin D, so make sure to stay within the recommended doses and test three months after high dosage. Too much vitamin D can interfere with vitamin A absorption and vice versa. Patient with certain conditions such as sarcoid need to consult their physician before supplementing with vitamin D.

DIM (diindolylmethane)

DIM is a compound generated when the body breaks down cruciferous vegetables such as broccoli, cabbage, and cauliflower. It is best known as a nutrient that supports healthy estrogen metabolism as well as the prevention of hormone-related cancers by its anti-estrogenic and anti-androgenic effects. It supports:

- phase 1 liver detoxification.
- the breakdown of estrogen into "clean" estrogens, not the antagonistic "dirty" ones
- a healthy balance of testosterone and estrogen by acting as an aromatase inhibitor, blocking some testosterone from converting to estrogen
- the cells from the damaging effects of oxidation

The Estrogen Reset Meal Plan is rich in cruciferous vegetables, but you'd have to eat about six pounds of crucifers each day to get enough DIM. That's just not doable for most people and is why a supplement is a good choice to consider.

DIM and Hormone Balance

DIM helps hormonal balance by supporting:

Liver detoxification and protection: DIM may support the liver in numerous ways, including lowering inflammation and promoting detoxification.

Balance of estrogen and testosterone: DIM has the ability to act as an aromatase inhibitor. This means it blocks the conversion of testosterone to estrogens, important for women who suffer from estrogen dominance.

Beneficial ratio of two forms of estrogen: DIM promotes the breakdown of estrogen into "clean" metabolites, not the potentially harmful "dirty" ones.

Blood sugar balance: DIM supplementation has also demonstrated some blood sugar lowering effects in animal models, showing decreased glucose and insulin. This may be an important development for people with diabetes or sugar-regulation issues.

Cancer prevention/protection/treatment: DIM supplementation has been shown to be therapeutic for breast and cervical cancer, as well as an effective helping agent when combined with the breast cancer drug tamoxifen. In a group of patients diagnosed with estrogen receptor positive breast cancer who were treated with tamoxifen, DIM helped to promote favorable changes in the metabolism of estrogen and related pathways.

Recommended Dosage

Anywhere from 100 mg to 300 mg daily has been determined as an effective and safe dosage. The recommended dose is 100 mg to 200 mg per day. Start with a lower dose (100 mg) if the supplement is suspended in oil and higher dose (200 mg) if in powder form.

Recommended Form

DIM is made up of a crystalline structure that makes it difficult for the body to absorb. The best DIM products are manufactured using an all-natural process which helps to optimize the absorption of this nutrient by the body—using a blend of MCT oils, non-soy-derived lecithin, and vitamin E, without the use of potentially harmful surfactants.

This delivery technology increases the absorption rate and reduces the absorption time for DIM,

DIM can be wonderful as it helps metabolize estrogen, especially "dirty" estrogens, which are the problematic metabolites that can cause so many of the estrogen dominance symptoms.

as a result it may allow for superior effects through lower dosages.

For brand recommendations, see Supplement Guide on page 361.

For brand recommendations, see Supplement Guide on page 361.

Precautions

Some research has shown DIM may affect blood sugar levels. For this reason, people with diabetes or hypoglycemia and those taking drugs, herbs, or supplements that affect blood sugar should be cautious when supplementing with DIM. Talk to your healthcare provider and make sure blood glucose levels are being monitored if you start taking DIM.

Sulforaphane

Sulforaphane is a mighty (and safe) compound I feel is highly underestimated and underused by both allopathic and functional professionals. I'm so smitten by it that I may sound like a snake oil salesman! In addition to helping aid in the body's detoxification, sulforaphane has been shown to have long-lasting antioxidant effects, offering protection from oxidizing free radicals and anti-estrogenic cancer properties. It is also the most powerful anti-inflammatory and is showing an impressive anti-carcinogenic potency.

Derived from broccoli and broccoli sprouts, it has similar characteristics to DIM but is not quite the same. Not only does this compound offer detoxification and antioxidant support, but it is protective for the cardiovascular as well as nervous systems.

Its benefits:

- phase 2 liver detoxification

- raises "good" estrogen (2-OH estrone)
- shrinkage of breast lumps and cancers
- powerful anti-inflammatory
- protects from free radicals
- strengthens the immune system

I'm a big fan of getting sulforaphane from broccoli sprouts (see page 88 for how to triple their sulforaphane content), but if you don't have the time or access, a supplement is a good option.

Sulforaphane and Hormonal Balance

Sulforaphane aids hormone balance in several ways.

Liver detoxification: Sulforaphane is directly involved in supporting liver detoxification, which is important not only for liver function itself but for the rest of the body as well. It targets biological pathways that both modulate Phase I enzymes and elevate Phase II enzymes, allowing for full and proper detoxification of unsafe chemicals along with "dirty" hormone metabolites, especially estrogens.

Anti-carcinogen and detoxifier: Research shows when it comes to supplementing with sulforaphane:

- Premenopausal breast cancer risk was decreased with higher broccoli consumption.
- Oral supplementation with sulforaphane reached the mammary glands of test subjects and increased activity of detoxification enzymes.
- There is potential for sulforaphane to protect from tumor resistance and relapse or recurrence of cancer. This nutrient has also been shown to be effective for thyroid cancer and is an anti-tumor agent.

- It raises OH-2 estrone, which is the protective form of estrogen

Chemoprotection: Sulforaphane is considered a chemoprotective agent for various types of cancers, including estrogen-receptive breast cancers.

Digestive health: A recent study determined sulforaphane supplementation decreased the overgrowth of pathogenic bacteria in the stool and improved daily bowel habits of the study participants.

Recommended Dosage

500 mg, 6 to 8% standardized extract

Recommended Form

Sulforaphane is a very unstable compound, therefore buying a supplement in a standardized form is key. It means that the supplement guarantees the active constituent amount. Sulforaphane should also contain myrosinase – an enzyme that improves sulforaphane availability by about eight times.

For brand recommendations, see Supplement Guide on page 361.

Precautions

If you are taking medications that are changed by the liver (Cytochrome P450 1A2 (CYP1A2) substrates), check with your provider before taking sulforaphane. Sulforaphane impacts the liver and these medications may act too fast or have side effects.

The Difference Between DIM and Sulforaphane (the clogged toilet analogy)

Since both DIM and Sulforaphane support liver detoxification, especially from the perspective of hormone clearance, what is the difference?

The one supplement that has established itself in the market as a "estrogen buster" is DIM. DIM can be wonderful as it helps metabolize estrogen, especially "dirty" estrogens, which are the problematic metabolites that can cause so many of the estrogen dominance symptoms.

Many women notice it helps at first and then it stops working. Some may have found it makes estrogen symptoms even worse.

Here is the reason: DIM upregulates phase 1 liver detoxification. Your liver also has phase 2 detoxification. Both of them need to work well for the junk to eventually get evacuated through your colon and kidneys (i.e., poop and pee).

To make it a little more graphic, imagine a toilet with a toilet bowl and a drain to carry the waste out. With DIM, you have just unclogged your toilet bowl but not the drain. In fact, the toilet bowl might be so open now that the drain can't cope, and the result is the toilet is still clogged up and overflowing.

So, back to your liver and estrogens. DIM has just helped you open up phase 1 detoxification, but if your phase 2 isn't working as well (which in most people it isn't), you won't feel better.

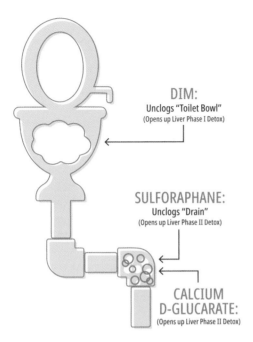

DIM:
Unclogs "Toilet Bowl"
(Opens up Liver Phase I Detox)

SULFORAPHANE:
Unclogs "Drain"
(Opens up Liver Phase II Detox)

**CALCIUM
D-GLUCARATE:**
(Opens up Liver Phase II Detox)

- the removal of harmful "dirty" estrogens
- liver detoxification
- a strong immune system
- lower inflammation
- lower LDL ("bad") cholesterol
- post-surgery and toxic exposure recovery

Calcium D-Glucarate and Hormone Balance

Calcium D-glucarate aids hormone balance by supporting:

Liver detoxification: Glucaric acid (which is what calcium d-glucarate is converted to) binds to toxins, which are then removed in the urine. Supplementation with calcium-D-glucarate has been shown to inhibit beta-glucuronidase, a specific enzyme produced by microflora in the large intestine and involved in phase 2 of liver detoxification that lowers the occurrence of breast, prostate and colon cancers. Removing toxins from the liver will increase liver function and promote a healthy metabolism. It will also allow your liver to flush out other toxins that would otherwise cause problems.

The good news: You can open up phase 2 liver detoxification with a beautiful substance called sulforaphane. I personally love sulforaphane because it's also a powerful antioxidant that supports estrogen detoxification in the liver and has anti-cancer properties.

Estrogen detoxification: Calcium d-glucarate removes the harmful "dirty" estrogens, which are the harmful metabolites of estrogen that may be responsible for conditions such as fibrocystic breasts, breast lumps, ER+ breast cancers, thyroid nodules, thyroid cancer endometriosis, fibroids, infertility, mood swings, and PMS. This research validates cancer prevention and estrogen metabolism.

Calcium D-Glucarate

Calcium D-glucarate, as an activator of the glucuronidation liver pathway, is a potent liver detoxifier that clears "dirty" estrogens and other harmful toxins. I also have found it to be very beneficial after several toxic exposures. For example, if you live in a polluted place or have been taking painkillers and antibiotics to prepare for a surgery, you may particularly benefit from calcium D-glucarate. It supports:

The Immune system: Furthermore, this study shows calcium d-glucarate decreases inflammation by activating the immune system and increasing the activity of the anti-inflammatory cytokines.

Lower LDL ("bad") cholesterol: One study showed the use of calcium d-glucarate lowers LDL cholesterol by 35%. Many women with low thyroid function suffer from high LDL cholesterol.

Recommended Dosage

Recommended dosage of calcium d-glucarate ranges from 150 mg to 300 mg per day, taken with meals.

Recommended Form

Pick a supplement free of gluten, soy, additives, and colorants.

For brand recommendations, see Supplement Guide on page 361.

Precautions

Calcium d-glucarate can speed up the metabolism of toxins and decrease the effectiveness of medications changed by the liver. If you are taking any medications, please speak to your doctor before adding calcium d-glucarate. If taking calcium d-glucarate, some patients take it four hours away from their medications.

Omega 3 Fatty Acids

The most common way to get your omega 3 is through a fish oil supplement. Although there are 11 different omega 3s in existence, the bulk of the research focuses on the main three: EPA, DHA, and ALA.

- Eicosapentaenoic Acid (EPA) and Docosahexaenoic Acid (DHA): Found in fish, fish oil, and krill oil, these long-chain fatty acids are key components of cell membranes, act as anti-inflammatory agents, are precursors for multiple metabolic processes, play an important role in healthy fetal development, as well as support overall health and wellness. EPA and DHA also support some of our most important organs: the heart, brain, and eyes.
- Alpha-Linolenic Acid (ALA): Different from the other two because, unlike EPA and DHA, it is mostly found in plant oils such as flax seed oil. It can also be found in chia seeds and walnuts. It's beneficial for heart and brain health, but unlike the other two, it cannot be directly used by the body and must first be converted into EPA and DHA. Sufficient levels of vitamins B_1, B_6, zinc and magnesium are needed for the conversion to happen. People who are deficient won't convert and might be still deficient in omega 3s.

Omega 3 Fatty Acids and Hormone Balance

Hormones and omega-3 fatty acids have an extremely important relationship. Omega 3s are involved in both the production and function of hormones. Omega 3 supplementation supports:

- Overall hormonal health: Research has shown not only are omega-3s essential for daily hormonal function, but they are also essential for preventing hormone-based health conditions, especially in women. These conditions include postpartum depression, menopause, postmenopausal osteoporosis, polycystic ovarian syndrome (PCOS), thyroid issues, adrenal insufficiency, and even breast cancer.
- Menopause: This study researched the effects of EPA on hot flashes, one of the

most common and frustrating symptoms of menopause. Results showed supplementation with an EPA-rich omega 3 reduced the frequency and intensity of the hot flashes. Another study observed supplementation with EPA containing omega 3 at 1 gram per day had beneficial effects on multiple symptoms, including libido, depression, anxiety, and sleep loss. All of these symptoms are closely associated with menopause. Further research confirms daily use of an omega 3 supplement can reduce the severity of menopause-associated depression.

- Hypothyroidism and Hashimoto's thyroiditis: This autoimmune form of hypothyroidism is largely due to an underlying level of inflammation. Studies have shown the anti-inflammatory properties of omega-3s may be useful in the management of inflammatory and autoimmune diseases.
- HPA-axis dysfunction: When we are under immediate or chronic stress our nervous and endocrine systems take a beating. Research has shown proper supplementation with an omega-3 fatty acid can help regulate the proper functioning of the hypothalamic-pituitary-adrenal (HPA) axis that oversees adrenal processes in the body.
- Lower inflammation: Studies have shown positive effects on inflammatory conditions, such as rheumatoid arthritis, Crohn's disease, ulcerative colitis, psoriasis, lupus erythematosus, multiple sclerosis, and migraine headaches.

Recommended Dosage

A proper omega 3 supplement will have both EPA and DHA forms totaling about 1 gram of fatty acids per serving.

Recommended Form

The best omega 3 supplements contain fish oil in triglyceride (TG) form, which is better absorbed and more readily available than other forms. It also matters where your fish oil is sourced to make sure you are getting it in its purest form, without mercury, or PCB toxicity. It should be molecularly distilled and filtered to ensure purity in order to maximize the removal of heavy metals, pesticides, solvents, PCBs, along with other contaminants.

For brand recommendations, see Supplement Guide on page 361.

Precautions

There have been some cases showing a possible interaction between fish oil and warfarin, an anticoagulant, but that has been mostly disproven in recent years. As a precaution, if you are taking a blood thinner along with a fish oil supplement, make sure you are being closely monitored by your doctor.

Vitamin B_6

Vitamin B_6 is found in a wide variety of both plant and animal foods but can easily be in short supply through poor food choices, stress, and environmental toxic burden. In 2016, the CDC reported 30 million Americans are deficient in vitamin B_6, that is 10% of the population!

The key issue with low levels of vitamin B_6 is elevated homocysteine levels result, which is a contributor to elevated inflammation in the body. High homocysteine has been linked to a number of conditions, including heart disease, stroke, macular degeneration, migraine, dementia, cancer, depression, and osteoporosis.

Vitamin B_6 also performs a host of functions in the body and is a required cofactor for the enzyme needed to convert certain neurotransmitters like L-Dopa to dopamine as well as 5-HTP to serotonin. These neurotransmitters help support balanced moods and are essential to feeling good.

Other roles for B_6 include healthy metabolism of proteins, proper immune function, proper hormone signaling, and synthesis of heme, the portion of hemoglobin that carries oxygen in the blood.

For these reasons, adequate B_6 levels may help maintain steady energy levels. Certain medications may interfere with the absorption of B_6 from foods, potentially increasing the need for supplementation. Among these are oral contraceptives and NSAIDs (non-steroidal anti-inflammatory drugs).

Vitamin B_6 and Hormone Balance

Vitamin B_6 aids hormone balance by supporting:

- phase 2 liver detoxification and the clearance of "dirty" estrogens
- optimal liver function, including the proper flow of fat and bile to and from the liver
- balanced blood sugar
- progesterone production
- lower histamine
- the production of neurotransmitters, such as dopamine and serotonin that support balanced moods, a positive outlook, and resilience to stress
- a lower risk of hormone-related cancers by binding to estrogen, progesterone, and

testosterone along with helping to detoxify excess amounts of these steroid hormones

Recommended Dosage

The optimal daily dose of Vitamin B_6 is 25 to 50 mg. Do not exceed the tolerable upper limit of 100 mg per day. Overdosing can cause:

- a lack of muscle control or coordination of voluntary movements (ataxia)
- painful, disfiguring skin lesions
- gastrointestinal symptoms, such as heartburn and nausea
- sensitivity to sunlight (photosensitivity)
- numbness
- reduced ability to sense pain or extreme temperatures

Recommended Form

Methylated B_6 with magnesium and zinc.

For brand recommendations, see Supplement Guide on page 361.

Precautions

Doses higher than 500 mg may be unsafe.

Bioidentical Progesterone (Topical)

Low progesterone is one reason you may be experiencing estrogen dominance. When progesterone levels drop below a certain level, estrogen becomes the dominant hormone, and this change in the balance between these two hormones leads to many of the symptoms you are experiencing. This is the "unbalanced partners" scenario. Topical bioidentical progesterone can be a good way to rebalance while bypassing the digestive system and liver.

Balanced progesterone levels support:

- better sleep
- calmer, better mood
- reduction in hot flashes and night sweats
- the relief of PMS
- higher libido
- more regular periods
- the relief of fibrocystic breasts, uterine fibroids, endometriosis, and pelvic pain
- bone building
- the conversion of fat to energy
- slowing down of the growth or shrinkage of breast cancer tumors
- lowering high blood pressure
- lowering LDL cholesterol
- growth of scalp hair
- reduction of water retention
- higher metabolism
- antidepressant actions
- creation of an anti-inflammatory response

Conventional doctors most often prescribe estrogens for women in peri-menopause and menopause without adding progesterone. This is a mistake because estrogen needs to be balanced out with progesterone, which most women underproduce, especially in older age.

Progesterone and Hormone Balance

Progesterone supports hormone balance by:

Balances estrogen: Progesterone helps balance estrogen and prevents it from developing into estrogen dominance, especially when supplementing with estrogens. Women suffering from fibrocystic breasts, endometriosis, fibroids, PMS, ER+ breast cancer, infertility, or heavy periods can benefit from progesterone a great deal.

Helps breast cancer: Numerous studies indicate progesterone helps ER+ breast cancers, including the fact it induces apoptosis (death of cancer cells).

Improves hot flashes: Studies have also demonstrated the effect of topical progesterone on the improvement of hot flashes, but more research still needs to be conducted in this area. Anecdotally, I have worked with many women who experienced an almost instant improvement from hot flashes and night sweats after using progesterone.

Aids sleeping: It can help regulate menstrual cycles and improve sleep, which is especially problematic in women with low progesterone.

Supports digestive health and regular bowel movements: Progesterone impacts gut motility. In one study, a low dose increased motility while a high dose slowed it down. Dosage definitely matters when it comes to supplementing with progesterone.

Supports thyroid health: Progesterone supplementation also has benefits for thyroid health, as research has shown it plays a hand in increasing levels of the free T4 hormone.

Recommended Dosage

Recommended dose is 20 to 40 mg per day. I recommend starting low and then dose up as needed. Consider using your body weight as a guide.

- Women under 150 pounds: start with 20 to 30 mg of bioidentical progesterone.
- Women over 150 pounds: start with 40 to 50 mg of bioidentical progesterone.

If you want to try a higher dosage, I recommend working with a skilled functional practitioner who knows the ins and outs of bioidentical hormones who will test your levels to provide guidance along the way.

Where to apply topical progesterone and why?

Rotate where you apply the topical progester- one to produce both immediate and sustained benefits. Switch between fatty and non-fatty areas. Whereas fat will store the progesterone and absorb it into capillary blood, progesterone applied to thinner areas will more readily be taken up into the body and metabolized. Uptake is best in the places where you blush, such as the face, neck, and chest.

When to use topical progesterone?

Menstruating women are advised to use topical progesterone during their luteal phase, days 14 to 28 of the cycle. Day one is the first day of your period. If your period is irregular or absent, start progesterone on day 14 and teach your body to

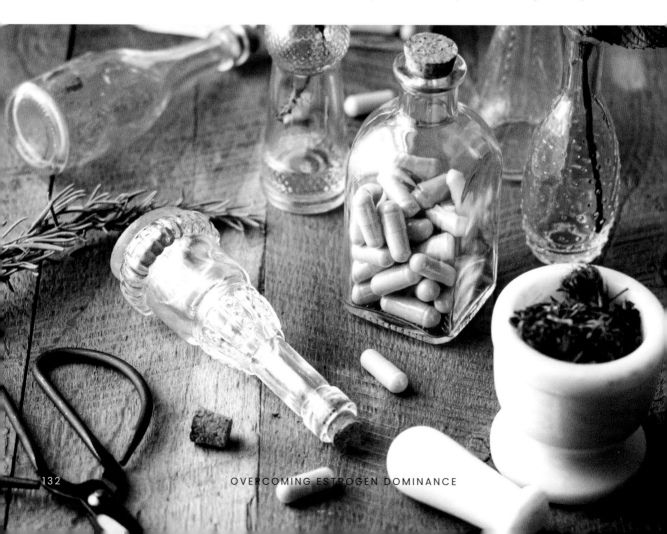

OVERCOMING ESTROGEN DOMINANCE

learn a new cycle. Stop when your period comes back.

Women going through peri-menopause, meno-pause, and post-menopause can use topical progesterone for 25 days out of a 30-day calendar, with five days off. Women in peri-menopause who are still menstruating should start progesterone five to seven days after the first day of your period and continue until the next period.

Women who are not ovulating, due to PCOS for example, can pick a day and start seven days after the first day of the period and continue until their period starts again.

Recommended Form

I do not recommend oral progesterone supplementation for two reasons. One, if you are taking other supplements, your digestion is already taxed with the absorption of the other compounds. Secondly, oral progesterone offers a very small dose of bioactive progesterone and works predominantly on the GABA receptors, therefore helping you feel calmer and sleep better, but without all the other benefits I mentioned.

I recommend a topical application using either oil or cream. When choosing a topical bioidentical progesterone, keep in mind that it should *never* contain:

- parabens (a xenoestrogen)
- mineral oil
- petroleum
- fragrance (they contain phthalates, another xenoestrogen)
- yams in their direct form (they are not harmful, just ineffective and a waste of money)

SHOULD I START ON PROGESTERONE RIGHT AWAY OR GIVE THE FOOD AND OTHER SUPPLEMENT RECOMMENDATIONS IN THE PROTOCOL TIME TO WORK FIRST?

As a medication, at the very top of the pyramid, progesterone is a "when needed" measure. First, try the food and supplement recommendations covered in the previous chapters to increase your progesterone levels and set your foundation. These may be enough for you but if they aren't, add progesterone. It's become a foundational supplement for me, especially when I travel or go through stressful periods (another depleter of progesterone). Supplementing with progesterone calms me and helps me sleep better. If your symptoms persist, I recommend trying topical progesterone next.

For brand recommendations, see Supplement Guide on page 361.

Precautions

Women with progesterone receptor-positive breast cancer should not use topical progesterone, even though progesterone is likely not the main culprit in this form of breast cancer. Women who have a personal history of breast cancer should work with a functional doctor to get clearance first. Additionally, if you are already on some kind of hormone treatment, it is best to speak to your doctor before switching or adding bioidentical progesterone. Progesterone raises blood sugar if not balanced with estrogen.

Can I start feeling worse before feeling better?

Yes, it can happen. Some women experience exacerbated symptoms of estrogen dominance (such as tender breasts and/or poor sleep) before they feel better. Functional practitioners recommend reducing the dose by half for a month before slowly increasing the dose.

Quick-Start Foundational Supplement Guide

SUPPLEMENT	SUPPORTS	RECOMMENDED DOSAGE	PRECAUTIONS
Magnesium	• liver detoxification • breast health (lumpy or fibrocystic breasts) • bone health • digestion and elimination • cardiovascular health • relaxation and sleep • blood sugar balance • kidney health Magnesium citrate has all of the benefits of magnesium, but this form also has a laxative effect and can ease chronic constipation. Topical magnesium is especially good for aches and pains.	The RDA is 320 mg per day but you may need a higher dose. To determine the best dose for you, try the "bowel tolerance test" on page 113.	• Caution should be taken in patients with kidney and heart problems. • Avoid taking magnesium with drugs that reduce urinary output. • May influence the absorption of the following drugs: Aminoglycosides, bisphosphonates, calcium channel blockers, fluoroquinolones, skeletal muscle relaxants, and tetracyclines. In these cases, always talk to your doctor first before supplementing with magnesium.
Vitamin C	• progesterone production • a strong immune system • detoxification	The RDA is 70 mg per day but you may need more, up to 2000 mg per day. To determine the best dose for you, try the "bowel tolerance test" on page 116.	• Consult your physician if you suffer from blood disorders, such thalassemia, G6PD deficiency, sickle cell disease, and hemochromatosis. • Avoid taking vitamin C immediately before or following angioplasty.

SUPPLEMENT	SUPPORTS	RECOMMENDED DOSAGE	PRECAUTIONS
Vitamin B Complex	• energy, brain, and nervous system health • optimal mental health, brain activity, and feelings of well-being • a healthy metabolism • estrogen balance • the production and maintenance of healthy blood cells and joints • a strong immune system • blood sugar balance • cell repair	• Thiamine (B_1): 25 to 50 mg • Riboflavin (B_2): 25 to 50 mg • Niacin (B_3): 25 to 50 mg • Pantothenic Acid (B_5): 25 to 50 mg • Pyridoxine (B_6): 25 to 50 mg, not to exceed 100 mg per day • Biotin (B_7): 30 to 100 mcg • Folate (B_9): 400 to 800 mcg • Cobalamin (B_{12}), in its most effective form, methylcobalamin: 50 to 100 mcg	• People with certain conditions should be cautious when taking niacin in high doses: jaundice, heart conditions, digestive issues, kidney failure and gout. • Vitamin B_6 should not be taken with the drug levodopa. • Women who are nursing should not take more than 50 mg per day of B_6 in order to maintain proper lactation. • Folate should always be avoided by anyone taking the drug methotrexate.
Zinc	• Essential in estrogen and progesterone production • cell growth and maintenance • gut health and repair • a strong immune system (like in Hashimoto's disease)	30 to 40 mg per day of zinc from both food and supplement sources	• Excess zinc inhibits copper absorption and can lead to a deficiency. • Excess zinc inhibits iron uptake and can lead to a deficiency. • Copper inhibits zinc absorption and can lead to a deficiency. • Iron interferes with the absorption of copper and zinc. • Take them separately, if using both.

SUPPLEMENT	SUPPORTS	RECOMMENDED DOSAGE	PRECAUTIONS
Vitamin D_3	• healthy bones and teeth • strong immune, brain, and nervous system health • blood sugar balance • cardiovascular health	If your blood lab result shows a deficiency, 5,000 IU to 10,000 IU is necessary to replete the vitamin in your body.	It's possible to overdose on vitamin D, so make sure to stay within the recommended doses and test three months after high dosage.
DIM	• phase 1 liver detoxification • the breakdown of estrogen into "clean" estrogens • healthy balance of testosterone and estrogen • cell protection from damaging effects of oxidation	Anywhere from 100 mg to 300 mg daily has been determined as an effective and safe dose. The recommended dose is 100 mg to 200 mg per day. Start with a lower dose (100 mg) if the supplement is suspended in oil and higher dose (200 mg) if in powder form (less effective).	If DIM makes you feel worse, reduce dose or stop and take sulforaphane instead
Sulforaphane	• phase 2 liver detoxification • shrinkage of breast lumps and cancers • protection from free radicals • improved immune system	500 mg per day, 8% standardized extract, contains myrosinase (an enzyme that aid conversion to sulforaphane)	If you are taking medications that are changed by the liver (Cytochrome P450 1A2 [CYP1A2] substrates), check with your provider before taking sulforaphane. Sulforaphane impacts the liver and these medications may act too fast or have side effects.

SUPPLEMENT	SUPPORTS	RECOMMENDED DOSAGE	PRECAUTIONS
Calcium D-glucarate	• removal of "dirty" estrogens • liver detoxification • a strong immune system • lower inflammation • lower LDL ("bad") cholesterol • post-surgery and toxic exposure recovery	Ranges from 150 mg to 300 mg per day, taken with meals	Calcium d-glucarate can speed up the metabolism of toxins and decrease the effectiveness of medications changed by the liver. If you are taking any medications, please speak to your doctor before adding calcium d-glucarate. If taking calcium d-glucarate, some patients take it four hours away from their medications.
Omega 3 Fatty Acids	• lower inflammation • improved mood • improved bone and joint health • better sleep • supple skin and hair	A proper omega 3 supplement will have both EPA and DHA forms totaling about 1 gram of fatty acids per serving.	There have been some cases showing a possible interaction between fish oil and warfarin, an anticoagulant, but that has been mostly disproven in recent years. As a precaution, if you are taking a blood thinner along with a fish oil supplement, make sure you are being closely monitored by your doctor.

SUPPLEMENT	SUPPORTS	RECOMMENDED DOSAGE	PRECAUTIONS
Vitamin B$_6$	• progesterone production • improved mood • better brain function • relief from all of the issues listed in the first column	The optimal daily dose of vitamin B$_6$ is 25 to 50 mg. Do not exceed the tolerable upper limit of 100 mg per day.	Doses higher than 500 mg may be unsafe.
Bioidentical Progesterone (topical)	• opposes excess estrogen • better sleep • calmer, better mood • higher libido • more regular periods • the relief of fibrocystic breasts • bone building • the conversion of fat to energy • a potential slowing down of the growth or shrinkage of breast cancer tumors	Recommended dose is 20 to 40 mg per day.	• Women with progesterone receptor-positive breast cancer should not use topical progesterone, even though progesterone is likely not the main culprit in this form of breast cancer. • Women who have a personal history of breast cancer should work with a functional doctor to get clearance first. • If you are already on some kind of hormone treatment, it is best to speak to your doctor before switching or adding bioidentical progesterone.

Optional Supplements You May Consider Depending on Your Needs

NAC and Glutathione

NAC (N-Acetyl-L-Cysteine) is the darling of the detoxification world because it gets converted to glutathione, the master detoxifier capable of preventing damage to important cellular components caused by free radicals, peroxides, lipid peroxides, and heavy metals. NAC also speeds up phase 2 liver detoxification (glutathione conjugation and sulfation pathway) and helps protect the liver. Studies show that NAC can help estrogen metabolism (by producing more of the "clean" estrogens) and protect the cells from estrogenic cancer growth. NAC is also an insulin receptor sensitizer; helping regular blood sugar levels and can therefore be helpful for women with PCOS. Recommended dose is 500 mg to 1500 mg per day.

Curcumin

A plant chemical found in turmeric, curcumin is a potent anti-inflammatory. It can help with the pain and inflammation caused by out of balance hormones, for instance menstrual cramps, achy joints from collagen loss in menopause, headaches, and overall inflammation. It also supports gut and liver health.

Recommended Dosage

There is no upper level of toxicity established for turmeric or curcumin. A range of 200 to 1,200 mg per day was used for various applications with significant benefits. The effective dose may depend on the severity of inflammation.

Recommended Form

Find a curcumin product that is a highly bioavailable formula containing these three types of curcurminoids: curcumin, bisdemethoxy curcumin, and demethoxy curcumin. Using a product with these three types of curcuminoids will ensure you get the strongest, most protective, and best researched compounds found in turmeric root. Find a formula that is concentrated to contain 70% curcumin because if you just use or take turmeric root powder it will only contain 5 to 7% curcumin. Also, it is important to find a formula containing sunflower lecithin, which acts as an emulsifier to enhance the absorption and bioavailability of the curcumin.

Precautions

Individuals on blood thinning therapy or anyone with gallstones (stimulates bile flow), ulcers, and GI inflammatory conditions should be monitored closely. Not recommended during pregnancy or breastfeeding. It inhibits growth of lactobacillus 1, so supplementation with probiotics is recommended.

Iron

If you have heavy periods because of fibroids, a non-constipating supplement can help restore your levels. Most iron supplements can cause constipation, which is exactly what we don't want when dealing with hormonal issues.

Recommended Dosage

I suggest 3 to 10 mg per day. Start low and go up if there is no constipation. Combining it with vitamin C improves absorption. Take four hours away from dairy, if consuming any (dairy is not recommended on this protocol), caffeine, antacids, and calcium supplements.

Recommended Form

The heme form of iron is preferred. It's derived from animal sources and has the highest bioavailability. Non-heme is plant derived but has a lower bioavailability and is suitable for vegetarians.

Precautions

People with hemochromatosis, ulcers, and gastritis should not supplement with iron.

Resveratrol

Occurring naturally in Japanese knotweed (and small amounts in red wine), this natural bioflavonoid is an effective antiviral, antioxidant, anti-inflammatory, and phytoestrogen. Studies show a daily 1 mg dose of resveratrol has favorable effects on estrogen metabolism and SHBG (Sex Hormone Binding Glubolin) by binding up excess testosterone. It also increases your levels of quinone reductase, a compound that protects DNA against the oxidative damage linked to raised cancer risk. Because of its anti-carcinogenic properties, resveratrol has been used as part of integrative breast cancer therapy in ER+ breast cancers.

Factoid: Red wine, marketed as a great source of resveratrol, only contains about 2 mg of resveratrol. That's not a medically significant dose (200 mg is) and drinking more wine will impair the liver. Enjoy the occasional glass of wine, but not with the excuse of it being a health food!

Recommended Dosage

200 mg.

Recommended Form

Derived from Japanese knotweed, as CO_2 extract is most viable.

Precautions

Anyone on medications changed by the liver should avoid resveratrol. It acts as a slight blood thinner and should not be taken with blood thinners.

Vitamin E

Vitamin E is more than just one nutrient; it's a collective name for a family of eight different fat-soluble vitamins used by the human body for a variety of cellular and metabolic processes. Vitamin E supports hormonal health by promoting the production of progesterone and inhibiting breast cancer: There has been a lot of research studying the effectiveness of vitamin E in ER+ breast cancer. One study showed vitamin E may play an important role in altering the cellular response to estrogen, thereby inhibiting estrogen receptor-positive cell growth that occurs in some types of breast cancer. Studies also suggest vitamin E is a natural pain reliever.

In a 2009 double-blind clinical trial of 150 women, 200 IU of vitamin E reduced breast pain by 70% in two months.

Recommended Dosage

The RDA of vitamin E in alpha-tocopherol form for adults is 15 mg or 22.4 IU.

Recommended Form

If you are sensitive to wheat or soy, read the label carefully to see if it has been derived from soy oil or wheat germ oil and if wheat or soy is used in the product.

Precautions

Always talk to your doctor if you are taking a medication that may be affected by vitamin E supplementation.

Special caution should be taken by people on anticoagulant medications, such as warfarin, because vitamin E may interfere with blood clotting. Another study suggests supplementation with vitamin E may interact with tamoxifen, a breast cancer drug, by interfering with its therapeutic effects on breast cancer cells. Additionally, antioxidant supplementation with the combination of simvastatin and niacin to treat cholesterol concerns can negatively affect the rise of HDL levels, which is considered the good, cardioprotective component of cholesterol.

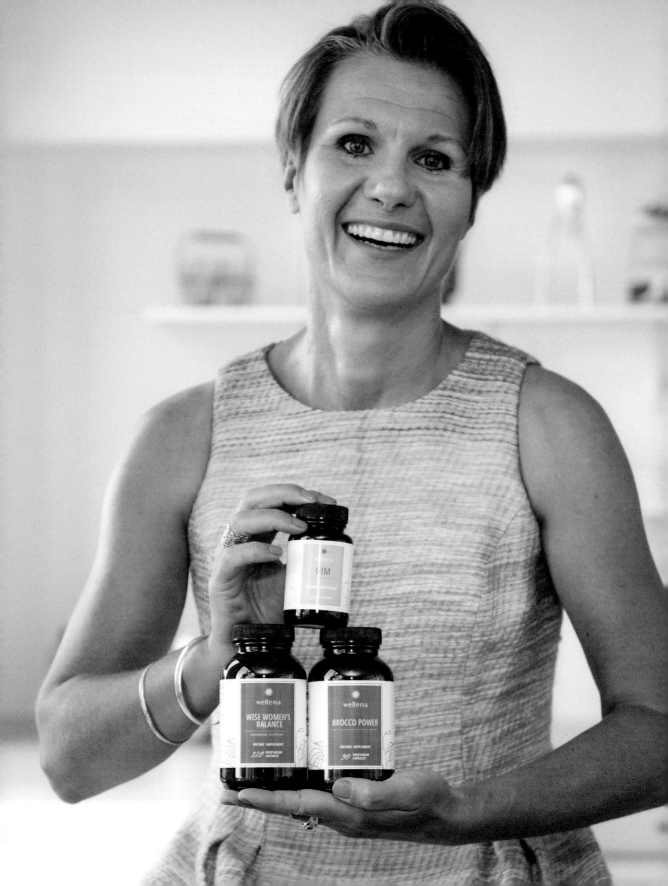

Chapter 8

Move Beyond Food Practices

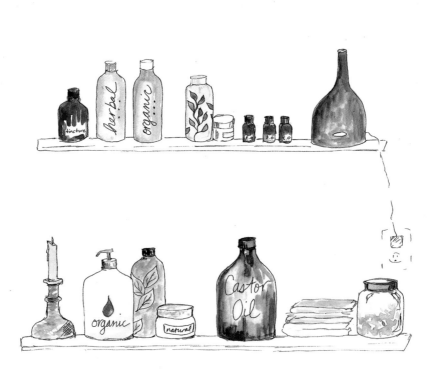

Over the last several chapters, I've talked a lot about food, herbs, and supplements. They are at the core of reversing your estrogen dominance. But, eating right isn't the only tool in our hormone-balancing toolbox. Reducing your exposure to the excess estrogens saturating our environment and making sure to get enough deep, restorative sleep are essential. Several other healing practices, such as castor oil packs, time in an infrared sauna, and lymphatic movement (such dry brushing or rebounding) can amp up liver detoxification, improve your digestive health, and reduce inflammation, among many other benefits. Making space in your life for these will accelerate your healing. The research, my own personal experience, and the experiences of so many of the women I hear from tell me so. These practices are real game-changers. I know you don't have time for anything less.

Clean Out the Xenoestrogens from Your Daily Life

Excess exposure to xenoestrogens, those man-made chemicals that disrupt your hormone balance by mimicking estrogen, throws off your hormonal balance in a huge way and contributes to estrogen dominance. We want to clear out as many of these excess estrogens from your daily life as possible and replace them with clean products.

I know detoxing your life can sound overwhelming. These chemicals, such as BPA, phthalates, and parabens, are in products likely filling your kitchen and bathroom cabinets. Don't get overwhelmed and paralyzed. The way to go is one step at a time. Commit to replacing one product during the 28-Day Foundation Protocol. Then, as your household and personal care products run out, replace them with cleaner options. Before you know it, you will have detoxed your life.

As you start looking at labels more closely, watch out for these frequent offenders:

- BPAs: found in plastics, often in ones that store food or beverages, such as water bottles and the linings of food and drink cans.
- Parabens: synthetic preservatives used in a lot of skincare products, but also found in cleaning products and some processed foods.
- Phthalates: make products smell nice and for a longer period. A personal care or cleaning product with the word "fragrance" on the label likely contains phthalates. Products scented with essential oil will say so. Also found in food packaging, plastic wrap, as well as some foods such as cream-based dairy products, poultry, and cooking oils.
- Triclosan: an antibacterial and antifungal agent found in toothpastes, soaps, body washes, and detergents. The FDA banned its use in antibacterial soaps in 2016 and other companies have started phasing it out from their products because of its dangers, including the damage it's been shown to do to our microbiome. This shows many toxins are widely used in products for decades before getting phased out.
- Aluminum: a lightweight metal found in antiperspirants to reduce wetness by blocking sweat ducts, astringents, cosmetics, some antacids and foods as an anti-caking agent. It's also used to make cans, foil, pots, and pans while also frequently found in tap water.
- Sodium Lauryl/Laureth Sulfate: a foaming agent used in shampoos, shower gels, facial cleaners, and dish soap.
- Fluoride: an antibacterial agent added to water, toothpaste, mouthwashes, and floss.

- Chlorine: a disinfectant found in bleach, other cleaners, and tap water.
- Formaldehyde: a bonding agent used in nail polish and remover, toothpastes, cosmetics, air fresheners, paints, glues, synthetic fabrics, wood composites/pressed wood, along with laminate flooring.
- Synthetic colors and dyes: added to make products look good, these are found in almost all processed foods.
- PFCs: these chemicals resist heat, oil, stains, grease, and water therefore are used in nonstick cookware, carpet cleaners, stain-resistant coatings, cleaning products, as well as food packaging (including microwave popcorn bags and pizza boxes).

These chemicals are bad news and not just for your hormones. They have been linked to everything from estrogen dominance, breast cancers, ovarian/uterine cancer, prostate cancer, inhibited thyroid function, thyroid nodules/cancers, infertility, child development issues, and low sperm count in men.

Kitchen Detox

The kitchen is a great place to start cleaning up your life.

Use this Out/In Detox Guide to help you identify the products to remove and ones to bring in.

OUT	IN
Non-stick cookware	Enamel, cast iron, glass, stainless steel, carbon steel
Plastic containers, for food storage	Glass containers
Canned food	Food in glass, especially tomatoes

Filter your water. Filtering your water is a must today, no matter where you live. Not only do you want to clear chlorine and fluoride from your drinking water, you also want to make sure you're not ingesting medications (such as antibiotics and antidepressants), heavy metals (such as aluminum and mercury), pesticides, along with the dozens of other potential contaminants. The contaminants in your water depend on where you live and where your water comes from. While Brita is a well-intending quality brand, it just

BEWARE OF GREENWASHING

This is one of the worst kinds of marketing spin: promoting a product as clean and safe with misleading information. Often, companies swap out harmful ingredients with "less bad" or completely untested ones. We have no idea how these new ingredients will impact us in the long term. That's not responsible or green. None of us have the time to play detective and chemist to research or figure out if a product is "really" green or just greenwashing green. What to do? Go back to basics. Use tried-and-true natural ingredients such as jojoba, almond, coconut oil, shea butter, honey, baking soda, vinegar, or ethanol for your personal care and cleaning needs instead of all of the toxic—and expensive—stuff out there. Go to go to chapter 11, The Estrogen Reset Recipes, for DIY recipes.

won't remove all of the necessary contaminants. Neither will the standard filter that comes built-in to your refrigerator.

Based on our current research and experience, you can find our most current brand recommendations on https://hormonesbalance. com/AllThingsWeLove/

OUT	IN
Tap water, water filtered with cheap or fridge filters. Avoid water in plastic bottles in the long-term.	Kitchen or house 3-stage filters that removes bacteria, fluoride, heavy metals. Reverse Osmosis filters if water source is highly contaminated.

Do a bathroom detox. Clear out cosmetics and personal care products. If it's from a major brand you've seen advertised on television or in magazines, odds are it contains one (or more) of the chemical offenders you are trying to avoid. This means soaps, body washes, lotions, and all of your cosmetics. The good news is, there are many brands that use only nontoxic and organic ingredients. Start looking at labels and check out some of my favorite brands on https://hormonesbalance.com/AllThingsWeLove. Don't forget, your local farmer's market and health food store are great resources for natural products, especially soaps.

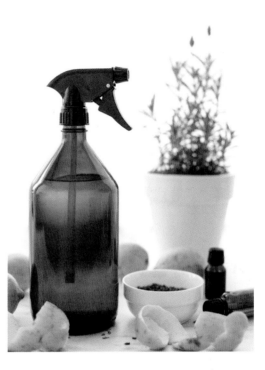

OUT	IN
Skincare products like body and facial creams and lotions from major brands	Coconut oil, almond oil, jojoba oil, sesame oil, rose hip oil
Body wash from major brands	Natural soaps made from organic oils, fats or glycerine

OUT	IN
Cosmetics, makeup from major brands	Cosmetic made with non-toxic and organic ingredients
Perfumes from major brands	Perfumes made with essential oils
Shampoos from major brands	Shampoos made with non-toxic and organic ingredients
Sunscreen containing retinyl palmitate (vitamin A), oxybenzone	Sunscreens containing mineral oils, zinc oxide and titanium dioxide

THE PROBLEM WITH PERFUMES

Perfumes from the major commercial brands are loaded with chemicals including xenoestrogens, such as phthalates to help the scent last longer. And where do you spray them? On your neck, usually directly onto your thyroid, potentially causing thyroid toxicity and dysfunction. Look for perfumes made with essential oils. They are wonderful. I often wear Love by Annmarie Gianni and I adore it!

- Get your coffee, tea, or other hot beverage to go in a porcelain mug with a silicone lid. Disposable cups are lined with plastic and when heated, xenoestrogens slip into the liquid and straight into your system.
- Maintain a dust-free home with a vacuum with an UltraHEPA/HEPA filter, microfiber cloths, and wet dusting instead of furniture polish.

Bathroom Detox

Do a daily item detox. Be more mindful of the items you use every day that could be adding to your toxic load. For example:

- Forget the commercial air fresheners and switch over to an essential oil ultrasonic diffuser.
- Use a stainless-steel or glass water bottle instead of plastic.

For products my team and I personally use in our lives, go to https://hormonesbalance.com/AllThingsWeLove.

Use this chart to start clearing things out and bringing better brands in.

OUT	IN
Laundry detergent from major brands	Detergents free of phthalates, optical whiteners, and bleach

OUT	IN
House cleaning products from major brands	Free of parabens, phthalates or "fragrances"
Fabric softener	1/2 cup of baking soda in wash water or wool dryer balls
New house products such as furniture, mattresses or carpet padding	Ask what fire retardant it contains. Be mindful of and/or avoid items containing PBDEs, antimony, formaldehyde, boric acid, and other brominated chemicals

Daily Items Detox

Go back to basics for your cleaning products. With a little ingenuity and some elbow grease, we can make and keep our homes perfectly clean using safe, affordable, effective, and easy to make DIY cleaners. Using nontoxic cleaners can give you deep satisfaction in knowing you're keeping your body toxin-free and your family safe in the best way possible. There is satisfaction in knowing you're creating a home that's truly a safe haven.

The three fundamental ingredients for home cleaning are:

- white distilled vinegar
- ethanol (contains 95.6% alcohol) or isopropyl alcohol (70% alcohol)
- baking soda

See the All-Purpose Cleaner recipe on page 358.

Go back to basics for your personal care products. These natural products have many nourishing health and beauty benefits. They can be used to make an array of personal care products from moisturizers and body washes to makeup removers, face masks, foot scrubs, lip gloss, as well as hair detanglers.

- castor oil: an inexpensive, shelf-stable, deeply penetrating and highly therapeutic oil
- coconut oil: antibacterial moisturizer for skin and hair
- almond oil: rich in vitamins D and E, this oil hydrates the hair and skin while reducing puffiness, additionally it helps reverse sun damage
- jojoba oil: a light, versatile moisturizer that absorbs easily into the skin which contains nutrients such as vitamins E and B
- sesame oil: beneficial to the skin as an antioxidant, antimicrobial, and anti-inflammatory; commonly used in Ayurveda as a highly therapeutic oil
- lanolin: a lightweight emollient, extremely effective at soothing dry, irritated skin
- rosehip oil: loaded with skin-nourishing vitamins and essential fatty acids, it hydrates, moisturizes, brightens, reduces inflammation, as well as protects against sun damage

- shea butter: a nourishing moisturizer that doesn't clog pores and helps reduce inflammation
- honey: raw, unpasteurized honey helps clear acne by balancing the bacteria on the skin, exfoliates, promotes healing, and reduces inflammation

Start adding these homemade products to your beauty routine. For recipes, go to chapter 24, The Estrogen Reset Recipes.

Get Good, Quality Sleep

I'm sure you don't need a hard sell on the benefits of sleep. Most of us know firsthand how much more energized, focused, and upbeat we feel after a good night's sleep—and how irritable, moody, and sluggish we feel after a restless, disturbed night. That's because sleep is essential for hormone balance.

Our hormones are produced to ebb and flow in sync with our bodies' circadian rhythm, the 24-hour internal clock that regulates most of our bodily functions, including when we sleep and wake. Our circadian rhythm is strongly influenced by sunlight and temperature. Different hormones rise and fall over the course of roughly 24 hours, making us feel tired as night falls or awake in the morning. When we are out of sync with this rhythm because of going to bed very late or checking emails and texts well after dark, we don't get enough sleep or enough of the deep, restorative REM sleep our hormones need to function. They get thrown off, such as ghrelin, the "hunger" hormone, which becomes elevated when we're sleep deprived, causing those carb and coffee cravings. (More sleep, fewer cravings.)

Modern life, filled with artificial lights, screens, and 24/7 demands on our time, makes getting good sleep a challenge. Once you understand the important role sleep plays in your health, I know you'll be compelled to make a good night's rest a priority. During sleep:

- Cells regenerate and heal.
- Energy is restored.
- Key hormones, such as melatonin, are produced. Melatonin promotes sleepiness while also anti-estrogenic and anti-inflammatory.
- The liver detoxifies between 1:00 a.m. and 3:00 a.m.
- The nervous system gets a reset.
- The mitochondria recover.
- The brain produces more gray matter.
- And much more.

Getting good sleep is critical for reversing estrogen dominance. If you're not sleeping and your energy is tanked, no amount of supplements or good-quality food is ever going to bring you back into balance. We live in a society that glorifies hard work and pushing yourself to the limit at

Modern life, filled with artificial lights, screens, and 24/7 demands on our time, makes getting good sleep a challenge the expense of sleep. We idolize people who boast they live on four hours of sleep per night. I want you to know: sleep is not laziness or indulgence. It is a *nonnegotiable* if you want to be healthy. I urge you to reflect on your perception of sleep and notice how much of your sleep deprivation is coming from trivializing its importance. Popping a sleeping pill is not the answer either. They do not give you the quality, deep sleep you need. But, I realize there are also some unique modern-day challenges to troubleshoot. Here's how to get good sleep and move the needle in a big way toward hormone balance:

In bed by 10:00 p.m., asleep by 10:30. Do this to stay in sync with your circadian rhythm.

Practice Sleep-Supporting Eating Habits

Eat to stabilize your blood sugar throughout the day. Start your day with a PFF breakfast and end it by not having sugary snacks or alcohol before bed. That glass of wine may make you sleepy but it will wake you up in the middle of the night. Elevated blood sugar levels are frequently the reason we get up in the middle of the night to urinate (It's rarely about your bladder being too full. Your bladder holds a lot more liquid than you think.). If you must snack, choose something savory like kale chips, nuts, or seeds.

Stop caffeine by 3:00 p.m. or even 12:00 p.m. Experiment and see how it impacts your sleep. You would be surprised to know how many women in the Hormones Balance community have been reporting better sleep when they stop caffeine early in the day.

Eat a light dinner, no later than 7:00 p.m. This allows you to digest your food in the evening and not tax the system while you are sleeping, which

could disturb your sleep. You'll sleep better after a light dinner. Remember the old Chinese saying: Make your breakfast your best friend, lunch your acquaintance, and dinner your enemy. The last meal of the day is not the best time for a lot of heavy foods. I try to eat dinner at home before 6:00 p.m. and when going out with friends, I typically meet them for dinner no later than 6:00 p.m. so we can eat before 8:00 p.m.

Create a Sleep-Ready Environment

Sleep in total darkness. This is a game-changer for most people. And I mean *total darkness*, so dark you can't see your hand when placed in front of your face. Cover the red "power" light on your TV, obscure street lamps with dark curtains, and cover your electronic clock. Once you start looking around the room, you'll find sneaky light sources everywhere. If this sounds like a lot of work, try a sleep mask. I like the ones that are fitted and don't touch your eye area.

No screens, from three hours to 30 minutes before bedtime. Do some experimenting to see how limiting your screen time influences your sleep. Some people are very sensitive and benefit from powering down a few hours before getting into bed while others only need to unplug for 30 minutes before bed. No screens means *all* screens: televisions, tablets, and phones. Why? These devices emit blue light which interferes with the production of melatonin, the hormone that prompts sleepiness. If you really must use a screen (I often work late too), consider a computer application called f.lux that blocks blue light (only somewhat effective) or blue light-blocking glasses (can be very effective if you get the right type). See my favorite brands in the Resources section, page 363.

Reduce electromagnetic field (EMF) exposure. Cell phones, Bluetooth devices, Wi-Fi routers, microwaves, computers, and other electronic appliances emit waves that create electric and magnetic fields (EMFs), or radiation, which may interfere with sleep. I recommend banishing these devices from your bedroom or at least turning everything off, especially your cell phone (or put it on airplane mode).

Promote a Restful State

Try a bedtime ritual to feel pampered and nourished before bed. Following a regular routine before slipping into bed can help relax you and promote good sleep by training your brain to recognize it's time to rest. There's no one ritual that works for everyone so find something which soothes you. These don't have to be complicated, either. Taking off your makeup, brushing your teeth, and putting on your pajamas may be all you need. Other activities to consider:

- soak in a warm bath or sauna time (if you have one at home)
- gentle stretching or yoga
- meditation
- reading a physical book (not on a screen)

Clear your mind. A busy mind filled with thoughts, worries, and to-do lists can sabotage sleep. Take a few moments before bed to get them out of your head and into a notebook. An evening mind dump can help create calm.

Soak in an Epsom salt bath. The magnesium in Epsom salt helps your body and brain relax. As you soak, your skin will absorb the magnesium. I recommend taking a bath with these salts twice weekly.

Increase progesterone level. If you are suffering from symptoms such problems falling and staying asleep, irregular periods, PMS, mid-cycle spotting, infertility, anxiety, depression, low progesterone could be the culprit. Increase your progesterone levels by either adding herbs such as vitex or try topical bioidentical progesterone.

Add melatonin. Supplementing with melatonin should be a last resort, after you've incorporated habits to promote good sleep. The reason is, we don't want to inadvertently turn off your body's ability to make melatonin naturally. This can happen if you take too much, so dosage is very important here. Research suggests that taking less than 5 mg of melatonin is safe and won't interfere with the body's own ability to produce it when you stop taking melatonin.

AN OVERACTIVE THYROID COULD BE TO BLAME

If you're experiencing anxiety, heart palpitations, sweaty palms, and a pounding chest, you may have an overactive thyroid. When I was hyperthyroid, I experienced all four. I'd lie in bed at 3 a.m. in the morning listening to my chest pound. Consider getting tested if this sounds like you.

Detoxify with Castor Oil Packs

The magic of castor oil is profound, especially its powers to reverse estrogen dominance by supporting healthy liver function, clearing out "dirty" estrogens and other toxins, while reducing inflammation. I was a skeptic at first, but now I'm a believer. Castor oil packs have made my PMS symptoms significantly less intense and boosted my gut healing. I encourage you to try them and feel the benefits for yourself.

Castor oil, made from extracting the oil from the seeds of the *Ricinus communis* plant has been used for medicinal purposes for thousands of years. It has a long history in ancient Egypt, India, Iran, Russia, and China. The seeds, known as castor beans, contain ricin, a toxic enzyme. During the refining process to produce the oil, the ricin is deactivated so the oil can be used safely.

Castor oil has many medicinal benefits:

- Acts as a natural laxative and "mover." It improves bowel movement regularity (key to reversing estrogen dominance and removing excess "dirty" estrogens), reduces straining, cramping, uncomfortable urgency, and leaves you with a feeling of complete evacuation. Castor oil doesn't have to be taken internally. It acts as a mild laxative when applied to the skin over your intestines.
- Reduces inflammation. Castor oil has a similar structure to prostaglandin, an anti-inflammatory agent.
- Supports the production of glutathione, an antioxidant necessary for both phase 1 and phase 2 liver detoxification.
- Improves the microbiome by breaking down the biofilm, a cluster of one or more microorganisms. Biofilms form a physical barrier to protect them from immune cells and they are hostile to antibiotics. Candida and other yeasts, bacteria, as well as fungi can hide in biofilms and thwart all of your efforts to eradicate them. Castor oil can get at them.
- Calms your intestines, known as improving their parasympathetic tone.

Anecdotally, I've seen over and over again how castor oil packs improve PMS symptoms and estrogen dominance in women.

How do you apply a castor oil pack? Here are the basics:

- Apply 2 to 3 tablespoons of castor oil to a cotton or flannel compress.
- Wrap the compress around your liver (located under your right rib cage).
- Leave it for a few hours or overnight (highly recommended).
- Placing a heating pad over the compress is great but not necessary if you are doing it overnight.
- Apply 3 to 4 times per week or 7 days on/7 days off.
- Proceed with caution during your period. Some experts advocate avoiding castor oil packs during your period because it may

HOW TO APPLY A CASTOR OIL PACK

For more on the benefits of castor oil packs and details on how to apply them, watch the demo videos on www.hormonesbalance.com/oed/downloads.

make your bleeding more intense. Others, like Dr. Marisol Teijerio, consider heavier bleeding as a form of detoxification that will only last for one period and then get lighter. One option is to use the 7 days on/7 days off method and apply a pack seven days before the start of your period so your "off" days occur when you are bleeding.

Restore with an Infrared Sauna

If your only experience has been a sweat session in a traditional sauna at the gym, have I got news for you: Infrared saunas provide a host of benefits which can ease the symptoms of estrogen dominance.

Unlike a traditional sauna that heats the air around you, an infrared sauna uses infrared lamps to warm your body. Because of this, they can operate at lower temperatures (140°F to 150°F) than traditional ones (160°F to 180°F). You do not have to sweat buckets to feel detoxified. The spectrum of an infrared sauna matters.

- Near-infrared: improves wound healing, cell health, and oxygenation of tissues.
- Mid-infrared: improves circulation, weight loss, and pain relief.
- Far infrared: supports detoxification and blood pressure balance.

Here are more reasons to consider an infrared sauna. It:

- reduces inflammation
- supports detoxification through sweating
- strengthens the immune system through

raised body temperature
- improves wound healing
- activates cell regeneration
- promotes weight loss
- increases blood flow
- improves athletic performance
- reduces pain
- fights cognitive decline
- lowers blood pressure

I use an infrared sauna at home and I absolutely love it. I typically go in thirty to forty-five minutes two or three times per week and set the temperature to between 140°F to 150°F. I consider it "me time," to read a book, meditate, or write in my journal. Relaxing in an infrared sauna is a healthy way of multitasking or taking time for yourself.

Move Your Lymphatic System

(Dry Brushing and Rebounding)

Your lymphatic system is a highway of lymphatic channels and lymph nodes that helps remove toxins along with waste from the body. Lymph nodes, small bean-shaped structures, filter substances that travel through the system. They are located throughout your body, including your neck, armpits, and groin. We want to encourage toxins to move through the lymph nodes. Both dry brushing and rebounding promote good circulation and detoxification.

Dry brushing. Dry brushing, brushing your full body with a bristled tool, encourages lymphatic drainage and circulation.

Dry brushing is easy.

- You'll need two brushes, one stiff and one softer for more sensitive areas (like your abdomen). Choose a stiff brush with a handle so you can reach your back.
- It's easiest when you are completely nude. I suggest you do it in shower so you can wash off any dead skin cells you've lifted right away. Your skin will be so soft and supple when you're done!
- Begin at your feet and move up your body, always stroking the brush toward your heart and repeating a stroke five times.
- Switch to your softer brush for more sensitive areas.
- It's important to do an especially thorough job under your arms to stimulate the lymph nodes located there.
- Remember to always brush toward your heart.

Rebounding. Rebounding on a trampoline is another great way to move and drain your lymphatic system. I particularly like it because you can do it for just 10 to 15 minutes in your own home, it does not strain your joints (like running), and it can be a pretty challenging cardio workout if you want it to be. The sheer power of gravity as well as the force with which you land opens the lymphatic system, promoting lymphatic drainage and detoxification.

HOW TO DRY BRUSH

To see how easy it is to dry brush, watch the video demonstration on www.hormonesbalance.com/oed/downloads.

4-7-8 Breathing Technique

This easy but powerful technique stimulates the vagus nerve along with the parasympathetic nervous system; promoting relaxation, lowering cortisol levels and reducing inflammation. The technique is simple: Breathe in for four seconds, hold the breath for seven seconds, and exhale for eight seconds. It takes just a few minutes a day to become an expert. You can see a demo on this page: www.hormonesbalance.com/oed/downloads. In my past life, advertising, I had a deeply insecure manager who would intimidate and bully people in meetings. As a newcomer, I couldn't do or say much at that point, but in order to manage my own sanity and emotional health in these toxic circumstances, I would go to the bathroom to use the 4-7-8 technique. It never ceased to amaze me how calm I felt each time I emerged from the bathroom. If you experience chronic stress in your life, I highly suggest to add this simple practice to your life. Stress contributes negatively to estrogen dominance.

Oxytocin and the Art of Self-Love

Oxytocin is the hormone of love, bonding, and connection. It's at its all-time high during childbirth and breastfeeding (creating that incredible connection between mom and baby), but it is also released during sex, orgasm, as well as when we cuddle or hug. Even when you don't have a partner, hugging your pet can release oxytocin. Bottom line: Whenever you do something that is highly pleasurable, you release oxytocin.

It is a fascinating hormone. It offsets the inflammation caused by excess cortisol (like during stress), which is why doing something that gives you pleasure even during stressful times, can help keep the equilibrium. Oxytocin release also speeds up the satiety process, making you feel full and not overeat. It also improves insulin sensitivity, helping you balance your blood sugar levels.

That's the science. My question for you is: What can you do daily and weekly to ensure regular oxytocin release? Schedule a massage, spend time in nature, cuddle with your partner or pet, call your favorite person for a heart-to-heart talk? It can be easy and inexpensive! All of them are an expression of self-love, which is essential on your healing journey.

One thing I've learned over the years of work is that yes diet, herbs, and supplements are fundamental in our healing journey. However, if you struggle with giving yourself permission to feel good, to eat well, you regularly sabotage your health, and you feel a lack of self-worth, then I urge you to go deeper into discovering the root causes. This is outside the scope of this book, but I just want to share with you I've seen many women feeling very stuck with their health journey until they addressed past or present unresolved trauma (physical or emotional) and stress. Let all that be a sign of self-love to yourself—a gift of healing you can give yourself.

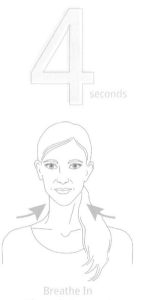
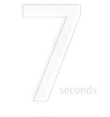
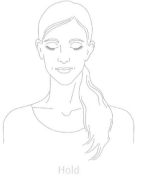
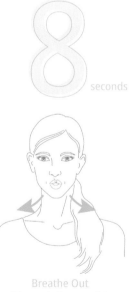

4 seconds

Breathe In
(through the nose)

7 seconds

Hold

8 seconds

Breathe Out
(through the mouth)

OVERCOMING ESTROGEN DOMINANCE

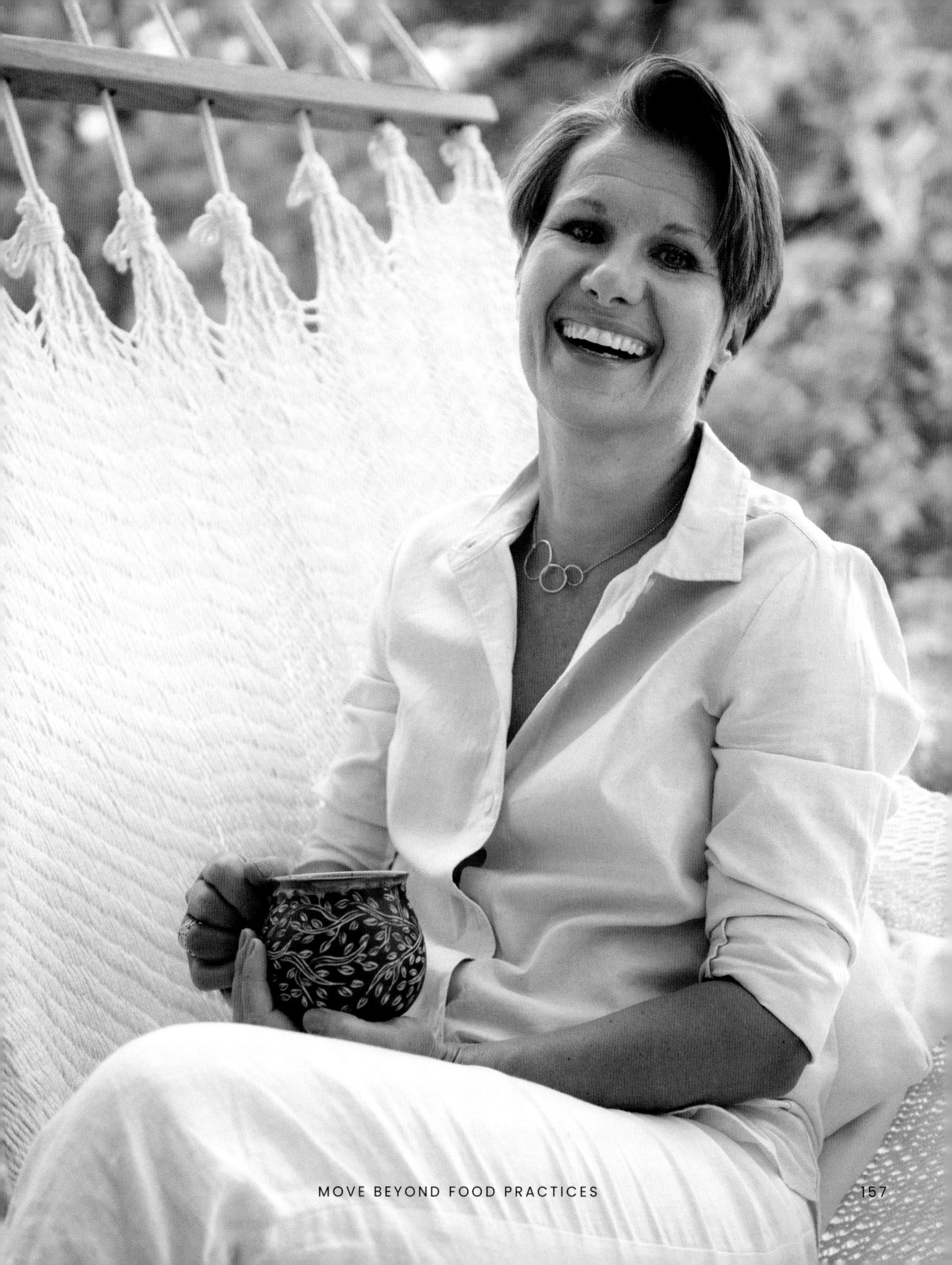

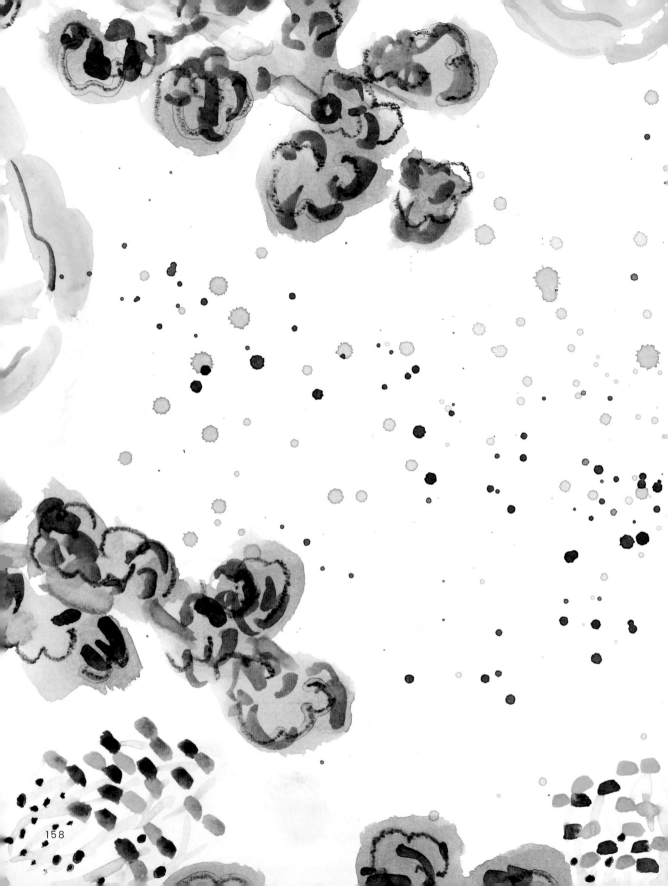

158

Part III

Personalized
Add-On
Protocols

Chapter 9

Fibroids Protocol

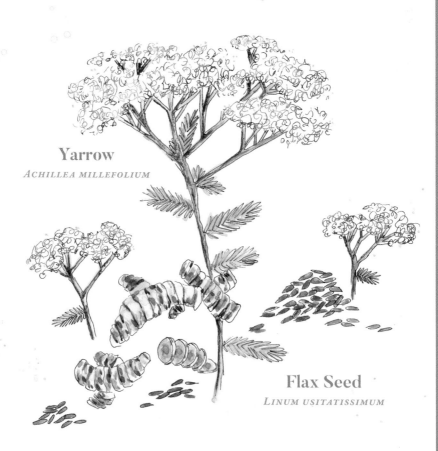

Yarrow
ACHILLEA MILLEFOLIUM

Flax Seed
LINUM USITATISSIMUM

Turmeric
CURCUMA LONGA

Uterine fibroids are the most frequent type of benign tumor found in women and a common challenge for many. Western, conventional medicine isn't very well prepared to shrink them in noninvasive and lasting ways. Understanding the presence of fibroids is early information for women that they might be experiencing estrogen dominance and, although fibroids are benign, they can lead to other, more serious health issues, such as estrogenic cancers.

In most cases, fibroids do not cause any symptoms—you may not even know you have them—but in others, they can lead to a wide range of issues, from heavy bleeding and severe cramps to low back pain and chronic vaginal discharge. The great news is it is possible to shrink them naturally.

Key Facts

Uterine fibroids, also known as uterine leiomyomas or myomas, are benign lumps or growths in and around the uterus (endometrium). They are made up of muscle and connective tissue.

There are several types of fibroids, classified by their location. These include:

Intramural: the most common type of fibroid is embedded in the muscles of the uterus.

Submucosal: these grow right underneath the mucus membrane that lines the uterus, the endometrium.

Subserosal: these grow on the outside of the uterus, much closer to your skin. You may be able to feel them.

Uterine Fibroids

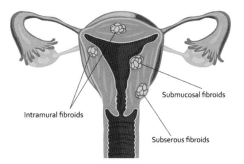

They are slow-growing. Fibroids can grow for as long as 10 years before making their presence known.

Each fibroid is unique, with varying shapes, textures, and sizes. They are usually round in shape. They can be soft or rock-hard to the touch. They can range in size from seedlings, undetectable to the naked eye, to as big as a pebble and larger than a grapefruit.

Fibroids may appear alone but are often found in groups.

They are most common in women in ages 40 to 44. This is not surprising because this is when our progesterone starts dropping and estrogen dominance becomes likely. Fibroids develop when estrogen levels are higher. Studies on the occurrence of fibroids show the following statistics: 20 to 40% women over age 35, 40% over age 40, and 70% of white women and 80% of black women by age 50. That's the majority of us!

Many women will not experience symptoms. It's estimated that 50 to 80% of women have no symptoms whatsoever and have no idea they even have a fibroid.

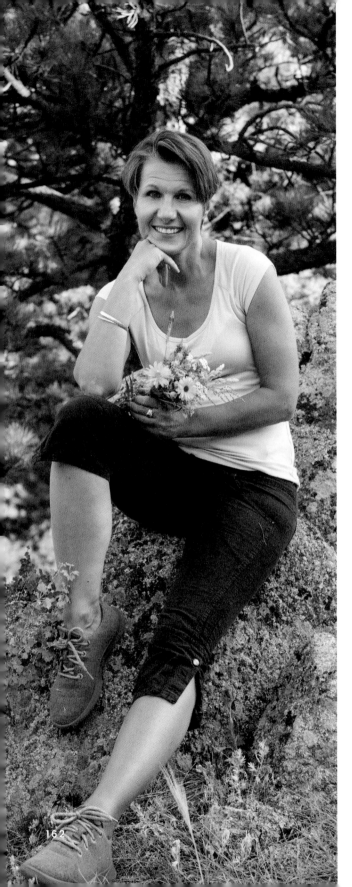

If fibroids don't shrink by menopause or are growing fast, they may become malignant. This is why I advocate for proactively addressing fibroids rather than adopt a "wait-and-see" attitude.

Symptoms of Fibroids

- increased menstrual bleeding
- anemia (due to heavy blood flow)
- abdominal bloating, pressure, and discomfort
- back pain
- excessive vaginal discharge
- pain or bleeding after intercourse
- irritation to the bladder, more frequent urination
- infertility, sub-infertility, and premature delivery

Diagnosis

It's important to get a proper diagnosis to rule out any form of ovarian tumor, abscesses in the fallopian tubes, endometriosis, or any adhesions to the pelvis. Fibroids are often found during a routine pelvic exam, but other diagnostic tests can detect them, such as:

- ultrasound
- MRI
- hysteroscopy, to examine the interior of the uterus
- laparoscopy, to examine the exterior of the uterus

Causes

- estrogen dominance (Fibroids have a large number of estrogen receptors and excess estrogen promotes the growth of fibroid tissue.)

- a high level of "dirty" estrogens and exposure to xenoestrogens (from personal skincare and house products; which add more excess estrogen to fuel endometrial tissue growth)
- progesterone deficiency (Remember, without enough progesterone to balance out estrogen, we have the "unbalanced partners" cause of estrogen dominance. Low progesterone allows estrogen to become dominant and the excess estrogen promotes the growth of the fibroid tissue.)
- hypothyroidism (often present with fibroids; low thyroid function goes hand-in-hand with estrogen dominance)
- high levels of IGF-1 (a growth hormone) due to high blood sugar levels
- melatonin deficiency
- excess body fat (Body fat, especially belly fat, produces estrogen, so overweight women are at a higher risk of estrogen dominance and developing fibroids.)
- There is some evidence linking fibroids to root canals.

Traditional Treatments

- "Wait and see" (especially if you are asymptomatic)
- gonadotropin-releasing hormone (GnRH) agonists, sold under the brand name Leuprolide, for example (Suppresses the production of estrogen and promotes progesterone production to slow the growth of fibroids; but these drugs with others on the market, have many side effects and don't treat the root cause. Symptoms will return when you stop taking the drugs.)
- myomectomy (a surgical procedure to remove fibroids)
- endometrial ablation (a procedure that destroys the lining of the uterus)

- uterine artery embolization, UAE (a minimally invasive procedure that shrinks fibroids by cutting off their blood supply)
- hysterectomy (a surgical procedure to remove the uterus and all of the attached fibroids)

The problem with all of these approaches is they don't address the root cause of the problem: estrogen dominance. Worse still, if left unaddressed, estrogen dominance can manifest in other conditions, such as thyroid nodules, fibrocystic breasts, or estrogenic cancers. That's why the best approach is to treat estrogen dominance and fibroids proactively. I've seen time and again how much fibroids can shrink when we address our estrogen-related imbalances.

The Fibroid Add-On Protocol

Step 1. Do the 28-Day Estrogen Reset Foundation Protocol, including the Foundational Supplements. See Part IV for everything you need to do it successfully. After doing the Foundation Protocol, you may not even need to implement Step 2, but if you feel you've mastered it and need to go deeper to address your fibroids, read on.

Step 2. Implement the Fibroid Protocol.

There are many proven tools in this section that may help you and it might get intimidating. Implement what you can. Some things may help and others won't. We are all different and will respond to changes in varied ways.

Add serrapeptase. This proteolytic enzyme, meaning it breaks down proteins into smaller components, dissolves fibroid tissue. It's also highly anti-inflammatory.

If you have heavy periods because of fibroids, add extra iron to your diet. This can come from food, such as liver, seaweed, or blackstrap molasses, or non-constipating iron supplements. In the Supplement Guide on page 361, I cover my favorite brands.

Lower inflammation. Inflammation is a common companion in women with fibroids. An anti-inflammatory diet (detailed out in chapters 10 and 11) and supplements which target inflammation, such as those containing curcumin, boswellia, or omega 3 can help a great deal.

Take two tablespoons of freshly ground flax seed per day. Even though flax seeds contain phytoestrogens and can be estrogenic, they are not bad for you. Flax seeds promote the breakdown of estrogen into "clean" estrogens, not the damaging "dirty" ones.

Try castor oil packs to support liver detoxification, clear out "dirty" estrogens, and reduce inflammation. If you haven't already tried castor oil packs, now is a good time to begin. For more on their benefits and how to apply a pack, see page 150. I've also created a recipe for you–the Uterine Oil Pack on page 352 combines castor oil with magnesium oil–a powerful topical application for your uterus and fibroids.

Implement herbal strategies. Work with a local herbalist to create an herbal formula that combines several different strategies: supporting the liver, boosting progesterone, and constricting blood flow to the fibroids. These herbs support the following strategies:

Cholagogues, liver detoxifiers to promote the flow of bile from the liver and binding up of "dirty" estrogens:

- dandelion root
- burdock root
- gentian
- andrographis

Hormone modulators to rebuild progesterone levels:

- chasteberry
- black cohosh

Uterine astringents to cut off the blood supply (a short-term strategy):

- yarrow
- cinnamon
- cranesbill
- red raspberry

Uterine tonics, herbs to promote overall balance:

- blue cohosh
- motherwort
- red raspberry leaf

Consider acupuncture. Some women have reported amazing results with acupuncture, including less pain, and overall, I'm a big fan of acupuncture as a way to promote balance in the body.

Take the DUTCH test. Testing is a good idea to establish a baseline before you begin any protocol. It's also helpful if you've been doing the Foundation and Fibroid Add-On Protocol for three to four months and your fibroids are not shrinking. I suggest DUTCH testing every three to six months while on this Add-On Protocol to assess your levels of estrogen metabolites, cortisol, and melatonin (with a few others) levels to help determine why those fibroids are not going away and where you may need extra support.

Consider saliva testing. I recommend saliva testing to check your progesterone levels. Progesterone cannot be measured in urine (DUTCH will only show you an approximation). Saliva is a great medium to understand your progesterone levels. Unfortunately, saliva testing won't show estrogen metabolites. At the time of writing this book, there is no provider offering both urine and saliva screening in one test. For providers and periodically updated information, see Recommended Labs on page 362.

Yarrow
ACHILLEA MILLEFOLIUM

Chapter 10
Endometriosis Protocol

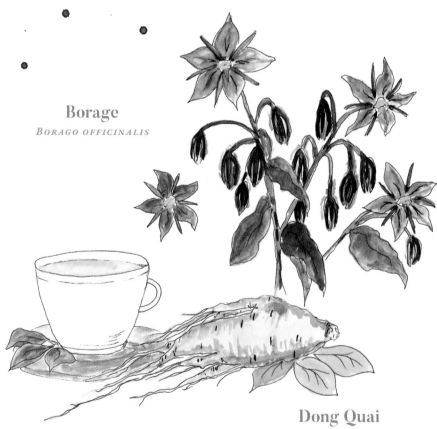

Borage
BORAGO OFFICINALIS

Green Tea
CAMELLIA SINENSIS

Dong Quai
ANGELICA SINENSIS

Endometriosis, affecting an estimated 10% of reproductive-age women, can be a debilitating and a life-altering condition. The pain can be off the charts, leaving every other type of pain you've ever felt in the dust. Know this: Endometriosis is not a life sentence. It can be treated naturally but may need a holistic, integrated approach. Be patient and kind to yourself throughout this journey.

Key Facts

Endometriosis occurs when tissue similar to the lining of the uterus or endometrium grows outside of it. Endometrial tissue is commonly found in the uterus, fallopian tubes, vagina, cervix, ovaries, bladder, and bowel but can grow almost anywhere, including the colon, lungs, nose, and brain.

ENDOMETRIOSIS

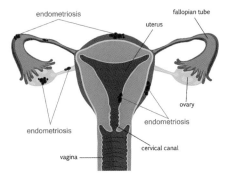

Endometriosis is characterized by intense, often incapacitating, pain. This is caused by the endometrial tissue swelling and bleeding in the same way the tissue lining your uterus does during your period. But in this case, the tissue has no way of leaving your body and becomes trapped. Inflammation, cysts (formed by trapped blood), scar tissue, and adhesions (a type of tissue that binds organs together) caused by expanding endometrial growths are also painful.

Scars and adhesions can prevent pregnancy. It is estimated that they are responsible for 25% of infertility cases.

Certain women are at higher risk for endometriosis. These include those who had an early onset of menstruation, use birth control pills or IUDs, have cycles longer than thirty days, no pregnancies, frequent vaginal and urinary infections, and a history of using immunosuppressants.

There may be a genetic connection. But this would only be a predisposition to endometriosis, not a "given" or guarantee of its development. Your diet, lifestyle, and stress levels all have a significant influence on the expression of your genes.

Toxic exposure may play a role. Carbon dioxide may influence the development of endometriosis. The same is true of mold.

Not all women with endometriosis experience symptoms. Half of those with an endometriosis diagnosis report few to no symptoms.

Symptoms

- pain before, during, and in-between menstruation (Keep in mind the severity of your pain does not necessarily correlate to the severity of your endometriosis.)
- unexplained pelvic pain
- irregular cycles
- infertility
- painful intercourse
- vomiting, nausea, and exhaustion
- bladder pain and urinary problems

Diagnosis

Diagnosis is typically done by doing a pelvic exam and ultrasound, and made definitively by laparoscopy, a surgical procedure in which a small, lighted viewing instrument is inserted in the abdomen or pelvis.

Causes

- estrogen dominance (Endometrial tissue has a large number of estrogen receptors and excess estrogen promotes its growth.)
- a high level of "dirty" estrogens and exposure to xenoestrogens (from personal skincare and house products; which add more excess estrogen to fuel endometrial tissue growth)
- progesterone deficiency (Remember, without enough progesterone to balance out estrogen, we have the "unbalanced partners" cause of estrogen dominance. Low progesterone allows estrogen to become dominant and the excess estrogen promotes the growth of the endometrial tissue.)
- magnesium deficiency
- imbalanced immune system (There could be an autoimmune element.)
- high toxic load, preventing adequate detoxification of "dirty" estrogens and fueling inflammation
- inflammation, caused by diet, alcohol, stress, and toxins, especially dioxide exposure, among many other sources that feed inflammation
- stress, often worsened by hypoglycemia, or low blood sugar
- too much coffee and alcohol (not causes but certainly contributors that will make symptoms worse)

Traditional Treatments

- "wait and see," especially if you are asymptomatic or mild (stage 1 or 2)
- laparoscopy, though there is a high recurring/regrowth rate
- hysterectomy, a surgical procedure to remove the uterus
- synthetic hormone replacement therapy, often birth control pills including progestin (synthetic progesterone)
- gonadotropin-releasing hormone (GnRH) agonists and antagonists, to induce menopause
- painkillers, which can have a detrimental effect on the gut lining, liver, and kidneys

The problem with all of these approaches is they don't address the root causes of the problem: estrogen dominance, poor immune system function, high inflammation, and toxicity. Worse still, if left unaddressed, estrogen dominance can manifest in other conditions, such as thyroid nodules, fibrocystic breasts, or estrogenic cancers. It doesn't go away—even with a hysterectomy. That's why the best approach is to treat estrogen dominance and endometriosis proactively, with holistic natural approaches that address what's causing the growth of the endometrial tissue in the first place.

Endometriosis Protocol

Endometriosis can be contained, but you must be patient and kind with yourself. Because it is a complicated condition, it takes longer to resolve than PMS or fibroids. Don't be frustrated if you don't see results right away. Chances are when you resolve endometriosis, many of your other health foes will vanish with it.

> The best approach is to treat estrogen dominance and endometriosis proactively, with holistic natural approaches that address what's causing the growth of the endometrial tissue in the first place.

Step 1. Do the 28-Day Estrogen Reset Foundation Protocol, including the Foundational Supplements. See Part IV for everything you need to do it successfully. After doing the Foundation Protocol, you may not even need to implement Step 2, but if you feel you've mastered it and need to go deeper to address your endometriosis, read on.

Step 2. Implement the Endometriosis Protocol.

Implement as much of the following as you can. Some things may help and others won't. We are all different and will respond to changes in varied ways.

Get off of synthetic hormone replacement therapy or birth control pills. If you are still on them, work with your healthcare provider to transition off of them. Copper IUDs can contribute to the inflammation. Hormonal IUDs (such as Mirena) may help initially but it won't address the underlying causes of endometriosis.

Address stress and reduce caffeine and alcohol consumption to an absolute minimum. I hope you are on top of this already but if not, know that making these changes will really help your endometriosis symptoms.

Add serrapeptase. This proteolytic enzyme, meaning it breaks down proteins into smaller components, dissolves endometrial tissue. Serrapeptase is used for many painful conditions as it has the ability to reduce inflammation and helps to dissolve old scar tissue and reduce adhesions.

Add curcumin, a potent anti-inflammatory. One of the active ingredients in turmeric, curcumin may destroy fibroid cells or stop them from reproducing. Its anti-inflammatory properties may help reduce pain.

Add borage oil (internally), a potent anti-inflammatory and pain reliever. It contains 20 to 26% gamma-linoleic acid (GLA), a fatty acid that converts into prostaglandins PgE1 and PgE3 (a natural painkiller) and suppresses PgE2 (the cause of the pain). The recommended dosage is 240 mg three to four times per day with meals, or as directed by your healthcare practitioner.

Try castor oil packs, to support liver detoxification, clear out "dirty" estrogens, and reduce inflammation. If you haven't already tried castor oil packs, now is a good time to begin. For more on their benefits and how to apply a pack, see page 150.

Implement herbal strategies. Work with a local herbalist to create an herbal formula that combines several different strategies: analgesics (painkillers), anti-inflammatories, antispasmodics (for immune support), adaptogens (to help the body resist stress), and hormone modulators. These herbs support the following strategies:

Analgesics (relieving pain)

- dong quai
- black cohosh
- white peony

Anti-inflammatories

- dong quai
- green tea
- licorice
- evening primrose (gamma-linoleic acid, or GLA)

Antispasmodics

- ginger
- wild yam
- cramp bark

Immune supporters and adaptogens

- dong quai
- ashwagandha
- echinacea
- eleuthero
- schisandra

Hormone regulators

- chasteberry (vitex)
- blue vervain

Consider acupuncture. Some women have reported amazing results, including less pain, with acupuncture and overall, I'm a big fan of acupuncture as a way to promote balance in the body.

Take the DUTCH test. Testing is a good idea to establish a baseline before you begin any protocol. It's also helpful if you've been doing the Foundation and Endometriosis Add-On Protocol for three to four months and you're still symptomatic. I suggest DUTCH testing every three to six months while on this Add-On Protocol to assess your levels of estrogen metabolites, cortisol and melatonin (with a few others) to help determine where you may need extra support.

Consider saliva testing. I recommend saliva testing to check your progesterone levels. Progesterone cannot be measured in urine (DUTCH will only show you an approximation). Saliva is a great medium to understand your progesterone levels. Unfortunately, saliva testing won't show estrogen metabolites. At the time of writing this book, there is no provider offering both urine and saliva screening in one test. For providers and periodically updated information, see Recommended Labs on page 362.

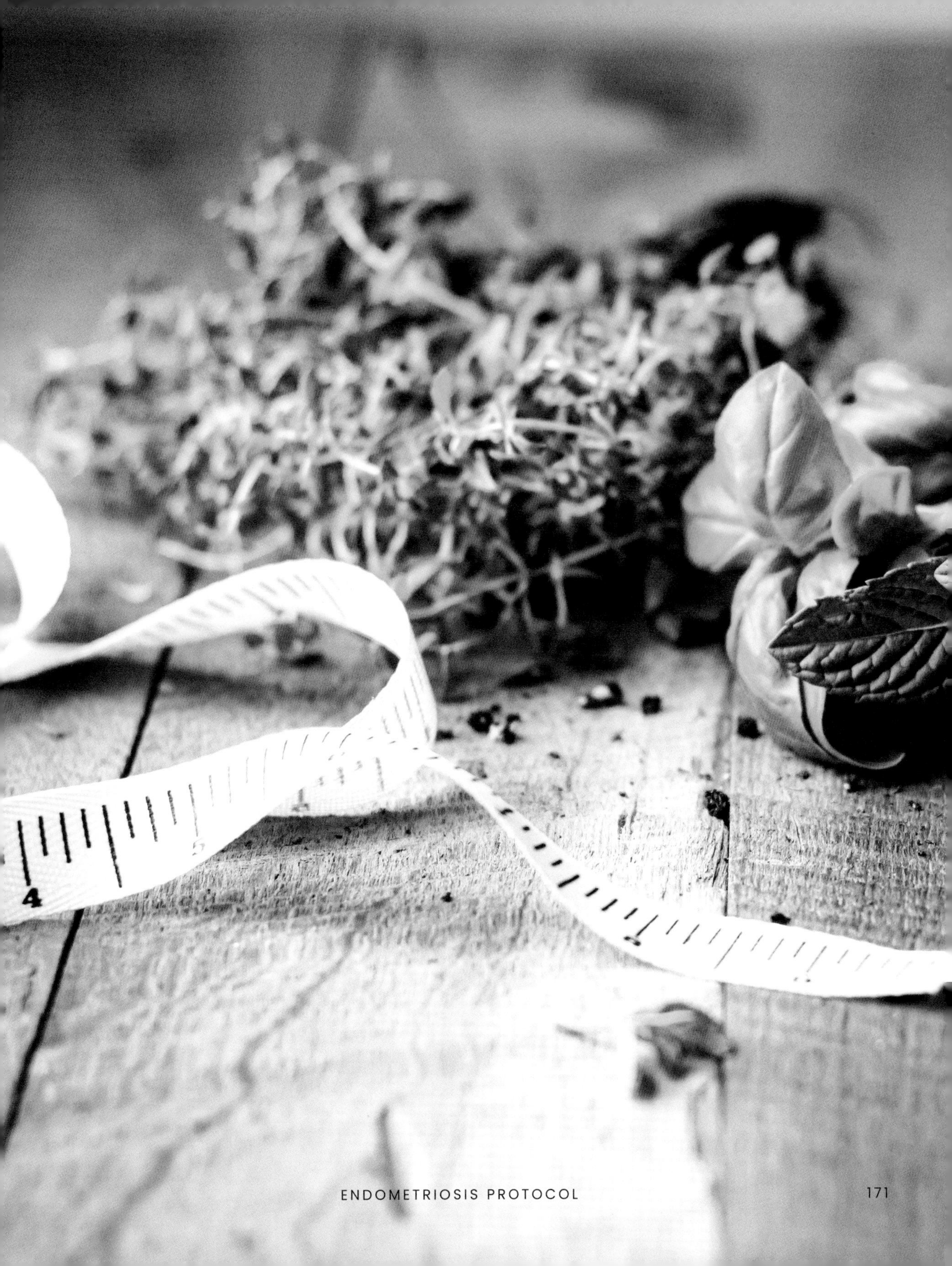
4
5

Chapter 11

Fibrocystic and Lumpy Breasts Protocol

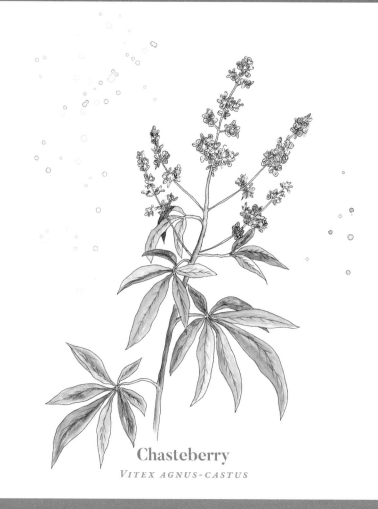

Chasteberry

VITEX AGNUS-CASTUS

Any woman who has found a lump on her breast knows the barrage of emotions that comes with the discovery: you're afraid and overwhelmed; you feel fear, confusion and perhaps experience paralysis. Healthy breasts are dependent on your hormone status. If your hormones are out of balance and you have estrogen dominance, your breasts may develop more lumps, feel tender, and sore. These changes though, known as fibrocystic breast changes, can be a thing of the past.

Key Facts

Breast texture is naturally irregular and changes with your monthly hormonal cycle. Breasts are made up of fatty tissue, milk-producing glands, ducts, and connective tissue, so their texture is not fixed. They change with the hormonal ebb and flow of your menstrual cycle. At times, your breasts can feel lumpier when ducts enlarge as they fill with fluid in anticipation of a possible pregnancy, then softer and smaller toward the end of menstruation when estrogen/progesterone are at their lowest.

Fibrocystic breasts develop when excess fluid isn't reabsorbed or adequately drained by the lymphatic system and turns into cysts surrounded by rubbery fibrous tissue. Cysts are fluid-filled lumps or sacs that may move around, appear, and disappear. In some cases, the fibrous tissue surrounding them can thicken and firm up, like scar tissue. These cysts inflame and enlarge the breast ducts, causing a lumpiness, discomfort, and pain in the breast.

Fibrocystic breasts are benign. Rarely do they indicate breast cancer, especially if the changes are bilateral (occurring in both breasts). And your risk of breast cancer does not increase if you have them.

They are very common. It's estimated that 60 to 90% of women have fibrocystic breasts. For this reason, medical professionals have stopped labeling the condition a disease. These breast changes are considered perfectly normal.

Fibrocystic breasts occur bilaterally. Meaning on both sides/in both breasts.

Normal

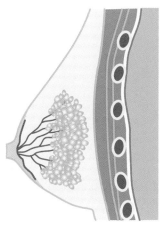

Fibrocystic

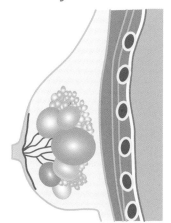

Fibrocystic breast changes can be cyclic or noncyclic. Cyclic changes alter with your period (fluctuations in size and level of pain, for example) while noncyclic ones are not impacted by the different stages of your menstrual cycle with pain persisting throughout the month.

Symptoms

- soft, tender, moveable cysts (Cysts are cyclic [more common] or noncyclic [less common], often painful, freely moveable, and multiple, and they vary in size and occur in both breasts.)
- lumpy, thickening of breasts caused by excess fibrous tissue
- breast swelling and soreness

Diagnosis

Your doctor can diagnose fibrocystic breasts by doing a physical breast exam. To get a closer look at your breast tissue, your doctor may order these diagnostic tests, best performed right after menses:

- ultrasound
- thermography, a test that uses an infrared camera to detect heat patterns and blood flow
- electrical resistance testing
- mammogram
- biopsy (a last resort)

Causes

- estrogen dominance, especially due to an excess of "dirty" estrogens (Excess estrogen can cause an increase in fluid and swelling of the breast ducts.)

CYCLIC AND NONCYCLIC BREAST PAIN

Cyclic

- typically generalized throughout both breasts
- connected to your period and hormone fluctuations
- may start somewhere after mid-cycle or the week before your period
- usually goes away when your period starts

According to Jerilynn Prior, MD, a Canadian clinician and professor of endocrinology at the University of British Columbia, here's what premenstrual soreness can tell you about your hormonal health.

Soreness on the sides of the breasts and under the armpit: Indicates ovulation has happened, therefore this type of pain is normal and acceptable.

Soreness on the front of the breasts and over the nipples: Indicates no ovulation, but the presence of estrogen dominance.

Soreness on the sides and the front of the breasts: Can indicate that ovulation occurred but not enough progesterone was produced three or four days after ovulation, thus estrogen dominance is occurring.

Noncyclic

Persistent throughout the month and is usually localized to one area of the breast. It can be caused by:

- estrogen dominance
- pregnancy
- hormone replacement therapy
- medications, including antidepressants
- mastitis or local infection/cysts
- rarely caused by breast cancer

- a high level of "dirty" estrogens and exposure to xenoestrogens (from personal skincare and house products, which add more excess estrogen to fuel the growth of those ducts)
- progesterone deficiency (remember, without enough progesterone to balance out estrogen, we have the "unbalanced partners" cause of estrogen dominance. Low progesterone allows estrogen to become dominant and the excess estrogen promotes fibrocystic breasts.)
- magnesium deficiency
- iodine deficiency
- sugar addiction (sugar promotes inflammation)
- chronic constipation, preventing the excretion of "dirty" estrogens
- high toxic load, preventing adequate detoxification of "dirty" estrogens and fueling inflammation
- inflammation, caused by diet, stress, and toxins, especially dioxide exposure, among many other sources that feed inflammation
- stress, often worsened by hypoglycemia, or low blood sugar
- smoking
- too much coffee and alcohol (not causes but certainly contributors that will make symptoms worsen)

Traditional Treatments

- loose-fitting clothes and bras
- decreasing caffeine
- quitting smoking
- getting off birth control pills (especially progestin)
- anti-estrogen medications (estrogen blockers)
- diuretics
- painkillers

- shedding fat, especially belly fat

The problem with all of these approaches is they don't address the root causes of the problem: estrogen dominance, high inflammation, and toxicity. Worse still, if left unaddressed, estrogen dominance can manifest in other conditions, such as thyroid nodules or estrogenic cancers. That's why the best way to treat estrogen dominance and fibrocystic breasts proactively with holistic natural approaches that address what's causing the development of breast cysts in the first place.

Fibrocystic and Lumpy Breasts Protocol

Step 1. Do the 28-Day Estrogen Reset Foundation Protocol, including the Foundational Supplements. See Part IV for everything you need to do it successfully. After doing the Foundation Protocol, you may not even need to implement Step 2, but if you feel you've mastered it and need to go deeper to address your fibrocystic breasts, read on.

Step 2. Implement the Fibrocystic and Lumpy Breasts Protocol.

Implement as much of the following as you can. Some things may help and others won't. We are all different and will respond to changes in varied ways.

Reduce caffeine and alcohol consumption to an absolute minimum. I hope you are on top of this already but if not, know that making these changes will really help your symptoms. My breasts get lumpy pretty quickly when I drink coffee or alcohol on a regular basis.

Apply bioidentical progesterone to breast tissue. I have found that applying progesterone topically makes a big difference, especially if you are in a lot of pain, for instance if you can't even put on your bra because your breasts hurts so much. Topical progesterone is an absolutely wonderful solution. Not only does progesterone help with fibrocystic breast and estrogen dominance, it also improves sleep, promotes a calmer, better mood, raises your libido, regulates your cycle for more predictable periods, builds bones, lowers LDL cholesterol, converts fat to energy, lowers your risk of developing estrogenic breast cancer, and reduces hot flashes.

Move your lymphatic system. I feel like the lymphatic system is underestimated given it's a highway of tunnels that evacuate junk from your body. It's easy to support your lymphatics-dry brushing and rebounding can be easily incorporated into your day and only take a few minutes. This is especially important in breast health. For more on the benefits, also how to dry brush and rebound, see page 154.

Add breast lymphatic massage. I was first made aware of this technique by a wonderful holistic breast health practitioner, Gaye Walden. She then introduced me to Dr. Bruce Rind, who teaches this profound method of massage around the world.

Massage in general has been shown to activate blood flow in the lymphatic system; however, there's a special kind of massage that targets the breast lymph system specifically. Breasts are very high in lymphatic channels and stagnation can manifest in the form of tender or fibrocystic breasts. I've recorded a video with a breast specialist, showing how to do the massage. You can find it at www.hormonesbalance.com/oed/downloads. If you prefer to get in-person help, there are trained therapists in MLD, or "manual lymphatic drainage" who use gentle pressure to promote lymph flow.

Lymphatic Breast Massage (do daily when you shower)

Massage tips:

- Massage in the shower when wet, soapy, and slippery.
- Use your open hand to sweep in the direction of the lymphatic flow (see arrow directions).
- Sweep from nipple toward 12:00, 2:00, 4:00, 6:00, 8:00, and 10:00, two times per breast.
- Go slow, about three to five seconds per sweep, and gently deep.
- Massage with your opposite side hand.
- Visualize the breast as being made of sponge containing thick honey. Slow, deep sweeps make the honey flow out.
- Visualize your breast being nourished, cleansed, and healed.

Infused oils. Topically, herbalists very successfully use oils infused with dandelion, violet and calendula flowers, or sometimes comfrey and poke root, to lower breast inflammation and to move the lymphatic system in the breasts. See Breast Massage Oil on page 348 on how to make it-it's simple and inexpensive. I've tried this oil many times and felt like my breast tenderness had reduced by 50 to 70% within hours. Use this oil when doing the breast massage described above.

Consider iodine. We have iodine receptors in our breasts, brain, thyroid, and ovaries. These organs need iodine to function properly. I've found that breast lumps can go away quickly, especially dense fibrocystic breasts, not just lumps, by adding iodine. I've seen many amazing results. Sensitivity improves significantly as well. Foods such as seaweed (kelp, wakame, hijiki), seafood, and eggs are good sources of iodine or

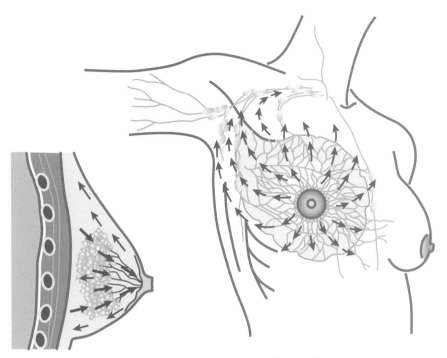

Lymphatic breast massage instructions.

try supplements, though only people found to be deficient in iodine through proper testing should take supplemental iodine. The preferred form of iodine supplementation is potassium iodide. Take 3 to 10 mg per day, start low. Some women report great results by applying iodine directly on their breasts.

Caution: Do not add iodine (internally or externally) if you have hyperthyroidism, Graves' disease, or Hashimoto's disease with elevated thyroid peroxidase (TPO) antibodies. Added iodine may cause a thyroid flare-up.

Add borage oil (internally), a potent anti-inflammatory and pain reliever. It contains 20 to 26% gamma-linoleic acid (GLA), a fatty acid that converts into prostaglandins PgE1 and PgE3 (a natural painkiller) and suppresses PgE2 (the cause of the pain). The recommended dosage is 240 mg three to four times per day with meals, or as directed by your health care practitioner.

Add vitamin E for pain relief. In a 2009 double-blind clinical trial of 150 women, 200 IU of vitamin E reduced breast pain by 70% in two months. Vitamin E promotes progesterone production and inhibits breast cancer.

Add an aromatase inhibitor. Natural aromatase inhibitors, such as chrysin and passionflower, lower estrogen levels by preventing the conversion of DHEA and testosterone into estrogen. The recommended dosage is 200 mg. Consult with your healthcare provider before taking one as there are precautions for medications for estrogen sensitive cancers (aromatase inhibitors) and medications changed by the liver (Cytochrome P450 1A2 [CYP1A2] substrates) such as clozapine. Pregnant and breastfeeding women should not take an aromatase inhibitor.

Take two tablespoons of freshly ground flax seed per day. Even though flax seeds contain phytoestrogens and can be estrogenic, they are not bad for you. Flax seeds promote the breakdown of estrogen into "clean" estrogens, not the damaging "dirty" ones.

Try castor oil packs to support liver detoxification, clear out "dirty" estrogens, and reduce inflammation. If you haven't already tried castor oil packs, now is a good time to begin. Alternate placement over your liver and breasts. Add essential oils for additional support (see box). For more on the benefits and how to apply a pack, see page 150.

Implement herbal strategies. Work with a local herbalist to create an herbal formula that combines several different strategies: hormone modulators, enhancing liver and bile production, in addition to relieving local congestions (lymphatics). These herbs support the following strategies:

Hormone modulators

- chasteberry
- dong quai
- red clover

Enhance liver health and bile production

- gentian
- dandelion root

Relieve local congestion (lymphatics)

- cleaver
- dandelion flower
- calendula flower
- comfrey root
- poke root

Take the DUTCH test. Testing is a good idea to establish a baseline before you begin any protocol. It's also helpful if you've been doing the Foundation and Fibrocystic and Lumpy Breasts Add-On Protocol for three to four months and you're still symptomatic. I suggest DUTCH testing every three to six months while on this Add-On Protocol to assess your estrogen metabolites, cortisol, and melatonin (with a few others) levels

HAPPY BREAST BLEND

Courtesy of Dr. Mariza Snyder, author of *The Essential Oils Hormone Solution*

To a 10 ml bottle add:

- 5 drops frankincense essential oil
- 5 drops lavender essential oil
- 3 drops tangerine essential oil
- 7 drops helichrysum essential oil
- 4 drops wild orange essential oil

Top up the bottle with fractionated coconut oil and apply to breasts and pulse points.

to help determine where you may need extra support.

Consider saliva testing. I recommend saliva testing to check your progesterone levels. Progesterone cannot be measured in urine (DUTCH will only show you an approximation). Saliva is a great medium to understand your progesterone levels. Unfortunately, saliva testing won't show estrogen metabolites. At the time of writing this book, there is no provider offering both urine and saliva screening in one test. For providers and periodically updated information, see Recommended Labs on page 362.

Chapter 12

Hot Flashes Protocol

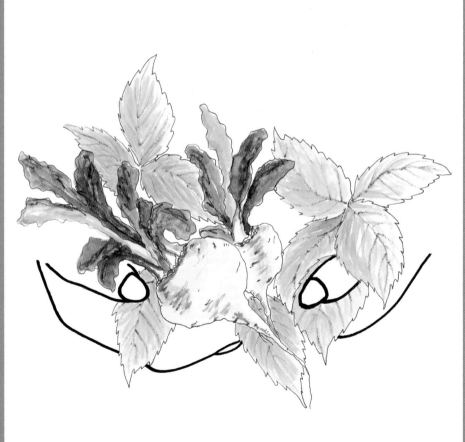

Maca

LEPIDIUM MEYENII

Hot flashes are one of the most common complaints for women in peri-menopause, especially those over age 45. It's estimated that 70 to 85% of peri-menopausal women have hot flashes so if this is you, know you are not alone. You can stop them. Figuring out your unique root causes and triggers will make it much easier for you to reduce or eliminate them.

Key Facts

The medical term for hot flashes is vasomotor flushing. Vasomotor refers to the vasomotor center, the part of the brain that regulates blood pressure by controlling the diameter of the blood vessels.

A hot flash is your body trying to cool itself off. When the body gets too hot, it lets off excess heat by opening up the blood vessels in the skin, allowing more blood to flow to the area. The additional blood flow is the reason for your reddish skin during a hot flash. The extra heat escapes your body through sweat, causing you to feel chilly and clammy once your temperature drops when the hot flash has passed.

The frequency and severity of hot flashes varies among women. Some women experience hot flashes several times throughout the day while others may get one every few weeks. Their intensity can vary, from mild to severe and last anywhere from one to five minutes.

In peri-menopausalwomen, hot flashes tend to occur before or during periods. Hot flashes can persist into menopause, for one to two years or much longer.

Night sweats are when a hot flash occurs during the night and the sweating that occurs to cool you off wakes you up. Some women lightly perspire while others may soak through their pajamas.

Symptoms

- sudden rush of intense heat, spreading over the body, especially the chest, neck, and face
- redness of the skin, especially of the neck, face, and nose
- perspiration
- increased heart rate
- tingling and crawling sensation under the skin
- nausea
- chills, once the hot flash has passed

Causes

- blood vessels opening up too much, causing a rush of blood to the surface of your skin
- dropping estrogen levels, expected during peri-menopause and especially menopause

It's estimated that 70 to 85% of peri-menopausal women have hot flashes so if this is you, know you are not alone.

- surging FSH, follicle stimulating hormone (Due to the slow-down of estrogen production in the ovaries during peri-menopause and menopause, the body pumps out more FSH in a last-ditch effort to kick the ovaries into producing more estrogen.)
- blood sugar imbalance (Riding the blood sugar roller coaster of surges and crashes is likely contributing to your hot flashes. Often a crash, a sudden drop in blood sugar, triggers them. This is why it's so important to follow the Foundation Protocol, balance your blood sugar, and eat a PFF breakfast.)
- high TSH (thyroid stimulating hormone), or low thyroid function (hypothyroidism)
- coffee and caffeine
- food sensitivities, especially gluten and dairy
- stress
- hot drinks, spicy food (not causes but certainly contributors that will make hot flashes worse)

Traditional Treatments

- synthetic estrogen hormone replacement therapy

This is the most common first-line treatment for hot flashes. The problem is synthetic hormone replacement therapy doesn't address root causes and can cause a range of serious side effects. This is why I recommend trying natural options first, then if necessary, explore bioidentical hormone replacement options with your healthcare provider.

The Hot Flashes Add-On Protocol

Step 1. Do the 28-Day Estrogen Reset Foundation Protocol, including the Foundational Supplements. See Part IV for everything you need to do it successfully. After doing the Foundation Protocol, you may not even need to implement Step 2, but if you feel you've mastered it and need to go deeper to address your hot flashes, read on.

Step 2: Implement the Hot Flashes Protocol.

Implement as much of the following as you can. Some things may help and others won't. Everyone is different and will respond to changes in varied ways.

Add topical progesterone. If you haven't already incorporated topical progesterone as part of the Foundational Protocol, now is the time. I have found that applying progesterone topically is an absolutely wonderful solution for hot flashes. It also improves sleep, promotes a calmer, boosts your mood, raises your libido, regulates your cycle for more predictable periods, builds bones,

KEEP A HOT FLASH JOURNAL

Take note of when you have a hot flash and what was happening before it occurred. Were you stressed? Did you have a breakfast high in carbohydrates and sugar? Did you have nothing but coffee three hours prior? Pay attention and you will likely see some patterns that can help you identify what's causing your hot flashes and what steps to take to curb them.

converts fat to energy, and lowers your risk of developing estrogenic breast cancer.

If stress is driving your hot flashes, try the 4-7-8 breathing technique. This technique stimulates the vagus nerve, promoting relaxation, lowering cortisol levels, and reducing inflammation. Breathe in for four seconds, hold the breath for seven seconds, and exhale for eight seconds. It takes just a few minutes a day to become an expert. You can see demo how to do it in this video: www.hormonesbalance.com/oed/downloads.

Try castor oil packs to support liver detoxification, clear out "dirty" estrogens, and reduce inflammation. If you haven't already tried castor oil packs, now is a good time to begin. For more on their benefits and how to apply a pack, see page 150.

Spending some time in an infrared sauna. Infrared saunas provide a host of amazing benefits, including lowering inflammation, promoting deep detoxification, and reducing pain. For more on the benefits of an infrared sauna, see page 154.

Implement herbal strategies. Work with a local herbalist to create an herbal formula that combines several different strategies: hormone modulators and tonics, adaptogens, as well as nervines (to promote calm). These herbs support the following strategies:

WHAT HAS WORKED FOR THE HORMONES BALANCE COMMUNITY

Poll Results: What has helped your hot flashes?

I've polled our community asking "What have you done to reduce hot flashes or night sweats? What has worked?" Of all the replies, this is what has produced the best results:

- reduced sugar consumption (This was the number one most effective method cited. Some women reported also reducing alcohol along with all processed carbohydrates such as pasta and bread.)

- reduced or eliminated coffee and caffeine

- started the elimination diet and reduced inflammation from foods such as gluten and dairy

- added herbs such as maca, black cohosh, and our Wise Women Balance

- added topical progesterone

As you can see, four out of five solutions are already covered in the Foundation Protocol in Part IV.

Hormone modulators and tonics

- black cohosh
- chasteberry (vitex)
- dong quai
- red raspberry leaf

Adaptogens

- ashwagandha
- schisandra
- rhodiola
- eleuthero
- licorice

Nervines, especially if you're very stressed

- skullcap
- oat straw
- passionflower

Take the DUTCH test. Testing is a good idea to establish a baseline before you begin any protocol. It's also helpful if you've been doing the Foundation and Hot Flashes Add-On Protocol for three to four months and your hot flashes aren't becoming fewer and less severe. I suggest DUTCH testing every three to six months while on this Add-On Protocol to assess your estrogen metabolites, cortisol, and melatonin (with a few others) levels to help determine where you may need extra support.

Consider saliva testing. I recommend saliva testing to check your progesterone levels. Progesterone cannot be measured in urine (DUTCH will only show you an approximation). Saliva is a great medium to understand your progesterone levels. Unfortunately, saliva testing won't show estrogen metabolites. At the time of writing this book, there is no provider offering both urine and saliva screening in one test. For providers and periodically updated information, see Recommended Labs on page 362.

Add bioidentical hormone therapy, if necessary. If natural solutions are not enough to relieve your hot flashes, bioidentical hormone therapy is an option. Bioidentical estrogen, DHEA, and testosterone may be right for you depending on your needs and health history.

Black cohosh
ACTAEA RACEMOSA

Chapter 13

Amenorrhea (Absent Periods) Protocol

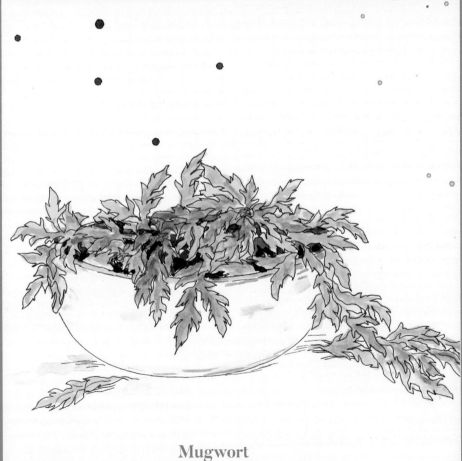

Mugwort

ARTEMISIA VULGARIS

When I first moved to the United States, I was surprised at how most women see periods as an inconvenient, unnecessary, and preventable event. I didn't know what I know now but intuitively, this way of thinking felt harmful.

And harmful it can be. Your period is *information*. An absent period is your body's way of telling you there is imbalance in your body preventing your period from happening. Acting upon this information cannot only fix your period but most likely a whole host of other medical issues such as chronic migraines, lumpy breasts, hair loss, chronic pain, frequent bouts of depression, and insomnia, among others. Address your lack of periods and you will probably address all of these other issues as well. Rest assured: You can start having regular periods again.

Key Facts

A regular menstrual cycle, involving a variety of hormones working together, is vital for good health. The four main hormones involved are estrogen, progesterone, LH (luteinizing hormone), and FSH (follicle stimulating hormone). On the first day of bleeding in a normal cycle (day one is the first day of bleeding), all of these hormones are low. That's part of the reason why a lot of us don't feel great at this time of the month. During ovulation, which occurs around day 14, a number of different hormones go up. Estrogen rises and LH reaches its peak, provoking FSH to increase, stimulating the follicles to thicken. After ovulation, progesterone steadily rises. Just before your period, all four hormones drop and the uterine lining sheds. That's part of the reason why, in days 26 to 28, two to three days before a period, you can be feeling pretty crummy.

As you can see, there's a lot going on here, with multiple hormone fluctuations dependent upon other hormone fluctuations. The menstrual cycle is a complex dance of hormones and if one (or more) of these hormones is deficient for any reason, the cycle can be thrown off, causing you to miss a period.

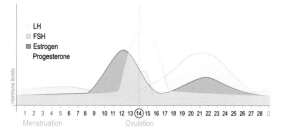

Ovulation is required for you to have a period. If you are not ovulating, you will not have a true period. Figuring out why you are not ovulating is key to getting your periods back.

There are two categories of amenorrhea.

Primary: Your menstrual cycle didn't occur by age 16.

Secondary: You have been having menstrual cycles but have not had one for three or more months (excluding pregnancy, breastfeeding, or menopause).

Symptoms

- Missing a period for three months or more if your cycle had been regular and six months or more if they had been irregular.

Causes

- estrogen dominance
- low estrogen and/or low progesterone
- stress (In order to make enough cortisol to support the body's stress response, pregnenolone is diverted or "stolen away" from

progesterone production to make cortisol. When this happens, you're producing so much cortisol to deal with a stressful situation that you have insufficient progesterone to support ovulation.)

- poor sleep and shift work (These situations interfere with the production and release of melatonin, the hormone that prompts sleep and plays a role in your menstrual cycle. Melatonin is anti-estrogenic and low melatonin can disrupt ovulation.)
- PCOS (polycystic ovarian syndrome)
- insulin resistance
- high testosterone
- ceasing hormonal birth control (It can take a few months for your hormones to return to normal when you stop taking hormonal birth control. Post-pill amenorrhea is when your period has not returned three months after stopping birth control.)
- toxin or radiation exposure
- over- or underactive thyroid
- autoimmune disease (such as Celiac or Hashimoto's)
- anemia (B_{12} or iron deficiency)
- anorexia or bulimia, low-fat diet, and/or low nutrient intake stress your body, prompting it to shut down all nonessential systems, like the reproductive
- overexercising (It's stressful to the body.)
- obesity
- hypothalamus dysfunction impacting your pituitary gland and hormone release
- adrenal tumor
- pituitary tumor or dysfunction
- elevated prolactin (most often due to pituitary tumor)

Traditional Treatments

- For secondary amenorrhea: birth control pills; synthetic estrogen or progestin hormone replacement therapy

These are the most common first-line treatments for missing periods. The problem is synthetic hormone replacement therapy doesn't address root causes and can cause a range of serious side effects. This is why I recommend trying natural options first and if necessary, explore bioidentical hormone replacement options with your healthcare provider.

Amenorrhea (Absent Periods) Protocol

Step 1. Do the 28-Day Estrogen Reset Foundation Protocol, including the Foundational Supplements. See Part IV for everything you need to do it successfully. After doing the Foundation Protocol, you may not even need to implement Step 2, but if you feel you've mastered it and haven't regained your period yet, read on.

Step 2: Implement the Amenorrhea (Absent Periods) Protocol.

Implement as much of the following as you can. Some things may help and others won't. We are all different and will respond to changes in varied ways.

Get quality sleep. Prioritizing sleep can be transformative when it comes to restoring and regulating your cycle by building up your levels of melatonin. If you haven't started practicing good sleep hygiene habits as part of your Foundation Protocol (switching off the electronic before bed, keeping your bedroom dark and cool, along with many more), start doing so now. See page 150 for how to improve your sleep.

Try seed rotation. Seed rotation is a technique to balance estrogen and progesterone levels by boosting estrogen levels in the first part of your cycle and progesterone levels in the second part. If you aren't menstruating, this simple food-based rebalancing technique can help your cycle return.

For two weeks, you will incorporate one of the following two seed combinations into your diet and then switch, alternating seed combinations every two weeks. Add these seeds to salads, smoothies, or a glass of water.

Seed combination #1, to boost estrogen: 1 tablespoon of freshly ground flax seed (do not use the pre-ground flax meal, it has little potency) and 1 tablespoon of freshly ground pumpkin seeds.

Seed combination #2, to boost progesterone: 1 tablespoon of freshly ground sesame seeds and 1 tablespoon of freshly ground sunflower seeds.

If you are not menstruating and peri-menopausal

Start any day and keep each seed combination (such as #1, flax seed and pumpkin) for two weeks, then switch to the other (#2, sesame and sunflower seeds). If you are going through peri-menopause, this may or may not bring back your period and that's okay. It's normal for your period to finally stop at this phase in your life. At least, the seed rotation method may help you feel more hormonally balanced.

Once you are menstruating, you can continue to seed cycle to help stay regular

In the Follicular Phase of your cycle (days 1 to 13): Add Seed combination #1, to boost estrogen.

In the Luteal Phase (days 14 to 28): Add Seed combination #2, to boost progesterone.

Add topical progesterone. If you haven't already started using topical progesterone as part of the Foundational Protocol, now is the time. Applying progesterone topically can raise progesterone levels so there's enough to balance out estrogen and create the right hormonal environment for the return of your period. It also improves sleep, promotes calm, boosts your mood, raises your libido, regulates your cycle for more predictable periods, builds bones, converts fat to energy, and lowers your risk of developing estrogenic breast cancer.

Try castor oil packs to support liver detoxification, clear out "dirty" estrogens, and reduce inflammation. If you haven't already tried castor oil packs, now is a good time to begin. For more on their benefits and how to apply a pack, see page 153.

Implement herbal strategies. Work with a local herbalist to create an herbal formula that combines several different strategies: emmenagogues (to bring blood supply to the uterus), hormone modulators, adaptogens and nervines, and PCOS support. These herbs support the following strategies:

Emmenagogues (bring blood supply to the uterus)

- dong quai
- mugwort
- motherwort
- ginger

Hormone modulators

- chasteberry (vitex)
- dong quai
- licorice

Adaptogens and nervines (especially if stress rules your life)

- ashwagandha
- schisandra
- rhodiola
- eleuthero
- skullcap, milky oats, passionflower

PCOS support

- chasteberry (vitex)
- peony
- licorice

Take the DUTCH test. Testing is a good idea to establish a baseline before you begin any protocol. It's also helpful if you've been doing the Foundation and Amenorrhea (Absent Periods) Add-On Protocol for three to four months and your period hasn't returned. I suggest DUTCH testing every three to six months while on this Add-On Protocol to assess your estrogen metabolites, cortisol, and melatonin (with a few others) levels to help determine where you may need extra support.

Consider saliva testing. I recommend saliva testing to check your progesterone levels. Progesterone cannot be measured in urine (DUTCH will only show you an approximation). Saliva is a great medium to understand your progesterone levels. Unfortunately, saliva testing won't show estrogen metabolites. At the time of writing this book, there is no provider offering both urine and saliva

screening in one test. For providers and periodically updated information, see Recommended Labs on page 362.

Add bioidentical hormone therapy, if necessary. If natural solutions are not enough to relieve your hot flashes, bioidentical hormone therapy is an option. Bioidentical estrogen may be right for you depending on your needs and health history.

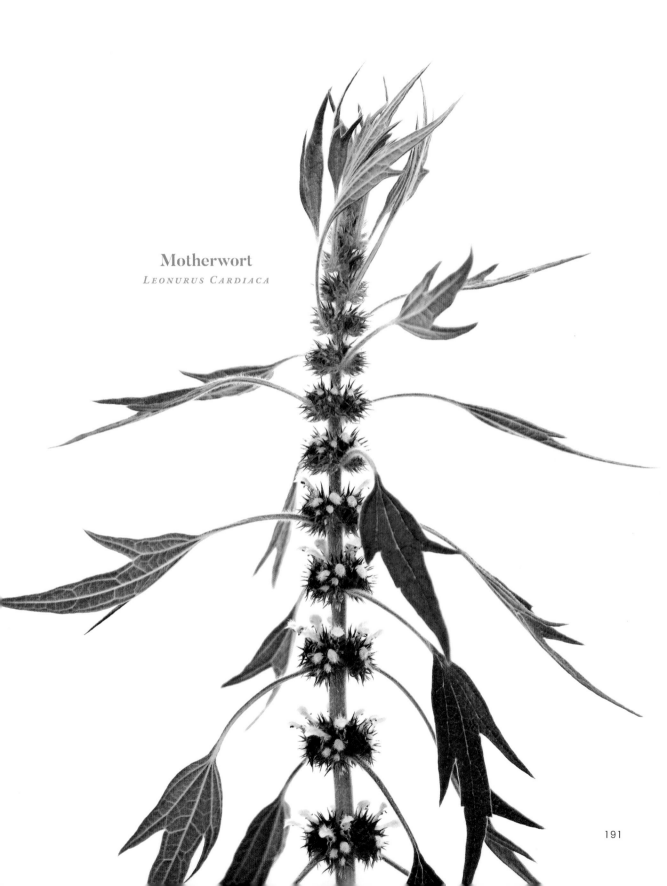

Motherwort
Leonurus Cardiaca

191

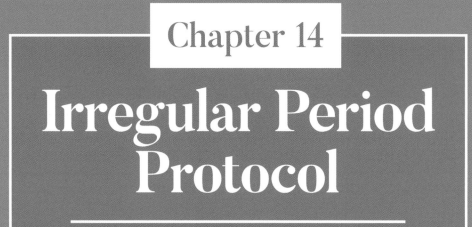

Chapter 14

Irregular Period Protocol

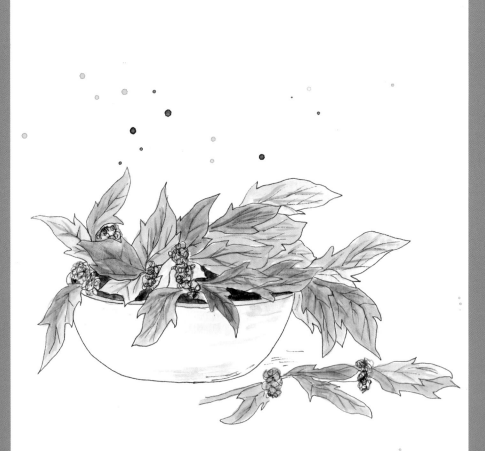

Motherwort

LEONURUS CARDIACA

Regular periods are a healthy part of being a woman, unless you're pregnant, lactating, in peri-menopause (when cycles naturally become irregular), or in menopause (when periods have stopped). That said, a lot of women assume just because they are in their mid-40s they must be in peri-menopause and that's the only reason for their irregular periods. Peri-menopause may be a part of what's going on, but there are often other factors contributing to the irregularity, such as stress, toxins and poor diet. Getting a handle on those and other root causes will help regulate your periods for longer during peri-menopause.

An irregular period, known as oligomenorrhea, indicates imbalances in the body that need to be addressed. If your period is erratic, you are most likely struggling with other issues, such as chronic pain, mood swings, weight gain, hair loss, and insomnia, among others. Rarely are irregular periods the only thing going on. The good news is when you follow my recommendations and improve the regularity of your periods, you will improve all of these other issues as well. You can start having regular periods.

An optimal menstrual cycle is between 28 to 30 days. An acceptable range is 21 to 35 days. Your period (bleeding) should last four to seven days.

A regular menstrual cycle, involving a variety of hormones working together, is vital for good health. The four main hormones involved are estrogen, progesterone, LH (luteinizing hormone), and FSH (follicle stimulating hormone). On the first day of bleeding in a normal cycle, (day one is the first day of bleeding), all of these hormones are low. That's part of the reason why a lot of us don't feel great at this time of the month. During ovulation, which occurs around day 14, a number of different hormones go up. Estrogen rises and LH reaches its peak, provoking FSH to increase, stimulating the follicles to thicken. After ovulation, progesterone steadily rises. Just before your period, all four hormones collapse and the uterine lining sheds. That's part of the reason why, in days 26 to 28, two to three days before a period, you can be feeling pretty crummy.

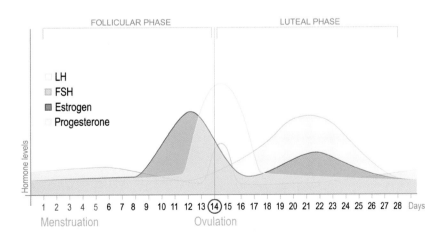

As you can see, there's a lot going on here, with multiple hormone fluctuations dependent upon other hormone fluctuations. The menstrual cycle is a complex dance of hormones and if one (or more) of these hormones is deficient for any reason, it can be thrown off, causing your periods to become irregular.

Ovulation is required for you to have a period. If you are not ovulating or are ovulating erratically, you will not have a true period. Figuring out why you are not ovulating is key to getting your periods back.

Symptoms

- going longer than 35 days without a period
- having fewer than nine periods in a year
- menstrual cycles that are irregular with unpredictable flow
- unusually light flow

Causes

- estrogen dominance
- low estrogen and/or low progesterone
- stress (In order to make enough cortisol to support the body's stress response, pregnenolone is diverted or "stolen away" from progesterone production to make cortisol. When this happens, you're producing so much cortisol to deal with a stressful situation that you have insufficient progesterone to support ovulation.)
- poor sleep and shift work (These situations interfere with the production and release of melatonin, the hormone that prompts sleep as well as plays a role in your menstrual cycle. Melatonin is anti-estrogenic and low melatonin can disrupt ovulation.)

- PCOS (polycystic ovarian syndrome)
- insulin resistance
- high testosterone
- ceasing hormonal birth control (It can take a few months for your hormones to return to normal when you stop taking hormonal birth control. Post-pill amenorrhea is when your period has not returned three months after stopping birth control.)
- toxin or radiation exposure
- over- or underactive thyroid
- autoimmune disease (such as celiac or Hashimoto's)
- anemia (B_{12} or iron deficiency)
- anorexia or bulimia, low-fat diet, and/or low nutrient intake stresses your body, prompting it to shut down all nonessential systems, like the reproductive
- overexercising (It's stressful to the body.)
- obesity
- hypothalamus dysfunction impacting your pituitary gland and hormone release
- adrenal tumor
- pituitary tumor or dysfunction
- elevated prolactin (most often due to pituitary tumor)

Traditional Treatments

- Birth control pills and synthetic estrogen or progestin hormone replacement therapy

These are the most common first-line treatments for missing or irregular periods. The problem is synthetic hormone replacement therapy doesn't address root causes and can cause a range of serious side effects. This is why I recommend trying natural options first and if necessary, explore bioidentical hormone replacement options with your healthcare provider.

Irregular Periods Protocol

Step 1. Do the 28-Day Estrogen Reset Foundation Protocol, including the Foundational Supplements. See Part IV for everything you need to do it successfully. After doing the Foundation Protocol, you may not even need to implement Step 2, but if you feel you've mastered it and need to go deeper to regulate your cycles, read on.

Step 2: Implement the Irregular Periods Protocol.

Implement as much of the following as you can. Some things may help and others won't. Everyone is different and will respond to changes in varied ways.

Get quality sleep. Prioritizing sleep can be transformative when it comes to regulating your cycle by building up your levels of melatonin. If you haven't started practicing good sleep hygiene habits as part of your Foundation Protocol (switch off the electronics before bed, keeping your bedroom dark and cool, along with others), start doing so now. See page 150 for how to improve your sleep.

Try seed rotation. Seed rotation is a technique to balance estrogen and progesterone levels by boosting estrogen levels in the first part of your cycle and progesterone levels in the second part. Rebalancing your cycle using this simple food-based technique can help regulate your cycle.

Over the course of your period, you will incorporate one of the following two seed combinations into your diet and then switch, alternating seed combinations depending on where you are in your cycle. Add these seeds to salads, smoothies, or a glass of water.

Seed combination #1, to boost estrogen: 1 tablespoon of freshly ground flax seed (do not use the preground flax meal, it has little potency) and 1 tablespoon of freshly ground pumpkin seeds.

Seed combination #2, to boost progesterone: 1 tablespoon of freshly ground sesame seeds and 1 tablespoon of freshly ground sunflower seeds.

If you are menstruating but your cycle is irregular

On day one of your period, start seed combination #1, to boost estrogen.

On day 14, around ovulation, switch to seed combination #2, to boost progesterone.

What if your cycle doesn't last 28 days? You'll always start seed combination #1 to boost estrogen on day one of your period and switch to seed combination #2 to boost progesterone at roughly the midway point of your current cycle. In a normal cycle, the midway point is day 14. Right now, your midway point may be day seven or day 19. Your cycle might be shorter or longer for now, but over time it will regulate as you continue to seed cycle and follow the Foundation Protocol along with the Irregular Period Protocol Add-On recommendations. Seed rotation may be a little harder to do when your periods are erratic. The bottom line: Go back to seed combination #1 the moment you get your period in the form of full bleeding (spotting doesn't count).

Seed rotation is yet another tool in the toolbox—it may work very well for you. If it doesn't, try the other suggestions in this chapter.

Add topical progesterone. If you haven't already started using topical progesterone as part of the Foundation Protocol, now is the time. Applying progesterone topically can raise progesterone levels so there's enough to balance out estrogen and create the right hormonal environment for a regular period. It also improves sleep, promotes a calmer, boosts your mood, raises your libido, regulates your cycle for more predictable periods, builds bones, converts fat to energy, and lowers your risk of developing estrogenic breast cancer. To restore your period, start progesterone 14 days after the first day of your period and stop it when your period starts.

Try castor oil packs to support liver detoxification, clear out "dirty" estrogens, and reduce inflammation. If you haven't already tried castor oil packs, now is a good time to begin. For more on the benefits and how to apply a pack, see page 153.

Implement herbal strategies. Work with a local herbalist to create an herbal formula that combines several different strategies: emmenagogues (to bring blood supply to the uterus), hormone modulators, adaptogens and nervines, and PCOS support. These herbs support the following strategies:

Emmenagogues (bring blood supply to the uterus)

- dong quai
- mugwort
- motherwort
- ginger

Hormone modulators

- chasteberry (vitex)
- dong quai
- licorice

Adaptogens and nervines (especially if stress rules your life)

- ashwagandha
- schisandra
- rhodiola
- eleuthero
- skullcap
- milky oats
- passionflower

PCOS

- chasteberry (vitex)
- peony
- licorice

Take the DUTCH test. Testing is a good idea to establish a baseline before you begin any protocol. It's also helpful if you've been doing the Foundation and Irregular Periods Add-On Protocol for three to four months and your period has not become more regular. I suggest DUTCH testing every three to six months while on this Add-On Protocol to assess your estrogen metabolites, cortisol, and melatonin (and a few others) levels to help determine where you may need extra support.

Consider saliva testing. I recommend saliva testing to check your progesterone levels. Progesterone cannot be measured in urine (DUTCH will only show you an approximation). Saliva is a great medium to understand your progesterone levels. Unfortunately, saliva testing won't show estrogen metabolites. At the time of writing this book, there is no provider offering both urine and saliva screening in one test. For providers and periodically updated information, see Recommended Labs on page 362.

OVERCOMING ESTROGEN DOMINANCE

Dong Quai
ANGELICA SINENSIS

Chapter 15

Dysmenorrhea and PMS Protocol

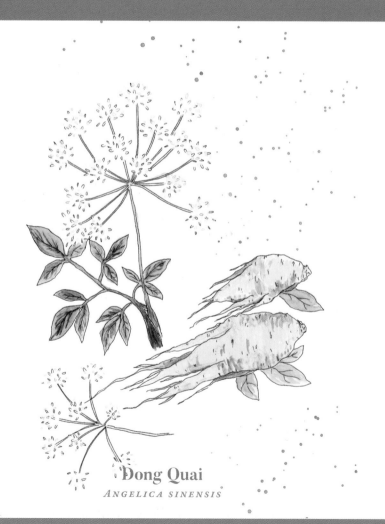

Dong Quai

ANGELICA SINENSIS

Dysmenorrhea, period pain, and PMS are not a given with every woman. That's right: Your period can be an uneventful occurrence. Our culture has led us to believe menstrual periods are unbearable and miserable, a time to be dreaded. Getting your period means canceling appointments and putting fun activities on hold, right? Wrong. Your period can be a gentle event, with most of the day passing without you affording it too much thought.

Key Facts

Dysmenorrhea is the medical term for pain occurring just before menstruation, marked by severe and frequent cramps. There are two types:

Primary: pain caused by cramping related to your period as your uterine muscles work to push menstrual blood out.

Secondary: pain caused by another condition impacting the reproductive organs, such as endometriosis, fibroids, or pelvic inflammatory disease (PID).

Premenstrual syndrome (PMS) refers to dozens of potential symptoms impacting a woman's physical and emotional health in the five to ten days leading up to your period. PMS can affect 80% of women to various degrees and about 5 to 10% of women say it is debilitating.

Symptoms

- pain (lower back and lower abdomen)
- anxiety
- depression
- tension and feeling edgy
- irritability and anger
- mood swings
- insomnia
- suicidal thoughts
- low self-esteem and self-doubt
- higher sensitivity to adversity
- feeling overwhelmed
- vomiting
- craving carbs ("comfort food") and sugar
- weight gain (through water retention)

Severe menstrual pain that compromises your daily life may indicate secondary dysmenorrhea or an infection. In this case, it's time to speak with your gynecologist or healthcare provider. Symptoms to look out for include:

- at least three painful periods
- passing blood clots
- cramping accompanied by diarrhea and nausea
- pelvic pain when not menstruating
- infection, fever, sudden and severe pelvic pain, or foul-smelling vaginal discharge

Diagnosis

A pelvic exam is the first step to determine if secondary dysmenorrhea and an underlying medical condition affecting your reproductive or pelvic organs is causing your pain. They may also order these diagnostic tests:

- ultrasound
- CT scan
- MRI
- laparoscopy

Causes

- estrogen dominance (especially high estrogen, particularly estradiol, as compared to progesterone)
- low progesterone

- stress (In order to make enough cortisol to support the body's stress response, pregnenolone is diverted or "stolen away" from progesterone production to make cortisol. When this happens, you're producing so much cortisol to deal with a stressful situation that you have insufficient progesterone to balance out estrogen.)
- high TSH (thyroid stimulating hormone) or low thyroid function (hypothyroidism, a.k.a. Hashimoto's)
- high testosterone
- inflammation, caused by diet, food intolerances, alcohol, stress, and toxins, among many other sources that feed inflammation
- synthetic hormones, such as estrogen and progestins
- high caffeine consumption (not a cause but will certainly make cramps and PMS worse)

Traditional Treatments

For Primary Dysmenorrhea

- painkillers
- antidepressants, for the mood swings associated with PMS
- birth control pills; synthetic estrogen or progestin hormone replacement therapy
- hysterectomy, in rare, very severe cases

For Secondary Dysmenorrhea

- Treatment options will depend on the underlying cause of your pain.

The most common first-line treatments for period pain don't address the root causes, including estrogen dominance and inflammation. Synthetic hormone replacement therapy can cause a range of serious side effects. That's why I recommend trying natural options.

The Dysmenorrhea and PMS Add-On Protocol

Step 1. Do the 28-Day Estrogen Reset Foundation Protocol, including the Foundational Supplements. See Part IV for everything you need to do it successfully. After doing the Foundation Protocol, you may not even need to implement Step 2, but if you feel you've mastered it and need to go deeper to address your period pain and PMS, read on.

Remember to see your doctor if you have any of the symptoms of secondary dysmenorrhea or suspect infection, endometriosis, fibroids, PID, or another underlying medical condition is the source of your pain.

Step 2: Implement the Dysmenorrhea and PMS Protocol.

Implement as much of the following as you can. Some things may help and others won't. Everyone is different and will respond to changes in varied ways.

Try seed rotation. Seed rotation is a technique to balance estrogen and progesterone levels throughout the month by boosting estrogen levels in the first part of your cycle and progesterone levels in the second part. Rebalancing your cycle using this simple food-based technique can help alleviate period pain and PMS in as little as one or two months.

You will incorporate one of the following two seed combinations into your diet and then switch, alternating seed combinations. Add these seeds to salads, smoothies, or a glass of water.

Seed combination #1, to boost estrogen: 1 tablespoon of freshly ground flax seed (do not use the pre-ground flax meal, it has little potency) and 1 tablespoon of freshly ground pumpkin seeds.

Seed combination #2, to boost progesterone: 1 tablespoon of freshly ground sesame seeds and 1 tablespoon of freshly ground sunflower seeds.

In the Follicular Phase of your cycle (days 1 to 13): Add Seed combination #1, to boost estrogen.

In the Luteal Phase (days 14 to 28): Add Seed combination #2, to boost progesterone.

Try essential oils in this PMS Salve. I've formulated the PMS Salve (see page 350 for the recipe) that acts as an anti-inflammatory, painkiller, and relaxer for the uterus. By using castor oil, you will benefit from deep penetration of this salve. I personally use it each time I get dysmenorrhea and find 70% of the pain eases within 30 minutes.

Add topical progesterone. If you haven't already started using topical progesterone as part of the Foundation Protocol, now is the time. I have found that applying progesterone topically is an absolutely wonderful solution for cramps and PMS. It also improves sleep, promotes a calmer, boosts your mood, raises your libido, regulates your cycle for more predictable periods, builds bones, converts fat to energy, and lowers your risk of developing estrogenic breast cancer.

Lower inflammation. Inflammation is a primary driver of cramps and PMS. An anti-inflammatory diet and supplements that target inflammation, such as those containing curcumin, can help a great deal.

Add borage oil (internally), a potent anti-inflammatory and pain reliever. It contains 20 to 26% gamma-linoleic acid (GLA), a fatty acid that converts into prostaglandins PgE1 and PgE3

(a natural painkiller) and suppresses PgE2 (the cause of the pain). The recommended dosage is 240 mg three to four times per day with meals, or as directed by your healthcare practitioner.

Try castor oil packs to support liver detoxification, clear out "dirty" estrogens, and reduce inflammation. If you haven't already tried castor oil packs, now is a good time to begin. For more on their benefits and how to apply a pack, see page 150. Use a compress large enough to cover your uterus and liver and be sure to apply it seven days before your period starts. You can add the PMS salve (page 350) to your castor oil packs for more support.

Implement herbal strategies. Work with a local herbalist to create an herbal formula that combines several different strategies: hormone modulators, liver support, analgesics (to relieve pain), as well as adaptogens and nervines (to promote calm). These herbs support the following strategies:

Hormone modulators

- chasteberry (vitex)
- dong quai
- ginger
- black cohosh

Liver support

- dandelion
- burdock

Analgesics

- cramp bark
- corydalis (headaches)
- kava kava (anxiety, stress, restlessness)

Adaptogens and nervines (especially if you have a lot of stress)

- ashwagandha
- schisandra
- rhodiola
- eleuthero
- skullcap
- milky oats
- passionflower

Take the DUTCH test. Testing is a good idea to establish a baseline before you begin any protocol. It's also helpful if you've been doing the Foundation and Dysmenorrhea and PMS Add-On Protocol for three to four months and your cramps and PMS aren't improving. I suggest DUTCH testing every three to six months while on this Add-On Protocol to assess your levels of estrogen metabolites, cortisol, and melatonin (and others) to help determine where you may need extra support.

Consider saliva testing. I recommend saliva testing to check your progesterone levels. Progesterone cannot be measured in urine (DUTCH will only show you an approximation). Saliva is a great medium to understand your progesterone levels. Unfortunately, saliva testing won't show estrogen metabolites. At the time of writing this book, there is no provider offering both urine and saliva screening in one test. For providers and periodically updated information, see Recommended Labs on page 362.

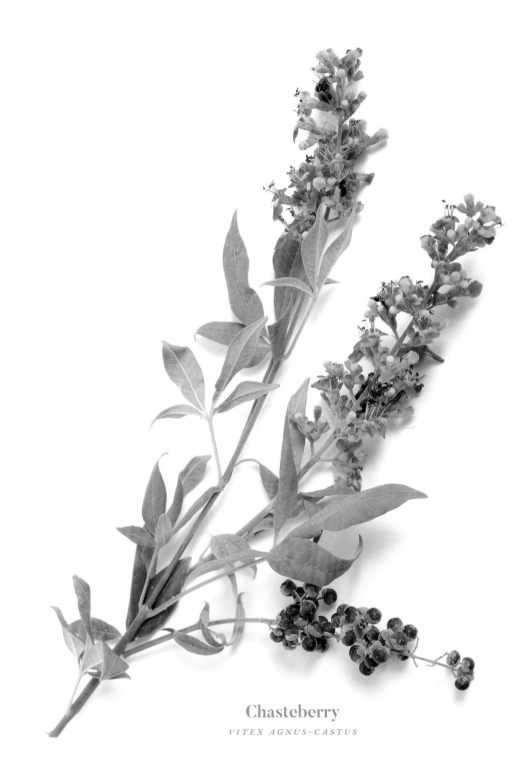

Chasteberry
VITEX AGNUS-CASTUS

Chapter 16

Menorrhagia (Heavy Period) Protocol

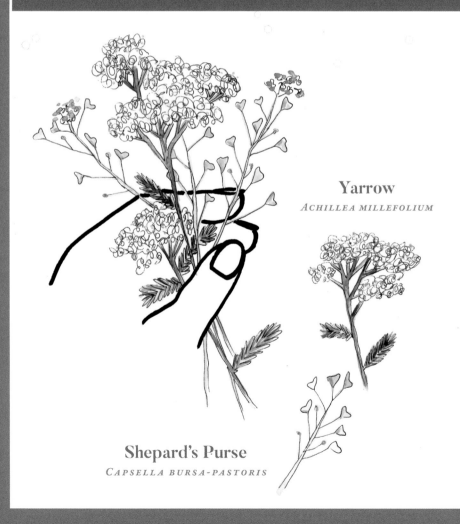

Yarrow
ACHILLEA MILLEFOLIUM

Shepard's Purse
CAPSELLA BURSA-PASTORIS

You should not live in fear of your period each month. If you are struggling with a heavy, extended flow that is depleting and keeping you from your daily activities, I want you to know it doesn't have to be this way. You can fix it.

Key Facts

Menorrhagia ("menstrual burst") is the medical term for abnormally heavy or prolonged flow during your period. It affects about 25% of women, most often at the beginning and end of their reproductive years. During these times, ovulation is often irregular, resulting in erratic progesterone levels.

"Heavy" means your flow lasts for more than seven days and you lose about 80 mg of blood, the equivalent of 16 fully soaked regular tampons or eight super tampons, throughout your cycle. If that doesn't seem like a lot (remember, those amounts are for the entirety of your cycle, not one day) consider most of us don't wait for a tampon to become fully soaked before changing it.

There are two types of menorrhagia

Primary: Caused by unidentifiable factors or disturbances in the release of prostaglandins, hormone-like substances that cause the uterus to contract.

Secondary: Related to identifiable clinical causes, such as fibroids, uterine polyps, or miscarriage.

Symptoms

- period lasting more than seven days
- going through 16 fully soaked regular tampons or eight super tampons over the course of one cycle

- soaking through one or more regular tampons every hour for several consecutive hours
- needing to wake up during the night to change your pad or tampon
- flow with blood clots larger than a quarter
- symptoms or diagnosis of anemia (iron-deficiency), such as tiredness, fatigue, or shortness of breath

Speak to your healthcare provider immediately if you experience any of these symptoms:

- bleeding so heavy it soaks at least one regular tampon an hour for more than two hours
- bleeding between periods or irregular vaginal bleeding
- any vaginal bleeding after menopause
- infection, including fever, sudden and severe pelvic pain, or foul-smelling vaginal discharge

Diagnosis

If you are experiencing symptoms of menorrhagia, see your doctor for a pelvic exam to rule out infections, miscarriage, fibroids, a clotting disorder, or another medical condition causing your heavy flow. They may also order these diagnostic tests:

- blood tests
- pap test
- biopsy
- ultrasound

Causes

- estrogen dominance (especially high estrogen, particularly estradiol, as compared to progesterone)

- low progesterone
- stress (In order to make enough cortisol to support the body's stress response, pregnenolone is diverted or "stolen away" from progesterone production to make cortisol. When this happens, you're producing so much cortisol to deal with a stressful situation that you have insufficient progesterone to balance estrogen.)
- high TSH (thyroid stimulating hormone), or low thyroid function (hypothyroidism, a.k.a. Hashimoto's)
- inflammation, caused by diet, food intolerances, alcohol, stress, and toxins, among many other sources that feed inflammation
- low iron (a cause and a result)
- uterine fibroids, polyps, adenomyosis
- medications, including anti-inflammatories and anticoagulants such as warfarin
- synthetic hormones, such as estrogen and progestins
- IUD

Traditional Treatments

- IUD
- birth control pills
- hysterectomy
- ibuprofen, an anti-inflammatory, reduces prostaglandins; 200 mg per day can reduce the flow by half but negatively impacts the liver and kidneys. It is an acceptable temporary solution.

These are the most common first-line treatments for heavy periods. The problem is none of them address the root causes and all come with a range of serious side effects. That's why I recommend trying natural options first.

Menorrhagia (Heavy Period) Protocol

Step 1. Do the 28-Day Estrogen Reset Foundation Protocol, including the Foundational Supplements. See Part IV for everything you need to do it successfully. After doing the Foundation Protocol, you may not even need to implement Step 2, but if you feel you've mastered it and haven't moderated your flow yet, read on.

Remember to first see your doctor to rule out an underlying medical condition as the source of your heavy flow.

Step 2: Implement the Menorrhagia (Heavy Period) Protocol.

Implement as much of the following as you can. Some things may help and others won't. Everyone is different and will respond to changes in varied ways.

Replenish iron levels, if low.

Symptoms of low iron:

- anemia, pallor (paleness), fatigue
- cold intolerance
- impaired cognition and behavior disturbances
- decreased productivity and work performance
- decreased immunity and resistance to infection
- sore tongue
- chewing on ice, paper, or clay
- advanced: thin, flat, or spoon-shaped nails

To replenish your iron levels with food, you'll need to eat iron in heme form (the highest bioavailable form) and it is only found in animal sources, especially in liver (chicken, veal, and pork). Vegetables are a source of non-heme iron, but it isn't highly absorbable by the human body.

To replenish your iron levels with supplements, proceed with care. Iron pills can be constipating, and constipation will just make your estrogen dominance even worse. Check out the Supplement Guide on page 361 for my recommended heme and non-heme iron brands.

Try seed rotation. Seed rotation is a technique to balance estrogen and progesterone levels by boosting estrogen levels in the first part of your cycle and progesterone levels in the second part.

For two weeks, you will incorporate one of the following two seed combinations into your diet and then switch, alternating seed combinations every two weeks. Add these seeds to salads, smoothies, or a glass of water.

Seed combination #1, to boost estrogen: 1 tablespoon of freshly ground flax seed (do not use the pre-ground flax meal, it has little potency) and 1 tablespoon of freshly ground pumpkin seeds.

Seed combination #2, to boost progesterone: 1 tablespoon of freshly ground sesame seeds and 1 tablespoon of freshly ground sunflower seeds.

What seeds to use when

In the Follicular Phase of your cycle (days 1 to 13): Add Seed combination #1, to boost estrogen

In the Luteal Phase (days 14 to 28): Add Seed combination #2, to boost progesterone.

Add topical progesterone. If you haven't already started using topical progesterone as part of the Foundation Protocol, now is the time. Applying progesterone topically can raise progesterone levels so there's enough to balance out estrogen and create the right hormonal environment for a normal flow. It also improves sleep, promotes a calmer, boosts your mood, raises your libido, regulates your cycle for more predictable periods, builds bones, converts fat to energy, and lowers your risk of developing estrogenic breast cancer.

Implement herbal strategies. Work with a local herbalist to create an herbal formula that combines several different strategies: astringents (to minimize blood supply to the uterus) and uterine tonics, hormone modulators, adaptogens and nervines. These herbs support the following strategies:

Astringents and uterine tonics

- yarrow
- witch hazel leaf
- stone root
- shepherd's purse herb
- partridgeberry herb
- cypress tip

Hormone modulators

- chasteberry (vitex)
- dong quai
- ginger

Adaptogens and nervines (especially with a lot of stress)

- ashwagandha
- schisandra
- rhodiola
- eleuthero
- skullcap, milky oats, passionflower

Take the DUTCH test. Testing is a good idea to establish a baseline before you begin any protocol. It's also helpful if you've been doing the Foundation and Menorrhagia (Heavy Period) Add-On Protocol for three to four months and your flow hasn't lessened. I suggest DUTCH testing every three to six months while on this Add-On Protocol to assess your levels of estrogen metabolites, cortisol, and melatonin (and others) to help determine where you may need extra support.

Consider saliva testing. I recommend saliva testing to check your progesterone levels. Progesterone cannot be measured in urine (DUTCH will only show you an approximation). Saliva is a great medium to understand your progesterone levels. Unfortunately, saliva testing won't show estrogen metabolites. At the time of writing this book, there is no provider offering both urine and saliva screening in one test. For providers and periodically updated information, see Recommended Labs on page 362.

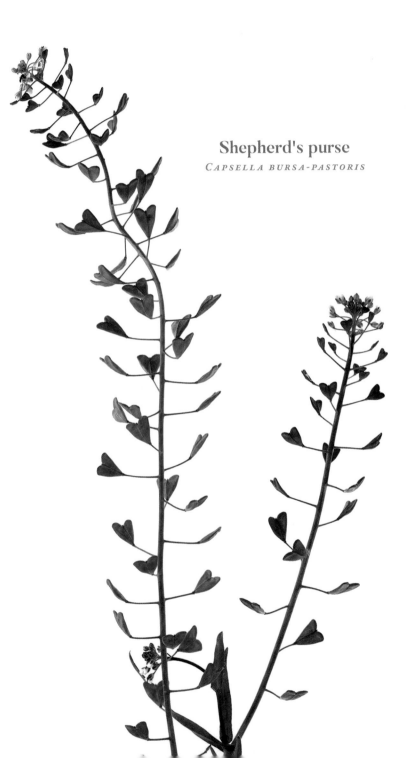

Shepherd's purse

CAPSELLA BURSA-PASTORIS

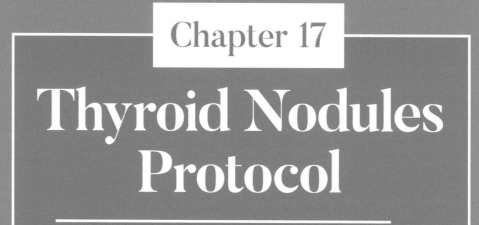

Chapter 17

Thyroid Nodules Protocol

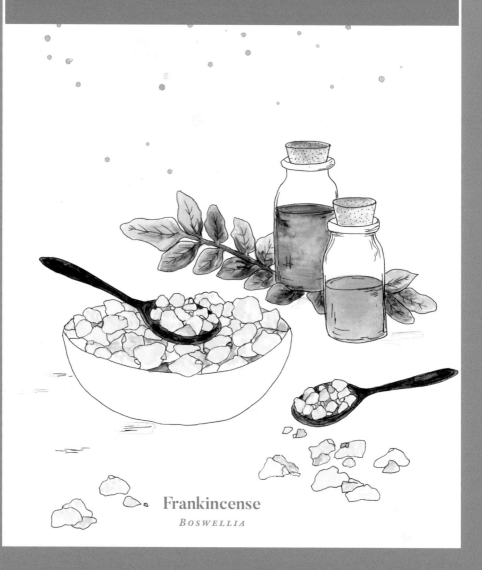

Frankincense

BOSWELLIA

This is a topic very close to me because I discovered three thyroid nodules about nine years ago that have since completely disappeared. So it is completely possible to eliminate them. Even if your thyroid nodules are small or benign, I encourage you to address them. Your doctor may have suggested a "wait-and-see" approach, but thyroid nodules are not okay. They indicate a hormone imbalance, such as estrogen dominance and high toxicity, among other damaging issues that need to be addressed for you to function at your best. Thyroid nodules won't go away on their own, but you can make them disappear by implementing the below protocol.

Key Facts

Your thyroid is a small butterfly-shaped endocrine gland located in the front of your neck. It produces hormones that regulate your metabolism, including your heart rate and body temperature, along with almost every other bodily process. Every human cell has thyroid hormone receptors so your entire body, from your brain and heart to your immune and digestive systems, requires thyroid hormone to function optimally.

The thyroid is believed to be the "sponge for toxins." This makes it vulnerable to nodules. People, especially women, who live near highly polluted or radioactive areas, tend to have a higher incidence of thyroid nodules and cancers.

A thyroid nodule is a lump in your thyroid gland. It can be a solid growth of thyroid tissue or a cyst filled with fluid. They can develop singly or in clusters, can be benign or malignant, though most are noncancerous.

Thyroid nodules are classified according to whether or not they produce thyroid hormone.

Cold nodules do not produce thyroid hormones.

Warm nodules act as normal thyroid cells.

Hot nodules overproduce thyroid hormones, causing hyperthyroidism.

In some cases, thyroid nodules develop in people with Hashimoto's disease. This autoimmune condition results in an underactive thyroid, or hypothyroidism.

Do not ignore thyroid nodules. Even if benign, they are not harmless. They can be an indication of estrogen dominance, which left untreated can lead to lumpy breasts, terrible PMS, and all of the other symptoms of this imbalance plus more serious concerns, such as breast and thyroid cancer. They may also indicate high toxicity in your life coming from food, skincare, cleaning products, air, water, and the environment. These issues should not be ignored. Thyroid nodules are your body's way of telling you it's struggling with toxicity. Nodules will not go away on their own but with the right approach, you can completely dissolve them.

Symptoms

- enlarged thyroid gland, known as a goiter
- pain at the base of your neck
- difficulty swallowing
- difficulty breathing
- hoarse voice

If you have a "hot" thyroid nodule producing excess thyroid hormones, you may experience symptoms of hyperthyroidism, an overactive thyroid. These include:

- fatigue or muscle weakness
- mood swings

This is a topic very close to me because I discovered three thyroid nodules about nine years ago that have since completely disappeared.

- nervousness or anxiety
- rapid or irregular heartbeat
- sweaty palms or excessive sweating
- trouble sleeping
- weight loss

Diagnosis

Many thyroid nodules go undetected because they are too small to cause symptoms. A doctor may be able to feel them during a routine physical exam or they may be discovered after an imaging procedure, such as a CT or MRI scan, to investigate another health concern.

If you suspect a nodule or have thyroid problems, I recommend seeing your doctor and insisting on a physical examination or sonogram. If your doctor suspects a thyroid nodule, they will probably refer you to an endocrinologist, an endocrine specialist who may order the following diagnostic tests:

- thyroid ultrasound
- thyroid CT scan
- fine-needle aspiration (to collect a sample of the nodule)
- blood tests (to check your hormone levels)

Causes

- estrogen dominance(especially excess "dirty" estrogens)
- low progesterone
- magnesium deficiency

- toxicity (from food, skincare, cleaning products, or the environment)
- inflammation, caused by diet, food intolerances, alcohol, stress, and toxins, especially dioxide (among many other sources that feed inflammation)
- stress (In order to make enough cortisol to support the body's stress response, pregnenolone is diverted or "stolen away" from progesterone production to make cortisol. When this happens, you're producing so much cortisol to deal with a stressful situation you have insufficient progesterone to balance out estrogen.)
- too much coffee and alcohol (not a cause, but will certainly contribute to the growth of thyroid nodules)

Traditional Treatments

- "wait and see" (if asymptomatic)
- partial or full thyroidectomy

These are the most common first-line treatment for thyroid nodules. The problem is they don't address the root causes of the problem: estrogen dominance, inflammation, and high toxicity.

Thyroid Nodules Protocol

Step 1. Do the 28-Day Estrogen Reset Foundation Protocol, including the Foundational

Supplements. See Part IV for everything you need to do it successfully. After doing the Foundation Protocol, you may not even need to implement Step 2, but if you feel you've mastered it and need to go deeper to address your thyroid nodules, read on.

Step 2: Implement the Thyroid Nodules Protocol.

Implement as much of the following as you can. Some things may help and others won't. Everyone is different and will respond to changes in varied ways.

Lower inflammation. Inflammation is a primary driver of thyroid nodules. An anti-inflammatory diet and supplements that target inflammation, such as those containing curcumin, can help a great deal.

Try castor oil packs, wrapped around your neck, to support liver detoxification, clear out "dirty" estrogens, and reduce inflammation. If you haven't already tried castor oil packs, now is a good time to begin. For more on their benefits and how to apply a pack, see page 153. Add essential oils, such as the Essential Thyroid Support Blend, for more support.

Apply essential oils topically. Many women in the Hormone Balance community have reported that applying essential oils has helped them shrink thyroid nodules and support the thyroid. Frankincense essential oil has anti-inflammatory, immune-boosting, and pain-relieving properties. Dilute it with a carrier oil such as jojoba, sweet almond, or fractionated coconut oil before applying to the skin over the thyroid or try the Essential Oil Thyroid Support Blend.

Implement herbal strategies. Work with a local herbalist to create an herbal formula that focuses

ESSENTIAL OIL THYROID SUPPORT BLEND

Courtesy of Dr. Mariza Snyder, author of *The Essential Oils Hormone Solution*

- 2 drops frankincense essential oil

- 1 drop lavender essential oil

- 1 drop chamomile essential oil

- 1 drop rose geranium essential oil

- 2 teaspoons jojoba, sweet almond, or fractionated coconut oil

Apply topically to the skin over the thyroid. Can be massaged into the skin before applying a castor oil pack.

on bringing the inflammation down. These herbs might be helpful:

Anti-inflammatories

- boswellia
- curcumin
- white willow bark

Take the DUTCH test. Testing is a good idea to establish a baseline before you begin any protocol. It's also helpful if you've been doing the Foundation and Thyroid Nodules Add-On Protocol for three to four months and your nodules haven't shrunk. I suggest DUTCH testing every three to six months while on this Add-On Protocol to assess your levels of estrogen metabolites, cortisol, and melatonin (and others) to help determine where you may need extra support.

Chapter 18

Infertility and Miscarriages Protocol

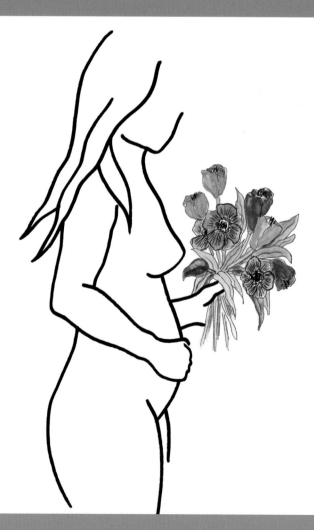

Infertility and miscarriage are Mother Nature's way of protecting us from unhealthy, problematic, dangerous pregnancies, or a health-compromised child. That said, infertility may result from an issue with either you, your partner, or it may be the result of a combination of factors. There is nothing simple about infertility or miscarriage. The number of people grappling with fertility issues speaks to that: one in five couples in North America. Knowing the causes is key to becoming pregnant and carrying to term.

Key Facts

Infertility is often defined as the inability to get pregnant despite having frequent, unprotected sex for at least a year. One in five couples in North America have fertility issues. In some infertile couples, no specific cause is found, which is known as unexplained infertility.

Female fertility relies on ovulation, the release of a viable egg from the ovaries. The reproductive tract must be clear, allowing the egg to pass into the fallopian tubes and join with sperm for fertilization. From there, the fertilized egg must be able to travel to the uterus and safely implant in the uterine lining, or the endometrium.

Miscarriage is the spontaneous loss of a pregnancy before the 20th week. Some women have a miscarriage before they even know they're pregnant.

Having two or more miscarriages in a row is known as having repeat miscarriages or recurrent pregnancy loss. Most women who have repeat miscarriages have an unknown cause and of those, most go on to have a successful pregnancy.

Symptoms

Of Infertility

- an inability to get pregnant
- in some cases, irregular or absent menstrual periods

Of Miscarriage

- vaginal spotting or bleeding
- pain or cramping in your abdomen or lower back
- severe stomach pain
- fluid or tissue passing from your vagina

Diagnosis

Of Infertility

A general physical exam and gynecological exam are the first steps. Before extensive infertility testing, your doctor would want to know your current sexual habits in order to make recommendations to improve your chances of getting pregnant. Infertility tests for women may include:

- ovulation testing
- hysterosalpingography, to evaluate the condition of your uterus and fallopian tubes
- ovarian reserve testing
- pelvic ultrasound
- laparoscopy

Of Miscarriage

- pelvic exam
- ultrasound
- blood tests
- tissue tests

Causes

Of Infertility

- hormonal imbalance, such as:

    - low thyroid, Hashimoto's
    - PCOS (high testosterone, insulin resistance)
    - estrogen dominance
    - low progesterone
    - low estrogen
    - high prolactin (a hormone produced by the pituitary gland with a role in lactation; high levels are often the result of a tumor in the pituitary)

- Ovulation is not happening. This can be checked by:

    - tracking your Basal Body Temperature (BBT)
    - an ultrasound of the ovaries at ovulation
    - testing LH levels
    - testing progesterone levels
    - a uterine biopsy

- Fallopian tubes are blocked due to:

    - infections
    - congenital abnormality
    - previous ectopic pregnancy
    - endometriosis
    - uterine fibroids
    - surgery
    - ruptured appendix

- Cervical mucus is unfriendly to sperm. Some women produce antibodies that work against their partner's sperm.
- emotional factors, such as:

    - past trauma
    - fear and hesitations

Of Miscarriage

- hormonal imbalance (25 to 50% of miscarriages), such as:

    - low thyroid
    - high testosterone combined with insulin resistance (as in PCOS)
    - estrogen dominance
    - low progesterone
    - high LH

- abnormalities, such as:

    - chromosomal issues (eggs, sperm)
    - abnormal placenta, uterus, or cervix; adhesions

- systemic issues, such as:

    - cardiovascular issues
    - inflammation
    - autoimmunity
    - diabetes
    - kidney disease
    - lupus

Traditional Treatments

For Infertility

Treatment will vary depending on the cause of the infertility (if it has been identified), your age, and your personal preference. If spontaneous pregnancy doesn't happen, you may be able to get pregnant through the use of assisted reproductive technology, such as in vitro fertilization (IVF).

Infertility and Miscarriages Add-On Protocol

Step 1. Do the 28-Day Estrogen Reset Foundation Protocol, including the Foundational Supplements. See Part IV for everything you need to do it successfully. After doing the Foundation Protocol, you may not even need to implement Step 2, but if you feel you've mastered it and need to go deeper to address your fertility issues, read on.

Step 2. Implement the Infertility and Miscarriages Protocol.

First, I recommend everyone take the DUTCH test. I suggest DUTCH testing before you begin to assess your levels of estrogen metabolites and progesterone. This will provide a comprehensive map of what's going on with your hormones. Recheck after three months on this protocol to determine where you may need extra support.

Also consider saliva testing. I recommend saliva testing to check your progesterone levels. Progesterone cannot be measured in urine (DUTCH will only show you an approximation). Saliva is a great medium to understand your progesterone levels. Unfortunately, saliva testing won't show estrogen metabolites. At the time of writing this book, there is no provider offering both urine and saliva screening in one test. For providers and periodically updated information, see Recommended Labs on page 362.

Next, determine the best step for you based on the underlying cause of your infertility or miscarriages.

- If estrogen dominance and/or low progesterone is suspected, follow the Amenorrhea (Absent Periods) Protocol.
- If endometriosis is the underlying cause, follow the Endometriosis Protocol.
- If high testosterone is the underlying cause, follow the High Testosterone (PCOS) Protocol.
- If you are not ovulating, follow the Amenorrhea (Absent Periods) Protocol.
- If your fallopian tubes are blocked, try castor oil packs. Castor oil packs reduce inflammation, support liver detoxification, and clear out "dirty" estrogens. If you haven't already tried castor oil packs, now is a good time to begin. For more on their benefits and how to apply a pack, see page 150. Use a compress large enough to cover your uterus, fallopian tubes, and liver.
- If you have low thyroid function or Hashimoto's, I recommend Dr. Izabella Wentz's books, such as *Hashimoto's Protocol* and *Hashimoto's Food Pharmacology,* for more targeted help.

For other causes of infertility and/or miscarriage, work with your trusted functional healthcare provider to determine the best way forward for you.

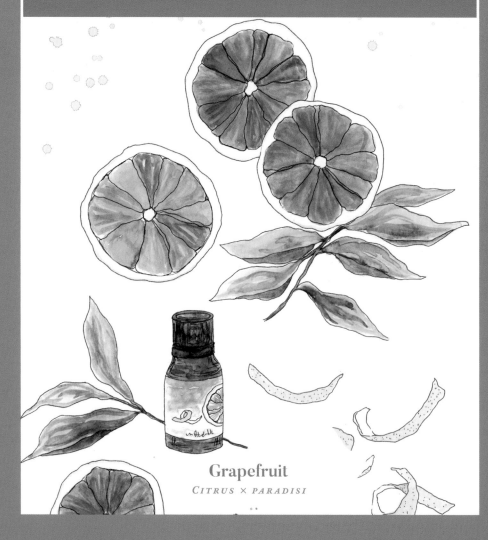

Chapter 19

Cellulite and Hip Fat Protocol

Grapefruit

CITRUS × PARADISI

Cellulite is most often the result of estrogen dominance, but it can also be due to high blood sugar levels. Remember the discussion about blood sugar balance in chapter 6? Excess sugar is converted to body fat. You may be tempted by those beautifully packaged anti-cellulite creams, but let me tell you, they don't work—no matter how expensive they are. Topical solutions may work for a few days, but then they stop working. For a lasting solution, heal the inside of the body instead of relying on topicals.

Key Facts

Cellulite is a fat deposit within the fibrous connective tissue that creates a puckered, lumpy, dimpled look to the skin. It is commonly found on the hips, thighs, buttocks, belly, upper arms, and breasts.

Some women are more predisposed to cellulite than others. Genes, body fat percentage, age, and skin thickness contribute to how much cellulite you have and how noticeable it is. People of all body types and weights can have cellulite.

Where we store fat and cellulite can be an indication of a hormonal imbalance. Women who are chronically stressed out with high blood sugar and insulin tend to have an apple shape. A pear shape indicates estrogen dominance.

Symptoms

- dimpled or bumpy skin, like the texture of cottage cheese or an orange peel, most commonly found on the hips, thighs, and buttocks and may also appear on the belly, upper arms, and breasts

Causes

- estrogen dominance
- high blood sugar levels
- high sugar consumption leading to increased fat storage
- systemic inflammation
- high toxicity

Traditional Treatments

- topical treatments, such as creams containing retinol (These may temporarily reduce the visibility of cellulite by tightening the skin, making it look smoother and firmer, but the fat cells remain. And retinol may cause allergic reactions, including dryness, redness, and peeling of the skin.)
- cryolipolysis (CoolSculpting)
- ultrasound
- laser and radiofrequency treatments

These are the most common first-line treatments for cellulite. The problem is none of them address the root causes and all come with a range of serious side effects. For long-lasting, healthy results, I recommend trying natural options.

Cellulite and Hip Fat Protocol

Step 1. Do the 28-Day Estrogen Reset Foundation Protocol, including the Foundational Supplements. See Part IV for everything you need to do it successfully. After doing the Foundation Protocol, you may not even need to implement Step 2, but if you feel you've mastered it and haven't seen a reduction in your cellulite and hip fat, read on.

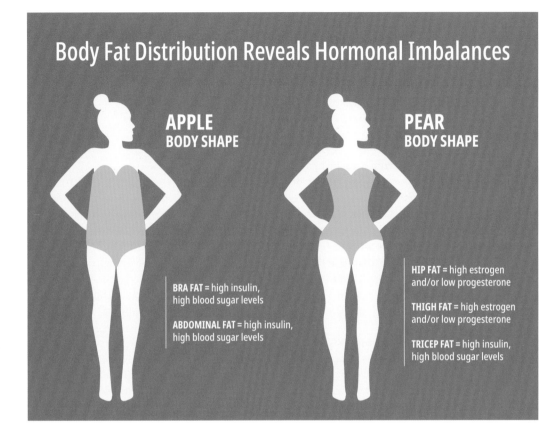

Body Fat Distribution Reveals Hormonal Imbalances

APPLE
BODY SHAPE

PEAR
BODY SHAPE

BRA FAT = high insulin, high blood sugar levels

ABDOMINAL FAT = high insulin, high blood sugar levels

HIP FAT = high estrogen and/or low progesterone

THIGH FAT = high estrogen and/or low progesterone

TRICEP FAT = high insulin, high blood sugar levels

Step 2: Implement the Cellulite and Hip Fat Protocol.

Implement as much of the following as you can. Some things may help and others won't. Everyone is different and will respond to changes in varied ways.

Make sure your blood sugar is balanced and, if necessary, take additional steps to get your blood sugar under control. Go back to chapter 6, Balance Your Blood Sugar, for a refresher on all of my recommendations for what you can do to keep your blood sugar in check, including supplement support.

Self-administer lymphatic massage (dry brushing), giving extra attention to areas with cellulite. Supporting lymphatic drainage and circulation is very beneficial, helping drain excess body fluid and increasing circulation while improving the appearance of cellulite. For more on the benefits and how to dry brush (it's very easy!), see page 154.

Apply essential oils topically. Many people in our community have reported positive results massaging with essential oils. The following essential oils are recommended:

- grapefruit
- cypress
- myrtle
- sage
- nutmeg
- geranium
- myrrh
- German chamomile

Add 10 drops of any of the essential oils listed above to a 10 ml glass bottle and top up with castor oil. I suggest castor oil because it penetrates deep into the tissue. (Never apply an essential oil directly to the skin.) Massage into the skin two to three times each week.

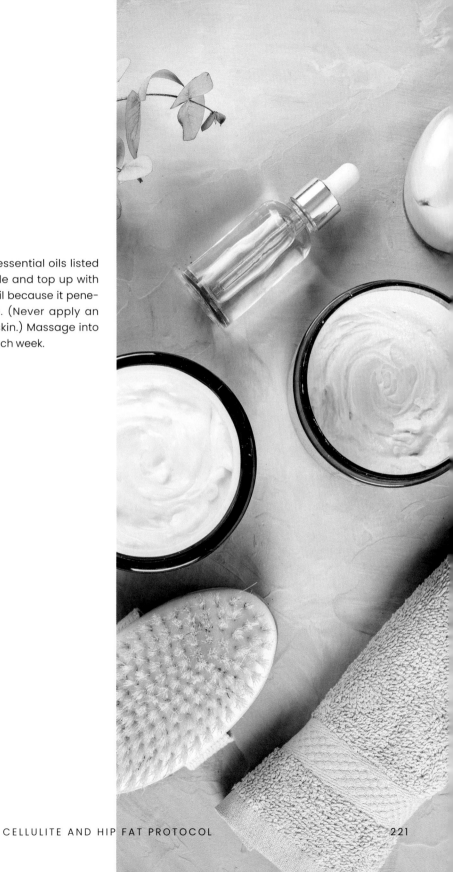

Chapter 20

Breast Cancer Protocol

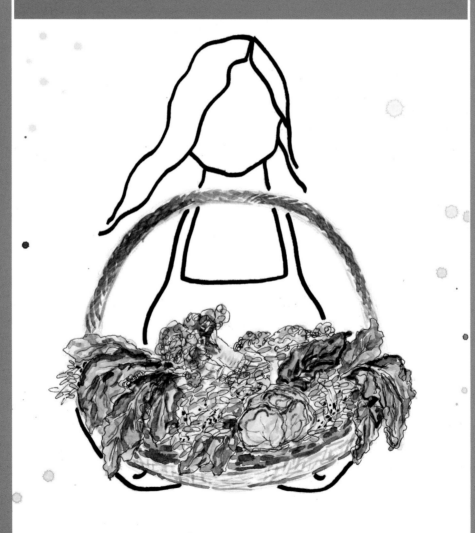

This protocol is for you if you are currently dealing with breast cancer, in remission, or interested in prevention. This is a topic very close to my heart because even though I have never had breast cancer, breast cancer and other estrogenic cancers run on both sides of my family. I've got all of the genetics that predispose me to being a statistic as well. Breast cancer is the leading cause of death in women ages 35 to 50. But as you know, genetics are only one piece to the puzzle. They do not dictate your health. By addressing estrogen dominance, we can help your body heal and lower your risk for these estrogenic cancers.

Key Facts

Breast cancer is a disease in which cells in the breast grows out of control, usually forming a tumor that can be seen on diagnostic tests or felt as a lump. There are two categories:

Noninvasive (in situ) cancer has not spread from the original tissue. This is stage 0.

Invasive (infiltrating) cancer has spread and is identified as stage 1, 2, 3, or 4, depending on the extent the cancer has been carried to other parts of the body.

Breast cancer can form in different types of tissue, influencing how the cancer behaves and the best course of treatment. Types of tissue include:

- the lining of the milk ducts, the most common source
- the lobules of the breast, where milk is produced
- the breast's connective tissue, very rare

Industrial development and "progress" play a role in breast cancer. Holland and the United States lead the world in the breast cancer epidemic, followed by Denmark, France, Australia, New Zealand, Belgium, Canada, and Sweden. In the United States one in seven and in Canada one in nine women will develop breast cancer. The lowest rates of breast cancer are found in most of the countries in Africa, Haiti, Mongolia, Korea, China, India, Costa Rica, and Japan.

Types of Breast Cancer

Cancer Cells Fueled by Hormones

Some breast cancers are sensitive to estrogen and progesterone thus have receptors for these hormones. These types include:

- **Estrogen receptor positive (ER+).** These breast cancer cells have receptors for estrogen that allow them to use this hormone to grow.
- **Progesterone receptor positive (PR+).** These breast cancer cells have receptors that allow them to use this hormone to grow.
- **Estrogen and progesterone receptor positive.** These breast cancers have receptors for both estrogen and progesterone.

Cancer Cells Fueled by Inherited Genetic Mutation

Certain inherited gene mutations increase the risk of breast cancer. In the United States, 5 to 10% of breast cancers are related to an inherited gene mutation. These include mutations to the following genes:

BRCA1 and BRCA2. Women who have a BRCA1 or BRCA2 gene mutation have an increased risk of breast cancer. BRCA1/2 mutations are thought to explain a large portion of hereditary breast cancers.

Women who have a BRCA1 mutation have an increased risk of triple negative breast cancer. These rare, very aggressive cancers are:

- estrogen receptor-negative (ER-)
- progesterone receptor-negative (PR-)
- HER2-negative (HER2-)

Cancer Cells Fueled by Somatic (Not Inherited) Genetic Mutation

Breast cancer can also be caused by gene mutations that are not inherited and develop after conception. These include mutations to the following gene:

- HER2. The Human epidermal growth factor receptor 2 (HER2) gene produces HER2 proteins that promote breast cell growth. If the HER2 gene is mutated, it causes an increase in the amount of HER2 proteins on the surface of the cells, causing cells to grow and divide out of control, potentially leading to cancer, called HER2-postive (HER2+).

Symptoms

- changes in the shape or appearance of the nipple
- an increase in size or change of shape of the breast
- nipple discharge from one breast that is clear, red, brown, or yellow
- general breast pain that doesn't go away after your next period
- a new lump on or inside the breast that doesn't go away after your next period
- skin changes, such as unexplained redness, swelling, itchiness, or rash, on the breast
- swelling or a lump around the collarbone or under the arm

It's important to remember other benign conditions may also cause these changes. Speaking with your doctor and seeking evaluation is the best way to determine if these changes are cause for concern.

Diagnosis

Visit your doctor if you are experiencing any of the symptoms of breast cancer or have breast cancer concerns. In addition to a physical exam with medical history, your doctor may also order these diagnostic tests:

- mammogram
- ultrasound
- MRI
- biopsy

Causes

- DNA changes caused by exposure to: chemicals, radiation, toxic compounds
- heavy metals
- EMF
- chronic inflammation, including from poor diet
- chronic stress and poor relationship with self
- nutritional deficiencies (a contributor rather than a cause)
- drugs, bacteria, viruses
- genetics (COMT, MAOA, VDR, MTHFR, CYP1A1, BRCA)
- poor gut microflora, estrobolome

What Drives Estrogen Receptor Positive (ER+) Breast Cancer

- Estrogen dominance caused by dropping progesterone, the estrogen-to-progesterone ratio (see chart below for a visual

MENOPAUSE HORMONE LEVELS

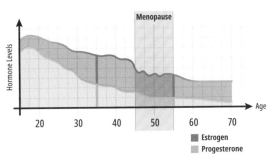

representation of how this disparity worsens with age and why older women are more prone to breast cancers), and estrogen being broken down into "dirty" estrogens
- How progesterone is broken down to "clean" and "dirty" metabolites (pregnene or pregnane formation)

Traditional Treatments

Treatment will depend on the type and stage of cancer, but some of the most common conventional practices associated with breast cancer include:

- lumpectomy
- mastectomy
- chemotherapy and the use of anticancer drugs
- radiation
- hormone and targeted therapy

I recommend combining conventional and natural treatments for the best results. Form a team that includes:

- an open-minded oncologist
- a naturopathic doctor
- a nutritionist (or use this program)
- an acupuncturist (a great add-on)

Breast Cancer Protocol

Step 1. Start with the 28-Day Estrogen Reset Foundation Protocol, including the Foundational Supplements. See Part IV for everything you need to do it successfully. After doing the Foundation Protocol, proceed to Step 2 to enhance your healing journey.

This protocol is designed to address cancers fueled by hormones. If you have or are concerned about any of the other types of breast cancer, speak with your healthcare provider about screening and treatment options.

Step 2: Implement the Breast Cancer Protocol.

Implement as much of the following as you can. Some things may help and others won't. Everyone is different and will respond to changes in varied ways.

Eat 1/2 to 1 cup of broccoli sprouts each day to support phase 1 and phase 2 liver detoxification, clear "dirty" estrogens, and fight cancer. Broccoli sprouts are rich in sulforaphane, an estrogen detoxification superstar. See the box on page 88 for how to triple the amount of sulforaphane in broccoli sprouts. Or consider adding it as a supplement.

Add an aromatase inhibitor such as chrysin or passionflower. Aromatase inhibitors lower estrogen levels by preventing the conversion of DHEA and testosterone into estrogen. They may be most beneficial to postmenopausal women with estrogenic breast cancer or those at high risk. The recommended dosage is 200 mg. Consult with your healthcare provider before taking one. There are precautions for medications for estrogen sensitive cancers (aromatase inhibitors) and medications changed by the liver (Cytochrome

P450 1A2 (CYP1A2) substrates) such as clozapine. Pregnant or breastfeeding women should not take an aromatase inhibitor.

Make sure your vitamin D levels are high enough. Several studies, including one from the Stanford University School of Medicine, have found vitamin D_3 inhibits the growth of breast cancer cells and stimulates apoptosis, the death of cancer cells.

Add iodine. The thyroid, ovaries, brain, and breasts all have iodine receptors that rely on this mineral to function optimally. Iodine helps the body get rid of "dirty" estrogens. A deficiency is a major contributor to estrogen dominance and an increased risk of estrogenic cancers. Foods such as seaweed (kelp, wakame, hijiki), seafood, and eggs are good sources of iodine. Or try supplements, though only people found to be deficient in iodine through proper testing should take supplemental iodine. The preferred form of iodine supplementation is potassium iodide. Take 3 to 10 mg per day, start low.

Caution: Do not add iodine (internally or externally) if you have hyperthyroidism, Graves' disease, or Hashimoto's disease with elevated thyroid stimulating immunoglobulin (TSI) antibodies or thyroid peroxidase (TPO) antibodies. Added iodine will cause a Graves' or Hashimoto's flare-up.

Add vitamin E. Vitamin E promotes progesterone production and inhibits breast cancer. There has been a lot of research studying the effectiveness of vitamin E in ER+ breast cancer. One study showed vitamin E may play an important role in altering the cellular response to estrogen, thereby inhibiting estrogen receptor-positive cell growth which occurs in some types of breast cancer.

Add resveratrol. Occurring naturally in red wine and Itadori tea/Japanese Knotweed, this natural bioflavonoid is an effective antiviral, antioxidant, anti-inflammatory, and phytoestrogen. It also increases your levels of quinone reductase, a compound that protects DNA against the oxidative damage linked to raised cancer risk. Because of its anti-cancer properties, resveratrol has been used as part of breast cancer therapy.

Lower inflammation. Make an anti-inflammatory diet a priority and add supplements that target inflammation, such as those containing curcumin.

Try castor oil packs to support liver detoxification, clear out "dirty" estrogens, and reduce inflammation. If you haven't already tried castor oil packs, now is a good time to begin. Apply packs on the breasts. For more on their benefits and how to apply a pack, see page 150. Add essential oils, such as the Essential Oil Breast Blend, for more support.

Add deep detoxification, such as time in an infrared sauna and lymphatic massage (dry brushing). Infrared saunas provide a host of amazing benefits, including lowering inflammation, strengthening the immune system, and reducing pain. For more on the benefits of an infrared sauna, see page 154. Lymphatic massage supports lymphatic drainage and circulation. For more on the benefits and how to dry brush (it's very easy!), see page 154.

Apply essential oils topically. Many people in our community have reported positive results from massaging with essential oils such as rosemary, lavender, and frankincense. Dilute essential oils with a carrier oil such as jojoba, sweet almond, or fractionated coconut oil before applying to your breasts or try the Essential Oil Breast Blend.

Take the DUTCH test. Testing is a good idea to establish a baseline before you begin any protocol. I suggest DUTCH testing before you begin to assess your levels of estrogen metabolites and progesterone, followed by a recheck after three months on this protocol to determine where you may need extra support.

Consider saliva testing. I recommend saliva testing to check your progesterone levels. Progesterone cannot be measured in urine (DUTCH will only show you an approximation). Saliva is a great medium to understand your progesterone levels. Unfortunately, saliva testing won't show estrogen metabolites. At the time of writing this book, there is no provider offering both urine and saliva screening in one test. For providers and periodically updated information, see Recommended Labs on page 362.

> ## ESSENTIAL OIL BREAST BLEND
>
> ---
>
> - 2 drops rosemary essential oil
>
> - 2 drops clary sage essential oil
>
> - 2 drops frankincense essential oil
>
> - 1 drop lavender essential oil
>
> - 1 drop clove essential oil
>
> - 3 teaspoons jojoba, sweet almond, or fractionated coconut oil
>
> Massage over the breasts before applying the castor oil pack.

Chapter 21

High Testosterone (PCOS) Protocol

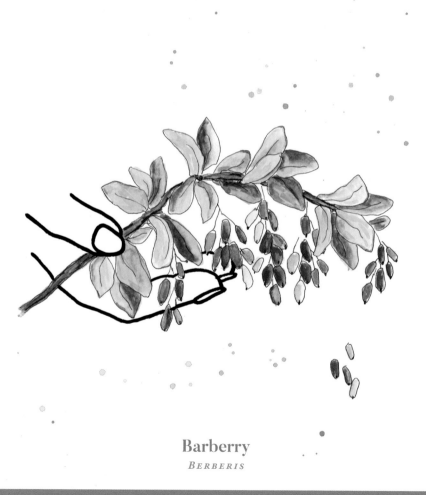

Barberry

Berberis

Testosterone gets converted to estrogens, therefore high testosterone levels can directly contribute to estrogen dominance. High testosterone, often present in PCOS, can disrupt a woman's menstrual cycle and make it harder to get pregnant as well as cause a host of unwanted symptoms, such as acne and unwanted hair growth. Women suffering from high testosterone or PCOS tend to have elevated sugar levels—caused by diet, stress, or inflammation—and insulin resistance. The good news is, these conditions are completely reversible.

Key Facts

PCOS is a "syndrome," or group of symptoms that affects the ovaries and ovulation. Its main features include, insulin resistance, small, fluid-filled sacs inside the ovaries, high levels of male hormones, and irregular or skipped periods.

An androgen is a hormone that regulates the development and growth of male characteristics, such as testosterone, DHEA, and/or DHT. Many women with PCOS produce higher than normal amounts of these hormones and have what's called androgen dominance. High levels of androgens disrupt the menstrual cycle and can prevent ovulation. When ovulation doesn't happen, the ovaries can develop small cysts which in turn produce androgens.

The term polycystic ovary syndrome (PCOS) describes the numerous small cysts that often form in the ovaries. However, not every woman with PCOS will develop cysts. And some women with cysts do not have PCOS.

Women with high testosterone levels (and often PCOS) can suffer from estrogen dominance, too. This is because testosterone is converted into estradiol in the aromatization process. Inhibiting this process can break the cycle of estrogen production and relieve symptoms of estrogen dominance.

Where we store fat and cellulite can be an indication of a hormonal imbalance. An "apple" body shape with fat stored around the belly is often a sign of high testosterone and PCOS.

Many women with PCOS have insulin resistance. It is important to get it under control right away and improve your insulin sensitivity. Insulin resistance causes systemic inflammation and can lead to several serious conditions including prediabetes, diabetes, elevated androgens, along with metabolic disorders which increase your risk for heart disease and stroke. If that's you, implement the sugar balancing protocol in chapter 6.

Symptoms

- irregular or missing menstrual periods
- delayed ovulation
- infertility
- excess or unwanted body or facial hair growth
- thinning hair on the scalp, especially in front
- weight problems, often including weight gain around the waist
- skin problems, including skin tags, darkening skin, and acne
- oily skin and hair
- polycystic ovaries visible on scan
- "Apple" body shape, characterized by abdominal fat

Diagnosis

Many women with PCOS go undiagnosed. In one study, up to 70% of women with PCOS hadn't

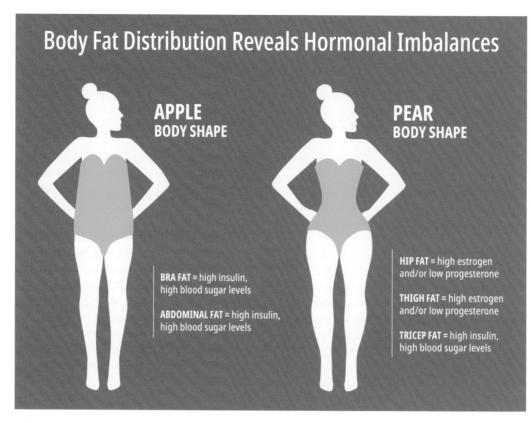

Body Fat Distribution Reveals Hormonal Imbalances

APPLE
BODY SHAPE

PEAR
BODY SHAPE

BRA FAT = high insulin, high blood sugar levels

ABDOMINAL FAT = high insulin, high blood sugar levels

HIP FAT = high estrogen and/or low progesterone

THIGH FAT = high estrogen and/or low progesterone

TRICEP FAT = high insulin, high blood sugar levels

been diagnosed. For a PCOS diagnosis, two of the following three criteria must be met:

1. insulin resistance

To determine if you have insulin resistance, your doctor will consider the following:

- high insulin levels (above 15)
- high HA1C (above 5.4)
- high glucose levels (above 90)
- belly fat, apple shape
- hunger after eating a meal
- tiredness after eating a meal
- cravings for sugar and processed carbohydrates

2. ovarian cysts

3. high androgens

Causes

A precise cause is unknown, but the following have all been linked to excess androgen production:

- genetics
- insulin resistance
- inflammation

Traditional Treatments

- birth control pills, to regulate ovulation
- diabetes drugs, such as Metformin, to improve insulin levels
- medications to treat symptoms such as acne or hair growth

The problem with these approaches is they don't address the root causes of the problem:

Hormone imbalance, high inflammation, and insulin resistance. The best approach is to treat PCOS proactively with holistic natural approaches that address what's causing it in the first place.

High Testosterone (PCOS) Protocol

Step 1. Do the 28-Day Estrogen Reset Foundation Protocol, including the Foundational Supplements. See Part IV for everything you need to do it successfully. After doing the Foundation Protocol, you may not even need to implement Step 2, but if you feel you've mastered it and need to go deeper to address your PCOS, read on.

Step 2: Implement the High Testosterone (PCOS) Protocol.

Implement as much of the following as you can. Some things may help and others won't. We are all different and will respond to changes in varied ways.

To lower inflammation and improve insulin sensitivity, make sure your blood sugar is balanced and, if necessary, take additional steps to get it under control. Go back to chapter 6, Balance Your Blood Sugar, for a refresher on all of my recommendations for what you can do to keep your blood sugar in check, including supplement support.

Look beyond diet to identify and reduce the other sources of inflammation in your life. Consider:

- stress
- trauma
- self-criticism, self-loathing

- birth control pills
- chemical or mold exposure

Consider supplements that target PCOS-related issues. These include:

- Berberine to help lower blood sugar. The recommended dosage is 500 mg per day.
- Chromium picolinate to improve insulin sensitivity and lower glucose levels. The recommended dosage is 300 mcg.
- Inositol, a B vitamin, can help increase insulin sensitivity and balance testosterone levels. Myo-inositol has been shown to be more involved with the health of the ovaries as well as overall reproductive and hormonal function, while D-chiro-inositol is a good regulator of insulin metabolism. The recommended dosage is 3.2 g per day.

Take the DUTCH test. Testing is a good idea to establish a baseline before you begin any protocol. It's also helpful if you've been doing the Foundation and High Testosterone (PCOS) Protocol for three to four months and your symptoms haven't eased. I suggest DUTCH testing every three to six months while on this Add-On Protocol to assess your levels of androgens, estrogen metabolites, cortisol, and melatonin to help determine where you may need extra support.

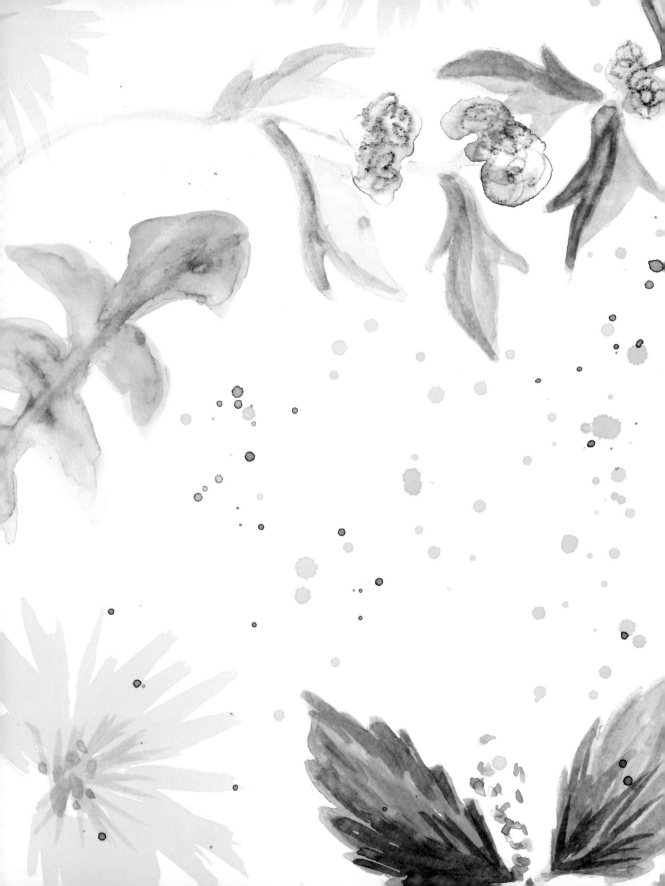

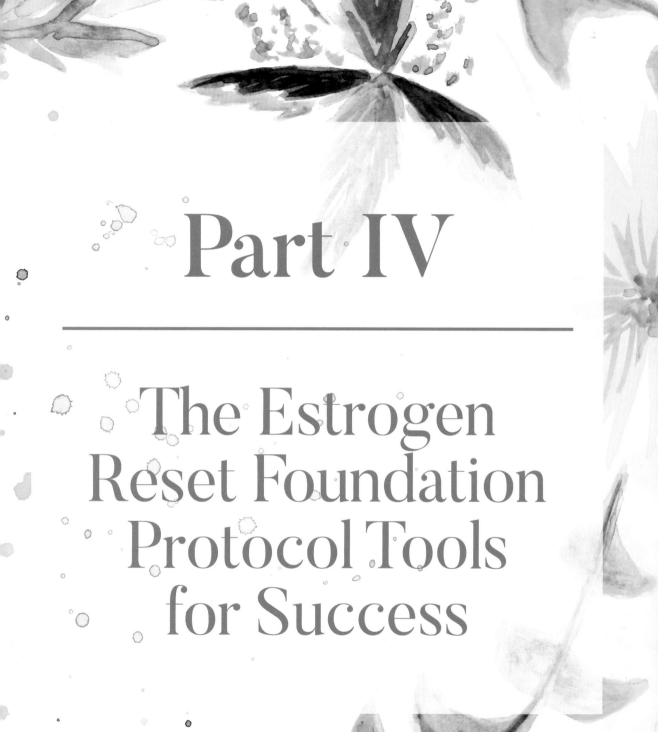

Part IV

The Estrogen Reset Foundation Protocol Tools for Success

Chapter 22

Get Going with Ease

A Quick-Start Overview

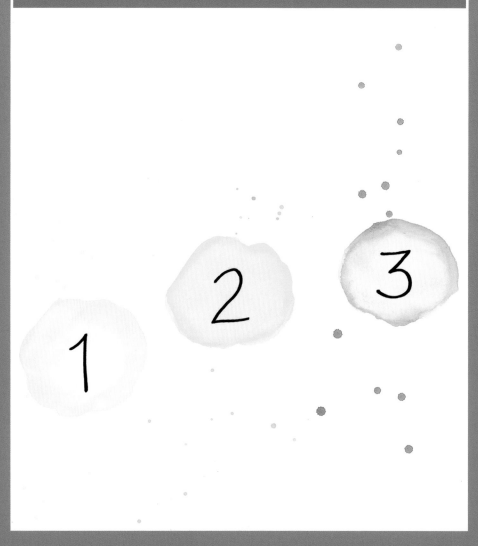

Add Healing Practices to Your Routine

There are many healing practices to restore your gut, support liver detoxification, balance your blood sugar, and encourage stress-reducing self-care. Over the next four weeks of the Foundation Protocol, make a commitment to start clearing out the xenoestrogens from your life while taking steps to get more and better sleep. Choose one suggestion from each section to get you started. I encourage you to try castor oil packs, an infrared sauna, dry brushing, or rebounding. Your plate may seem pretty full right now, but keep these suggestions in mind as you continue your hormone-balancing journey.

Ready to take a major step on your healing journey? The 28-Day Estrogen Reset Foundation Protocol is designed to reverse your estrogen dominance and support your body's own power to heal. We'll use food, herbs, supplements, and daily habits to restore your gut, detox your liver, and balance your blood sugar, which are the three legs of your hormone-balance stool.

What does that look like day-to-day?

Here's what you'll be doing:

- You will eat an abundance of nutrient-dense, delicious meals, snacks, and beverages. The Meal Plans and Recipes provided in the chapters 10 and 11 are simple, meal-prep friendly, flavorful, and nourishing. Eating this way will balance your estrogen, boost your energy, mood, immune system, ease cravings and digestive issues like constipation, bloating, and gas. You will feel like a new woman—not deprived or hungry.
- You will bridge the gaps in your nutrition with supplement support.
- You will incorporate more natural, toxin-free cleaning, and personal care products into your daily routine.
- You will get better sleep.

As you go through the Foundation Protocol, you may realize you are already doing some of the things I recommend. That's great! Stick with them and keep an eye out for new elements you may not have implemented yet. One rule though: *Please don't cherry pick*. The Foundation Protocol works best when you do *all* of it. Let's say you are already following a good diet, but you're highly reliant on caffeine, or still eat eggs, or only sleep five hours each night. In that case you won't experience the benefits of the protocol. It's as simple as that. We often get emails which read, "I'm so healthy, but I can't shrink my fibroids," and when we ask a few questions, the person hasn't been following half of what I recommend in the protocol. Commit to following the Foundation Protocol for four to eight weeks, do the work, and you will see the results. Thousands of women have done it and you can too. You're worth it and I know you can do it.

> The Foundation Protocol works best when you do *all* of it

Quick-Start Overview

This Add/Remove chart summarizes the action steps of the Foundation Protocol. Don't worry. By following the Meal Plans and Recipes, you'll add in all of the right foods and take out all of the bad ones. If our recipes and meal plans contain foods to which you are sensitive, please avoid them.

Want to find out more about a specific step? Check out the relevant chapter in Part II.

Here is an overview of what you will be doing when you eat according to the Estrogen Reset 28-day Meal Plan.

ADD (+)	REMOVE (-)
To Restore Your Gut **Whole Foods** • Organic, non-GMO, and pasture-raised meat • Digestive bitters • Probiotics and fermented foods • Good bowel movement (daily!)	**Inflammatory** **Foods** • Gluten, dairy, eggs, corn, soy, nightshades • Processed/conventionally grown vegetables, grains, meat, and fish • Coffee and caffeine • Sugar (limited quantities only)
To Detox Your Liver • Liver-supporting foods (pages 85–92 for the complete list) • NAC and glutathione • Liver herbs	Avoid inflammatory and fried foods, coffee, as well as alcohol. They take up a lot of liver resources to clear out.
To Balance Your Blood Sugar • A Protein, Fats, Fiber (PFF) breakfast • Supplements, such as berberine and chromium picolinate, if needed	• Excess sugar. Limit sugar to no more than 20 g (5 teaspoons) per day. • Excess alcohol. Limit to a maximum of 3 drinks per week.

ADD (+)	REMOVE (-)
To Amplify Your Healing Foundational Supplements • Magnesium (glycinate or citrate) • Vitamin C • Vitamin B Complex • Zinc • Vitamin D$_3$ • DIM • Sulforaphane • Calcium D-glucarate • Omega 3 • Vitamin B$_6$ • Bioidentical Progesterone (Topical)	• Poor quality supplements, use the five rules on page 52. • Birth control pills and synthetic hormone replacement therapy (HRT)
To Move Beyond Food Practices • Natural, toxin-free household and personal care products • Good sleep • Melatonin supplement, if needed • Castor oil packs • Infrared sauna • Dry brushing • Rebounding	Xenoestrogens from your daily life: cleaning, household, personal, and beauty products • Stress, past trauma • Sleep deprivation

Quick Start Foundational Supplement Guide

Supplements are a great way to bridge the gaps and amplify your healing when done in conjunction with solid diet changes. These supplements are included as part of the Foundational Protocol because I've found they benefit most women. Each of these supplements is covered in detail in chapter 7, but below is an overview.

To see the brands I personally use and recommend to the Hormones Balance community, please see Supplement and Herbs Guide on page 361.

If you choose to use your personal favorite brand of supplements, please read "Getting Started with Supplements" in chapter 3, page 52, for how to evaluate the quality of your supplements. It is an unregulated industry, therefore the quality of supplements can vary from highly efficacious and clean to harmful junk.

Magnesium	Vitamin C	Vitamin B Complex
Zinc	Vitamin D_3	DIM
Sulforaphane	Calcium D-glucarate	Omega 3 Fatty Acids
Vitamin B_6	Bioidentical Progesterone (topical)	

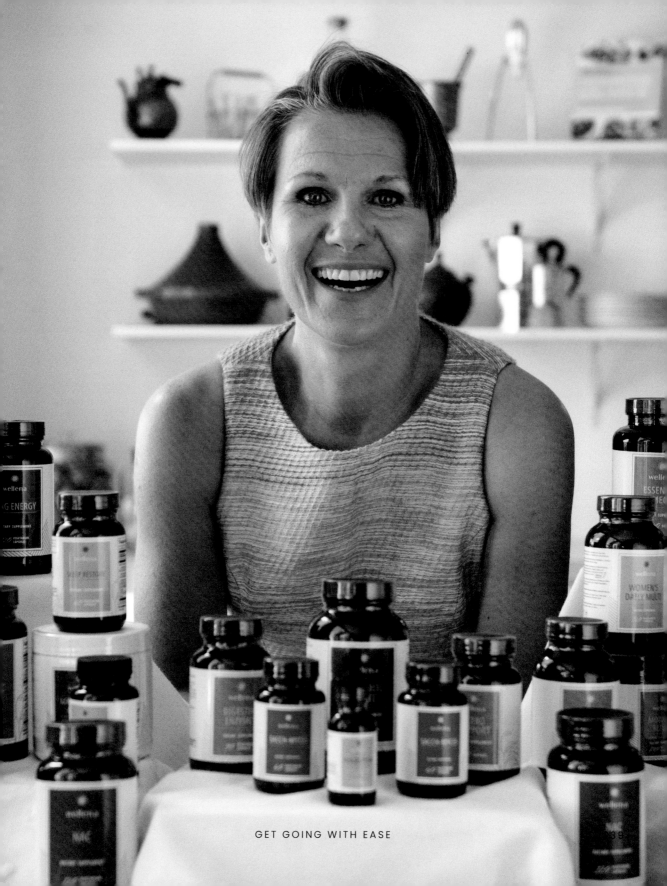

GET GOING WITH EASE

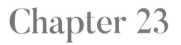

Chapter 23

The Estrogen Reset 28-Day Meal Plan

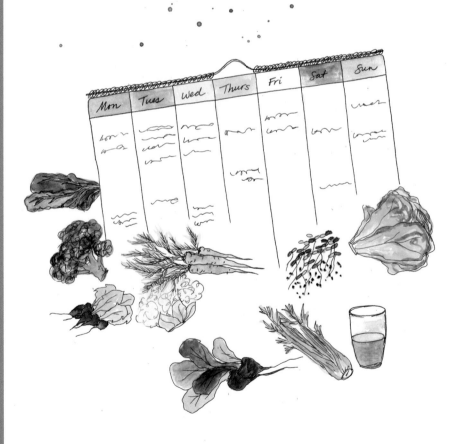

I've provided a meal plan and shopping list for the first two weeks of the program. Simply repeat those weeks to complete the full four-week Foundation Protocol.

About the Meal Plan and Recipes

Making these recipes as simple, easy, and quick has been my priority from the start. A lot of cookbooks promise "quick-and-easy recipes in 30 minutes or less". What they actually deliver is recipes calling for 20 to 30 ingredients and take a whole lot longer than 30 minutes to put together after you've done all the necessary prep, not to mention hours of soaking. Not so "easy," right?

The Foundation Protocol Recipes deliver as promised. Most involve about five ingredients, don't require multiple steps or pots, and take very little time, 20 minutes max for weekday meals. These recipes are basic enough to make every day. They may not be fancy, but they are satisfying, packed with nutrients, and delicious. These meals get the healing done! You won't even be cooking every day. Batch cooking cuts down on this plus most days you'll just be pulling together simple ingredients, like nut butter spread on an apple slice and sprinkled with cinnamon, for a very no-fuss treat. Or, using a spread, such as pestos, drizzles, and vinaigrettes to amp up the flavor of steamed vegetables or baked fish.

I'm a big fan of the Instant Pot. It's an incredible time-saver. Many dishes have an Instant Pot (or slow cooker) option as well as stovetop directions.

MY WORD OF CAUTION ON THE DARLING OF THE HEALTH WORLD … COCONUT!

Coconut, the darling of the health world. Yet you won't find many recipes in this cookbook containing coconut oil, milk, flakes, or coconut water. Why? When I first saw studies linking coconut to increased LPS, aka endotoxins, which increase gut permeability and disrupt the microbiome, I really didn't want to believe it. Subsequently, I noticed after having a daily latte with a coconut creamer, I would get phlegm and have to clear my throat for a good 20 minutes. When I quit coconut for good (in all forms), I noticed a number of immediate improvements: my gut was much happier, no more phlegm, and, the biggest one, my candida was GONE. I've struggled with candida for years and no treatments have ever worked. When I shared this revelation in our online group, many similar stories poured in.

I don't want to vilify coconut-it could be that you can tolerate it just fine. My belief is there is a potential genetic component. People of South Asian, Caribbean, and Polynesian descent may tolerate coconut very well because it's been part of their ancestral diet.

I know many of you substitute dairy with coconut milk and cream, but if you have been dealing with lingering, chronic issues that won't go away in spite of having committed to eating clean, do look into cutting coconut for a while. I've switched to almond and cashew yogurt, along with making my own nut and seed milks. If you can't tolerate nuts and seeds, try tigernuts; they are hypoallergenic tubers (not nuts) and can be purchased on Amazon.

And what about treats? We've got you covered, plus we have several different lattes for you to enjoy as well.

The foods you will be eating plenty of. The Meal Plan is packed with recipes rich in fresh, delicious, satisfying ingredients:

- whole foods
- organic, non-GMO foods, including meat
- fermented foods (unless you have histamine problems)
- liver-supporting foods

The foods you won't find here. All of the most inflammatory foods have been removed from the Meal Plan and Recipes of the Foundation Protocol. These are:

- gluten (wheat, barley, rye, farro, along with products containing processed gluten-containing grain flours like breads, pastas, cookies, and muffins)
- dairy (milk, yogurt, cheese, butter)
- eggs (both the yolk and whites)
- corn
- soy (in all forms, including soy sauce and tempeh)

- nightshades (tomatoes, white potatoes, eggplants, peppers, chili, goji berries)
- processed or packaged foods including protein powders
- coffee and caffeine (except an occasional green tea or matcha)
- sugar (in limited quantities only)
- coconut

DON'T USE PLASTIC IN THE MICROWAVE!

Certain chemicals in plastic, such as external estrogens, called xenoestrogens, can leach into your food and beverages. Heat the plastic, for example by microwaving it, and you speed up the leaching process. Disaster. If you must use a microwave, only use glass or ceramic containers.

Week One
Shopping List

Common Items

Before you go shopping—check your supply, you may have some of these staples in your kitchen.

- ☐ 6 tablespoons ground cumin
- ☐ 5.5 tablespoons sea salt
- ☐ ½ teaspoon onion powder
- ☐ 26 garlic cloves
- ☐ 3 teaspoons dried oregano
- ☐ 2.5 teaspoons black peppercorns
- ☐ 2 bay leaves
- ☐ ¼ cup ground coriander
- ☐ ¼ cup ground thyme
- ☐ 1 teaspoon dried rosemary
- ☐ 5 cups extra virgin olive oil
- ☐ ⅓ cup tahini
- ☐ 1.5 cups ghee
- ☐ 4 tablespoons raw honey
- ☐ 1.5 cups apple cider vinegar
- ☐ 1 teaspoon aluminum-free baking powder

Vegetables

- ☐ ⅓ cup kalamata olives
- ☐ 2 sweet potatoes
- ☐ 4 red onions
- ☐ 4 cups microgreens
- ☐ 4 cups Brussels sprouts
- ☐ 2 cups butternut squash

- ☐ 5 carrots
- ☐ 4 celery stalks
- ☐ 3 cups kale
- ☐ 5.5 cups broccoli sprouts
- ☐ 2 cups mixed greens (arugula, mizuna, baby kale, or baby spinach)
- ☐ ⅓ cup wakame
- ☐ 3 cups arugula or bitter greens
- ☐ 1 medium turnip
- ☐ 4 shallots
- ☐ 7 cups collard greens
- ☐ 6 cups baby arugula
- ☐ 2 medium heads cauliflower
- ☐ 2 cups broccoli florets
- ☐ 1 cup shiitake mushrooms
- ☐ 1 cup bok choy
- ☐ 1 small purple cabbage
- ☐ 2 cups sauerkraut

Fruit

- ☐ 7 lemons
- ☐ 7 avocados
- ☐ 4 limes

Meat

- ☐ 1 pound 85% lean grass-fed ground beef
- ☐ 4 large pieces bone-in skin-on chicken thighs
- ☐ 6 pounds beef, chicken, pork, or lamb marrow bones/knuckle bones/short ribs

- ☐ 2 8-ounce bone-in pork chops
- ☐ 1 pound ground beef, lamb, bison, turkey or a combination of any of them
- ☐ 3 ounces pasture-raised uncured bacon
- ☐ 2 6-ounce strip steaks
- ☐ 1 pound boneless skinless chicken thighs

Seafood

- ☐ 1 pound salmon
- ☐ 2 ounces smoked salmon

Herbs/Spices

- ☐ 4.5 cups cilantro
- ☐ 8 cups fresh parsley
- ☐ 5 sprigs fresh thyme
- ☐ 8 tablespoons fresh ginger
- ☐ 8 inches kelp strips
- ☐ 3 sprigs fresh rosemary
- ☐ ¼ cup sumac or ground dried lemon peel
- ☐ 1 teaspoon smoked sea salt
- ☐ ½ cup fresh tarragon
- ☐ 1 cup fresh basil
- ☐ 1.5 pounds fresh turmeric OR 3 tablespoons dried turmeric
- ☐ 1 tablespoon chives
- ☐ 2 tablespoons fresh dill
- ☐ 2 tablespoons calendula

- ☐ 2 tablespoons peppermint
- ☐ 4 tablespoons chamomile
- ☐ 2 tablespoons plantain
- ☐ 3 teaspoons licorice
- ☐ 1 tablespoon California poppy
- ☐ 1 tablespoon passionflower
- ☐ 1 tablespoon skullcap OR lemon balm
- ☐ 1 teaspoon lavender buds
- ☐ 2 tablespoons red clover
- ☐ 2 tablespoons red raspberry
- ☐ 2 tablespoons nettles
- ☐ 1 teaspoon hibiscus
- ☐ 1 tablespoon dandelion OR burdock root
- ☐ 1 tablespoon milk thistle
- ☐ 1 tablespoon turmeric root
- ☐ 1 teaspoon schizandra berry

Oils/Vinegar/Sauce

- ☐ 1.5 cups coconut aminos
- ☐ 6 tablespoons toasted sesame oil
- ☐ 2 cups chicken stock (or bone broth)
- ☐ 1.5 cups unsweetened almond milk
- ☐ 2 tablespoons rice vinegar

Flour/Powder

- ☐ 1 teaspoon coconut sugar
- ☐ 1 teaspoon rice flour
- ☐ 1 cup gluten-free flour
- ☐ 2 cups sprouted or regular chickpea flour

Grain/Lentils

- ☐ 4.5 cups raw buckwheat groats
- ☐ 1 can chickpeas
- ☐ 3 cups white beans (canned beans are OK if from non-BPA can or glass jar)
- ☐ 4 cups brown rice

Seeds/Nuts

- ☐ 6 tablespoons pumpkin seeds
- ☐ 3 tablespoons ground fennel seed
- ☐ 9 tablespoons sesame seeds
- ☐ 1 tablespoon carraway seeds
- ☐ 2 tablespoons shelled sunflower seeds
- ☐ 1 cup pomegranate seeds
- ☐ 4 tablespoons fennel seeds
- ☐ ½ cup raw walnuts
- ☐ 7 tablespoons flax seed

Other

- ☐ 2.5 cups mineral water

Optional

- ☐ ½ cup unsweetened tart cherry juice
- ☐ 3 tablespoons kudzu root powder
- ☐ ½ teaspoon almond extract
- ☐ 9 tablespoons pure maple syrup
- ☐ 2 ⅔ cups extra unsweetened almond milk
- ☐ ½ cup raw sliced almonds
- ☐ ½ cup pitted and halved cherries
- ☐ 1 cup dried figs
- ☐ ½ cup sunflower seed butter
- ☐ 3 tablespoons raw cacao nibs
- ☐ 2 tablespoons hemp hearts
- ☐ 1 cup blanched almond flour
- ☐ ½ cup extra gluten-free flour blend
- ☐ ½ cup unsweetened cacao powder
- ☐ 2 teaspoons extra aluminum-free baking powder
- ☐ 2 teaspoons vanilla extract

Week One

Meal Plan for 2 people

[NR] No recipe   ACV—Apple Cider Vinegar
[LO] Leftovers   DIB - Digestive Bitters
[MA] Made ahead   Morning Ritual—available on
[DB] Double the recipe   www.wellena.com
EVOO—Extra Virgin Olive Oil

	MORNING RITUAL & BREAKFAST	SNACK (OPTIONAL)	LUNCH	DINNER	BEDTIME RITUAL (OPTIONAL)
DAY 1	Warm lemon water or Morning Ritual Southwest Breakfast Bowl [DB] (page 284) DIB	Digestive Tea (page 346)	Fresh Herb Hummus (page 262) with carrot sticks [NR] Start on Polish Sourdough Buckwheat Bread (page 254) DIB	Garlicky Lemon Chicken (page 296) Vegetable Medley with Pomegranate and Pumpkin Seeds (page 300) DIB	Sleepytime Tea (page 346) Start on Bone Broth (page 260). Freeze 2 quarts, for next week.
DAY 2	Warm lemon water or Morning Ritual Southwest Breakfast Bowl [LO] (page 284) DIB	Avocado Sprout Smoothie (page 274)	Mediterranean Buckwheat Bowl (using LO chicken from Garlicky Lemon Chicken) (page 294) Dollop of Fresh Herb Hummus [LO] DIB	Honey Rosemary Pork Chops (page 290) Roasted Vegetable Medley [LO] DIB	Sleepytime Tea [LO] Cherry Almond Pudding (page 324) [MA]
DAY 3	Warm lemon water or Morning Ritual Farmer's Wife's Breakfast (page 276) DIB	Women's Daily Tea (page 345) Cacao Fig Balls—2 per person (page 316)	Japanese Powerhouse Salad (page 288) DIB	Sardinian Herb Soup (page 308) A slice of Polish Sourdough Buckwheat Bread [MA] (page 254), drizzled Sesame Tahini Drizzle [LO] DIB	Bone Broth [LO] with dash of ACV and sea salt Cherry Almond Pudding [LO]

	MORNING RITUAL & BREAKFAST	SNACK (OPTIONAL)	LUNCH	DINNER	BEDTIME RITUAL (OPTIONAL)
DAY 4	Warm lemon water or Morning Ritual 2 patties from Farmer's Wife's Breakfast [LO] with 1 cup sautéed collard greens and 1 cup sauerkraut [NR] DIB	Women's Daily Tea [LO] Cacao Fig Bliss Balls—2 per person [LO]	Sardinian Herb Soup [LO] (page 308) A slice of Polish Sourdough Buckwheat Bread [LO], drizzled with EVOO DIB	Roasted Pesto Salmon (page 302) Cilantro Lime Cauliflower Rice (page 266) DIB	Bone Broth [LO] with dash of ACV and sea salt Handful of nuts and seeds
DAY 5	Good Morning Elixir (page 334) Avocado Sprout Smoothie (page 274) DIB	Cacao Fig Bliss Balls—2 per person [LO]	2 patties from Farmer's Wife's Breakfast [LO] Fresh Herbs Hummus [LO] Bed of arugula, EVOO and ACV [NR] DIB	Roasted Pesto Salmon [LO] Cilantro Lime Cauliflower Rice [LO] DIB	Digestive Tea (page 346) Handful of nuts and seeds Start on Chimichurri Steak (page 292)
DAY 6	Good Morning Elixir [LO] Chimichurri Steak [MA] Cilantro Lime Cauliflower Rice [LO] DIB	Avocado Cacao Muffins—1 per person (page 282)	2 toasted slices Polish Sourdough Buckwheat Bread [LO] ½ avocado drizzled with Chimichurri Sauce [LO] DIB	Rainbow Chicken Stir Fry (page 304) DIB	Digestive Tea [LO] Handful of nuts and seeds Start on Liver Detox Tea (page 345)
DAY 7	Good Morning Elixir [LO] Salmon & Chives Over Waffles (page 272) Start on Easy Sourdough Focaccia (page 256) DIB	Avocado Cacao Muffins—1 per person [LO]	2 toasted slices Polish Sourdough Buckwheat Bread [LO] ½ avocado drizzled with Chimichurri Sauce [LO] DIB	Rainbow Chicken Stir Fry [LO] DIB	Liver Detox Tea [MA] Handful of nuts and seeds

Week Two
Shopping List

Common Items

Before you go—check your supply, you may have some of these staples in your kitchen.

- ☐ 1 tablespoon ground turmeric
- ☐ 4 tablespoons sea salt
- ☐ 2 teaspoons ground black pepper
- ☐ 1 teaspoon ground ginger
- ☐ 28 garlic cloves
- ☐ 1 teaspoon dried oregano
- ☐ 1.5 teaspoons ground coriander
- ☐ ¼ cup apple cider vinegar
- ☐ 7 teaspoons raw honey
- ☐ 2 cups plus 1 tablespoon extra virgin olive oil
- ☐ ⅔ cup ghee
- ☐ ⅓ cup tahini
- ☐ 4 teaspoons ground cumin

Fruit

- ☐ 5 lemons
- ☐ 3 avocados
- ☐ 5 limes

Vegetables

- ☐ ⅓ cup kalamata olives
- ☐ 10 carrots
- ☐ 1 bunch collard greens, kale or chard
- ☐ 6 ounces asparagus
- ☐ 5 cups arugula
- ☐ 3.5 cups broccoli sprouts
- ☐ 2 cups shiitake mushrooms
- ☐ 2 cups celery
- ☐ 2 cups white onion
- ☐ 1 red onion
- ☐ 2 cups kale
- ☐ ⅓ cup wakame
- ☐ 1 turnip
- ☐ 2 shallots
- ☐ 2 beets
- ☐ 1 can chickpeas
- ☐ 6 cups sweet potatoes
- ☐ 2 heads cauliflower
- ☐ 1 cup sauerkraut

Meat

- ☐ 4 strips bacon
- ☐ 2 pounds beef stew meat
- ☐ 4 large bone-in, skin-on chicken thighs
- ☐ 2 8-ounce bone-in pork chops
- ☐ 2 6-ounce strip steaks

Seafood

- ☐ 1 pound salmon
- ☐ 2 6-ounce cod filets
- ☐ 6 ounces sockeye smoked salmon
- ☐ 4 anchovies

Herbs/Spices

- ☐ 5 teaspoons whole cumin
- ☐ 2 cups fresh cilantro
- ☐ 2 sprigs fresh rosemary
- ☐ 3 sprigs fresh thyme
- ☐ 3 cups fresh parsley
- ☐ 1.5 cups fresh basil
- ☐ 3 tablespoons fresh ginger
- ☐ 3 tablespoons chamomile
- ☐ 1 tablespoon California poppy
- ☐ 1 tablespoon passionflower
- ☐ 1 tablespoon skullcap or lemon balm
- ☐ 1 teaspoon lavender buds
- ☐ 1 tablespoon dandelion root or burdock root
- ☐ 1 tablespoon milk thistle
- ☐ 1 tablespoon turmeric root

- ☐ 1 teaspoon schizandra berry
- ☐ 2 tablespoons red clover
- ☐ 2 tablespoons red raspberry leaves
- ☐ 2 tablespoons nettles
- ☐ 1 teaspoon hibiscus
- ☐ 2 teaspoons licorice root
- ☐ 1 tablespoon calendula
- ☐ 1 tablespoon peppermint
- ☐ 1 tablespoon plantain

Oils/Vinegar/Sauce

- ☐ 1 quart + 3 cups chicken stock (or bone broth)
- ☐ 2 cups beef bone broth
- ☐ 1 cup coconut aminos
- ☐ 3 tablespoons toasted sesame oil
- ☐ 2 tablespoons rice vinegar
- ☐ ½ cup unsalted and unsweetened creamy cashew or almond butter

Flour/Powder

- ☐ 3 tablespoons gluten-free flour
- ☐ 2 scoops collagen

Grain/Lentils

- ☐ 1.5 cups red lentils

- ☐ 2 cups raw buckwheat groats
- ☐ ½ cup uncooked quinoa

Seeds/Nuts

- ☐ ¾ cup sesame seeds
- ☐ 5 tablespoons flax seeds
- ☐ 1 tablespoon carraway seeds
- ☐ 2 tablespoons sunflower seeds
- ☐ ½ cup cashews
- ☐ ½ cup raw walnuts
- ☐ 2 teaspoons fennel seeds

Other

2.5 cups mineral water

Optional

- ☐ Preserved lemon
- ☐ 4 cups unsweetened dairy-free milk (like almond milk)
- ☐ ¼ cup chia seeds
- ☐ 2 tablespoons pure maple syrup or extra raw honey
- ☐ 1 cup mixed berries (blueberries, blackberries, strawberries, raspberries)
- ☐ ½ cup unsweetened tart cherry juice

- ☐ 3 tablespoons kudzu root powder
- ☐ ½ teaspoon almond extract
- ☐ 3 tablespoons pure maple syrup
- ☐ 1 cup raw sliced almonds
- ☐ ½ cup pitted halved cherries
- ☐ 12 ounces dark chocolate chips (over 70% cacao)
- ☐ ½ teaspoon dong quai root powder
- ☐ 1 tablespoon extra sesame seeds
- ☐ 1 tablespoon pumpkin seeds
- ☐ 2 tablespoons dried cherries or cranberries
- ☐ 32 ounces fresh strawberries
- ☐ 1 inch extra fresh ginger
- ☐ 2 extra limes
- ☐ 3 tablespoons gelatin

Week Two

Meal Plan for 2 People

[NR] No recipe   ACV—Apple Cider Vinegar
[LO] Leftovers   [DIB] - Digestive Bitters
[MA] Made ahead   Morning Ritual—available on
[DB] Double the recipe   www.wellena.com
EVOO—Extra Virgin Olive Oil

	MORNING RITUAL & BREAKFAST	SNACK (OPTIONAL)	LUNCH	DINNER	BEDTIME RITUAL (OPTIONAL)
DAY 8	Good Morning Elixir [LO] Salmon & Chives Over Waffles [LO] DIB	Avocado Cacao Muffins—1 per person [LO]	Red Lentil Stew with Greens (page 310) A piece of Easy Sourdough Focaccia [MA] Drizzle of Chimichurri (page 258) for dipping DIB	Sesame-Ginger Crusted Cod with Asparagus (page 306) Bed of arugula with EVOO, ACV and sea salt [NR] DIB	Sleepytime Tea (page 346) Handful of nuts and seeds Start on the Liver Detox Tea (page 345)
DAY 9	Good Morning Elixir [LO] Fisherman's Breakfast (page 278) DIB	Chia Pudding (page 322)	Red Lentil Stew with Greens [LO] A piece of Easy Sourdough Focaccia [LO] Chimichurri [LO] for focaccia dipping DIB	Hearty and Warming Beef Stew (page 312) A piece of Easy Sourdough Focaccia [LO] Sesame Thyme Drizzle [LO] DIB	Liver Detox Tea [MA] Cherry Almond Pudding (page 324)
DAY 10	Good Morning Elixir [LO] Fisherman's Breakfast [LO] DIB	Chia Pudding [LO]	Hearty and Warming Beef Stew [LO] A piece of Easy Sourdough Focaccia [LO] Sesame Thyme Drizzle for focaccia dipping [LO] DIB	Garlicky Lemon Chicken (page 296) Bed of bitter greens (like arugula, watercress) [NR] Chimichurri [LO] as salad dressing DIB	Liver Detox Tea [LO] Cherry Almond Pudding [LO]

	MORNING RITUAL & BREAKFAST	SNACK (OPTIONAL)	LUNCH	DINNER	BEDTIME RITUAL (OPTIONAL)
DAY 11	Good Morning Elixir [LO] Mediterranean Buckwheat Bowl (page 294) DIB	2 pieces Dong Quai Dark Chocolate Bark (page 318)	Japanese Powerhouse Salad (page 288) DIB	Honey Rosemary Pork Chops (page 290) Bed of bitter greens (like arugula, watercress) with EVOO, ACV and sea salt [NR] DIB	Women's Daily Tea (page 345) Handful of nuts and seeds
DAY 12	Good Morning Elixir [LO] Avocado Sprout Smoothie (page 274) DIB	2 pieces Dong Quai Chocolate Bark [LO]	Beet and Hummus Sandwich (page 298) [DB] DIB	African Sweet Potato Stew (page 314) DIB	Women's Daily Tea [LO] Handful of nuts and seeds
DAY 13	Good Morning Elixir [LO] Beet and Hummus Sandwich [LO] DIB	2 pieces Dong Quai Chocolate Bark [LO]	Chimichurri steak (page 292) [DB] DIB	African Sweet Potato Stew [LO] DIB	Start on the Strawberry Jellies (page 332) Digestive Tea (page 346)
DAY 14	Good Morning Elixir [LO] Sweet Potato Quinoa Patties (page 280) DIB	Strawberry Jellies [MA]	Chimichurri steak [LO] with a side of sautee greens and ½ cup sauerkraut DIB	Roasted Pesto Salmon (page 302) DIB	Digestive Tea [LO] Handful of nuts and seeds

Simply repeat Week One and Two for the complete 28-day Foundation Protocol.

Chapter 24

The Estrogen Reset Recipes

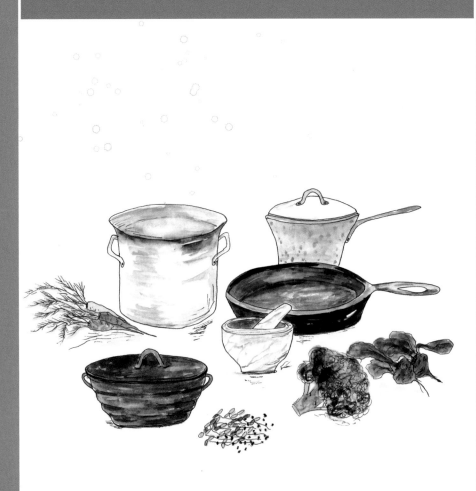

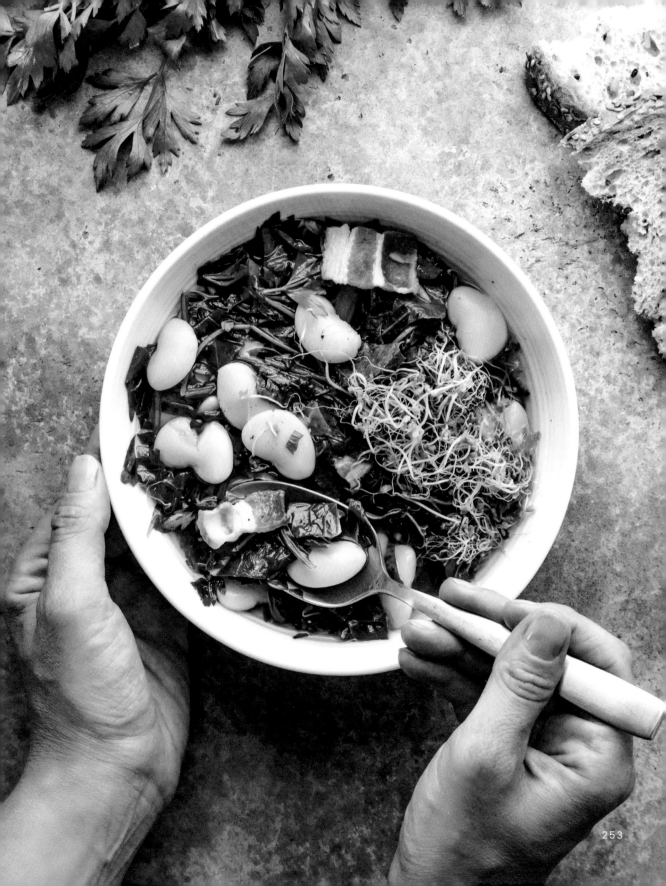

Polish Sourdough Buckwheat Bread

Unlike most sourdough recipes, this bread requires no sourdough starter, which can be an intimidating and time-consuming undertaking. It's simple and deeply nourishing. This bread is a staple in my house, and it saves me each time I need a quick meal and have no time to cook. Toast it, spread some sardines and avocado on top, sprinkle with some great herbs, and voilà! Lunch is served.

This bread requires time for the fermentation to do its magic. It is through this process that you will reap the benefits of making this loaf into a gut-healing food. Fermentation also makes grains such as buckwheat more digestible. In spite of its name, buckwheat does not contain wheat and is, therefore, free of gluten.

This loaf is packed with a lot of fiber, magnesium, and manganese.

2½ cups raw buckwheat groats (not roasted)

2½ cups mineral water (if using filtered, be sure it is chloride- and fluoride-free)

Extra virgin olive oil

1 tablespoon caraway seeds

1 tablespoon fine sea salt

2 tablespoons raw shelled sunflower seeds

2 tablespoons sesame seeds

Equipment: 9 x 5 x 2½-inch loaf pan, glass bowl, and food processor or blender

---

Makes: 1 loaf, about 12 servings
Prep time: 10 minutes
Soaking and fermentation time: 32 hours
Cooking time: 1 hour 30 minutes
Total time: 33 hours 40 minutes

1. Place the groats in a colander and rinse them under cold water. Place the rinsed groats in a large bowl (I like to use Pyrex so I can see the batter) and fill with water to cover. Place a lid or plate over the bowl and let soak at room temperature for 8 hours.

2. Transfer the groats and the soaking liquid to a blender or food processor and pulse several times until groats and water are well combined but still coarse. Do not overblend.

3. Return the mixture to the large bowl, cover again, and let the groats ferment at room temperature, ranging from 72°F to 76°F, for 12 to 24 hours or until the batter becomes slightly bubbly. The batter might have a somewhat unpleasant sour smell—that's normal.

4. Preheat the oven to 350°F. Line a loaf pan with parchment paper and grease with olive oil.

5. Stir the caraway and salt into the batter and transfer it to the prepared pan.

6. Sprinkle the sunflower and sesame seeds over top and bake, uncovered, for 1 hour and 30 minutes or until a toothpick comes out clean. Cool the bread on a wire rack before slicing.

This bread keeps well in the refrigerator for up to 5 days. It tastes best when toasted. If freezing, slice the bread first.

Easy Sourdough Focaccia

This simple recipe for a spongy, satisfying, grain-free focaccia is a great substitute for the grain-based version. The sourdough develops through fermentation and naturally raises the bread without the need for yeast or baking powder. I get the best sourdough when I ferment it at a consistent room temperature of 75°F for 12 to 24 hours or until the batter thickens and starts to bubble.

A practical tip: On cooler days, leave the batter in a warm place, such as in an oven with the light on or under a microwave light, to achieve a consistent temperature of 75°F.

2 cups sprouted or regular chickpea flour

2 cups filtered water
(chloride- and fluoride-free)

2 tablespoons extra virgin olive oil, plus more for the pan

1 teaspoon dried rosemary

½ teaspoon fine sea salt

Equipment: 9 × 5 3/4 × 2-inch baking pan, parchment paper

—————————————

Makes: 1 loaf, 6 to 8 servings
Prep Time: 10 minutes
Fermentation Time: 12 to 24 hours
Cooking Time: 50 minutes
Total Time: 25 hours

1. In a large bowl, mix the chickpea flour and water to form a smooth batter. Cover with a clean kitchen towel and let it sit on the counter for 12 to 24 hours, or until it becomes thick and bubbly.

2. Preheat the oven to 400°F.

3. Whisk the olive oil, rosemary, and salt into the chickpea batter.

4. Line a baking pan with parchment paper and grease it with a small amount of olive oil.

5. Pour the batter into the prepared pan and bake for 40 minutes or until the top becomes solid and a toothpick comes out clean.

6. Grab the sides of the parchment paper and lift the bread out of the pan. Let it cool on a wire rack before slicing and serving. It's best served warm with a dollop of ghee or a drizzle of olive oil. Cool completely and then store in an airtight container at room temperature for up to 3 days.

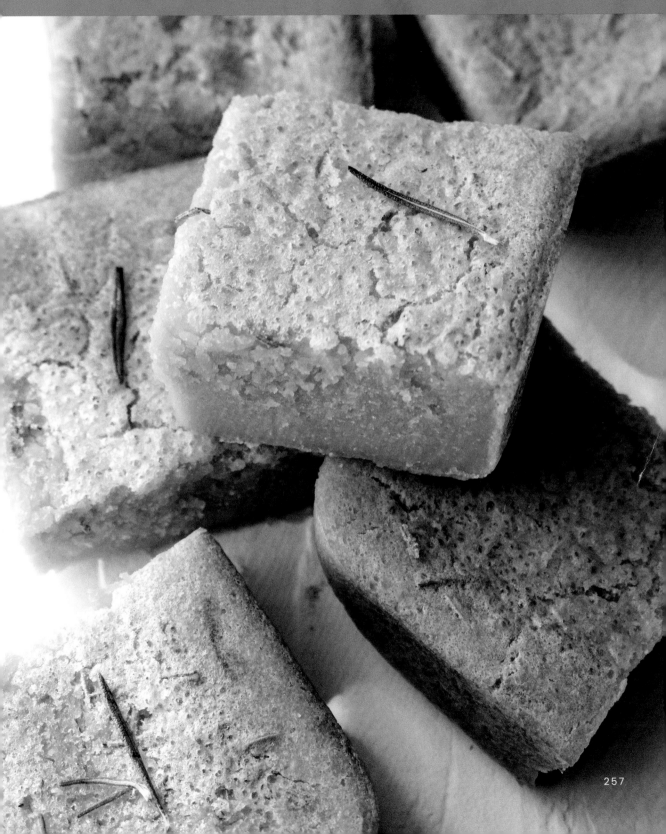

Bases

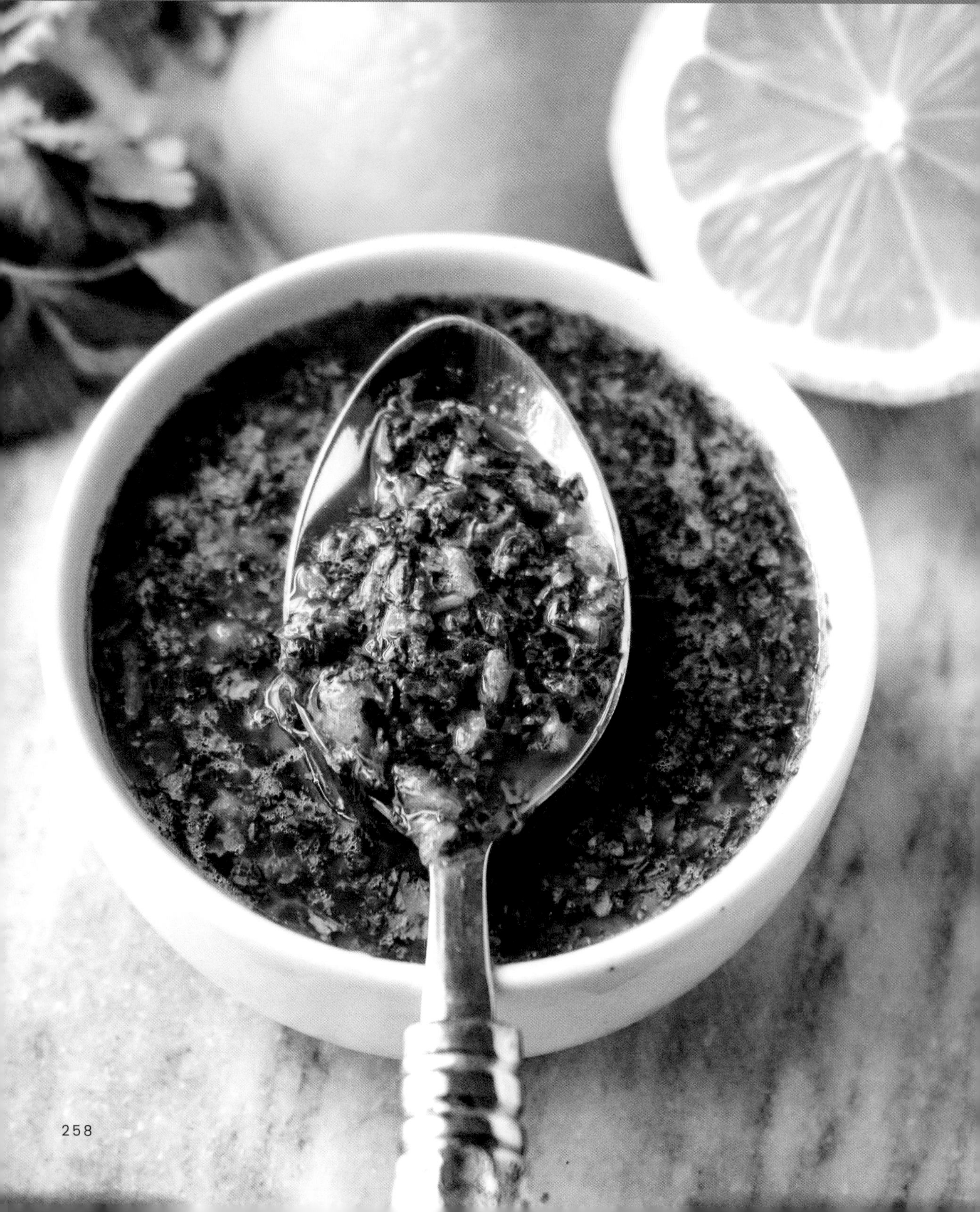

Chimichurri Sauce

Drizzle this bright and tangy sauce over fish, steak, or vegetables. Alkalize and load up your body with vitamin C with freshly squeezed lemon juice and support your liver with the lemon peel. Cilantro and parsley aid digestion with their slightly bitter qualities, boost the immune system, and flood your cells with countless phytonutrient goodness. If you don't like cilantro, substitute it with parsley, basil, or arugula.

2 cups firmly packed fresh cilantro, coarsely chopped

2 cups firmly packed fresh parsley, coarsely chopped

2 tablespoons dried oregano

1 shallot, chopped

Freshly grated zest of 2 lemons

½ cup freshly squeezed lemon juice

1 teaspoon fine sea salt

1 cup extra virgin olive oil

Equipment: High-speed blender, 24-ounce glass jar

1. Place cilantro and parsley in a high-speed blender and pack them down.

2. Add remaining ingredients and, starting slowly, begin to pulse the mixture. Use the tamper to push the herbs to the bottom. If necessary, increase the speed slightly, but not too high. Continue to pulse until smooth.

3. Transfer to a 24-ounce glass jar and label it.

Store in the refrigerator for up to 2 weeks or freeze for up to 3 months. If freezing in a jar, leave a 1-inch headspace, but I suggest freezing the sauce in ice-cube trays or flat in a zip-top bag, squeezing out as much air as possible.

Makes: 3 cups
Prep time: 15 minutes

Bases

6 pounds beef, chicken, pork, or lamb marrow bones, knuckle bones, and/or short ribs

2 medium onions, unpeeled and coarsely chopped

2 carrots, coarsely chopped

4 celery stalks, coarsely chopped

½ cup apple cider vinegar

2-inch piece fresh ginger, unpeeled and coarsely chopped

1 (8-inch) kelp strip

2 dried bay leaves

Several thyme sprigs

2 rosemary sprigs

1 teaspoon black peppercorns

6 quarts filtered water

1 bunch parsley

Equipment: 10-quart stockpot or larger (a multicooker, a pressure cooker, or a slow cooker will also work), parchment paper, rimmed roasting pan, fine-mesh sieve, wide-mouth funnel, and six (1-quart) mason jars

---

1. Preheat the oven to 450°F. Line a roasting pan with parchment paper. Arrange bones in a single layer on the pan. Roast for 20 minutes, until the bones are browned. Turn bones and turn on the broiler. Roast 10 minutes longer.

2. Transfer the roasted bones to the stockpot. Save any fat that has run off to use later or discard. Add bones to the pot with the onions, carrots, celery, apple cider vinegar, ginger, kelp, bay leaves, thyme, rosemary, and peppercorns. Add the water, cover with a lid, and bring to a boil over high heat. Reduce heat to low and simmer for 1 hour.

3. Remove any scum that has risen to the top of broth and simmer another 12 to 72 hours. The slower and longer the simmer, the more nutrient-dense the bone broth will be. If using a 10-quart stock pot, after 12 hours, remove melted fat with a large spoon. Add parsley 10 minutes before finishing.

4. Remove all the solids with tongs and discard. Strain broth through a fine-mesh sieve and transfer to mason jars.

5. Once broth has cooled to room temperature, store in the refrigerator.

Keeps well in the refrigerator for up to 10 days and in the freezer for up to 6 months. If freezing, leave 1-inch of headspace in the jars.

Makes: 6 quarts
Prep Time: 15 minutes
Cooking Time: 13 hours, 30 minutes
Total Time: 13 hours, 45 minutes

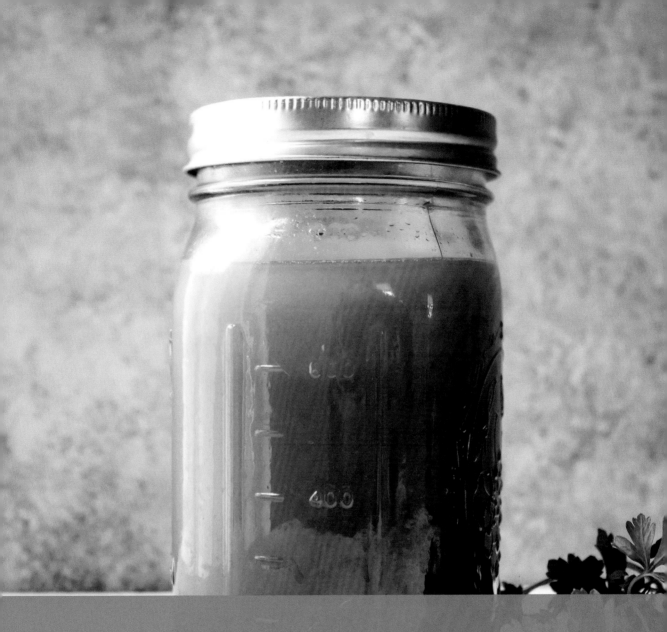

Bone Broth

Add gut-protecting collagen to your favorite soups and stews with this beefy bone broth. Collagen is rich in glycine, an amino acid that helps restore skin, joints, and connective tissue, helping them maintain elasticity. Sea kelp is rich in iodine, and fresh herbs like rosemary and thyme add a dose of antioxidants, anti-inflammatories, and complexity to the flavor of the broth.

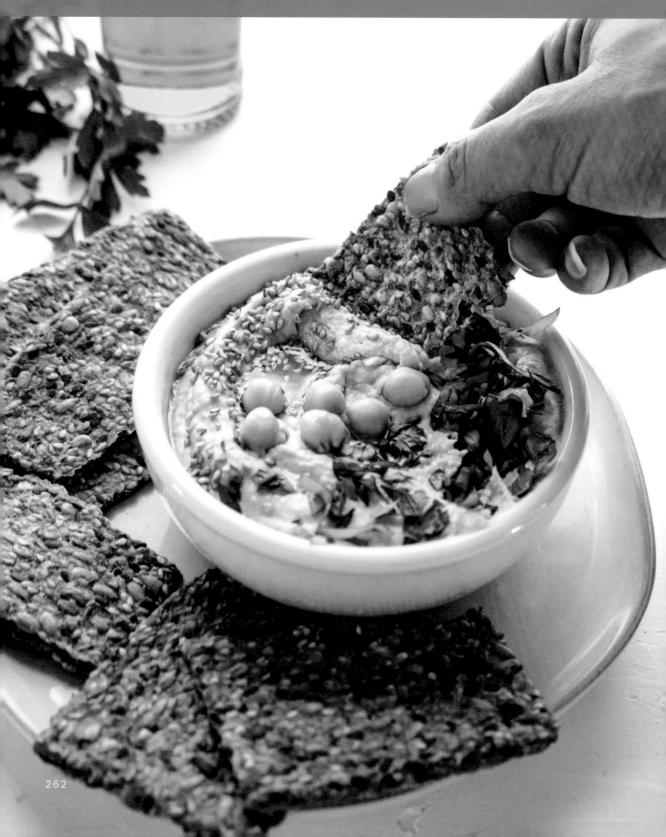

Fresh Herb Hummus

This quick and flavorful hummus is the perfect snack alongside seedy crackers or fresh vegetables. It also makes a wonderful sandwich spread, adding protein, healthy fats, fiber, and antioxidants. Best of all, it's whipped up in a blender for easy cleanup.

The base for this hummus is versatile and can be enhanced with any of your favorite herbs that you have on hand, like thyme, cilantro, or basil, for a no-waste way to use fresh herbs.

1 (15.5-ounce) can drained chickpeas

⅓ cup tahini

¼ cup extra virgin olive oil

¼ cup filtered water

2 tablespoons freshly squeezed lemon juice

2 garlic cloves

1 teaspoon ground cumin

1 teaspoon sea salt

For The Topping

Extra virgin olive oil

1 teaspoon toasted sesame seeds

2 tablespoons chopped fresh basil

2 tablespoons chopped fresh parsley

Equipment: High-speed blender or food processor

1. Add the chickpeas, tahini, olive oil, water, lemon juice, garlic, cumin, and sea salt to a high-speed blender.

2. Blend on medium-high speed until smooth and creamy, using the tamper to stir as you blend.

3. Transfer the hummus to a bowl and drizzle with additional olive oil. Top with sesame seeds, basil and parsley.

Store in an airtight container in the refrigerator for up to 1 week.

Prep time: 15 minutes
Serves: 6

Basil Walnut Pesto

Perfect for topping cooked vegetables, chicken, or fish, this dairy-free herb pesto is rich in flavor and aroma. Toasted walnuts add healthy fats and the texture of Parmesan cheese without the use of dairy.

½ cup raw walnuts

1 cup fresh basil leaves

1 cup fresh flat-leaf parsley leaves

½ cup extra virgin olive oil

1 tablespoon freshly grated lemon zest

2 teaspoons freshly squeezed lemon juice

1 teaspoon minced garlic

½ teaspoon sea salt

Equipment: Food processor or high-speed blender, 16-ounce mason jar

_____

Makes: ~ ¾ Cup

1. In a dry pan over medium-low heat, heat the walnuts for 8 to 9 minutes, or until lightly browned, stirring occasionally. Transfer walnuts to a bowl and cool completely before making the pesto.

2. Combine all of the ingredients in a food processor and pulse until the walnuts are finely ground and ingredients are thoroughly mixed, scraping the sides of the bowl as needed.

3. Transfer to a 16-ounce mason jar.

Store in the refrigerator for up to 1 week or freeze in a zip top bag or ice cube tray for up to 2 months.

Bases

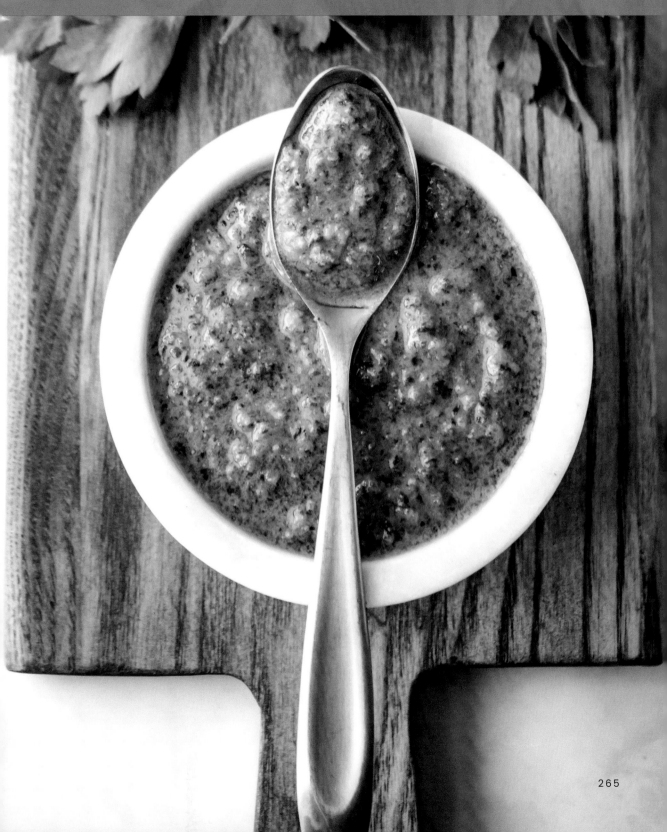

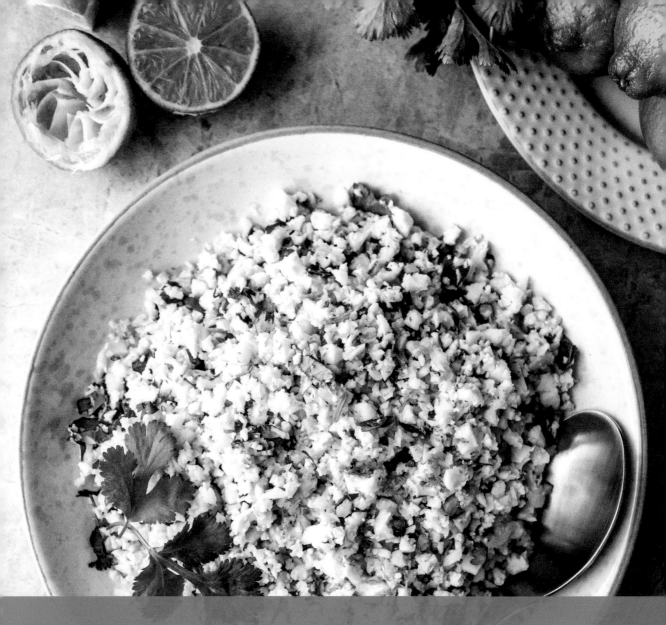

Cilantro Lime Cauliflower Rice

Bright lime and fresh cilantro come together in this easy cauliflower rice packed with a hefty dose of vitamin C. The recipe can be made ahead of time and refrigerated until cooking for easy preparation on busy days. It's the perfect alternative to traditional rice when you want to lighten things up.

Bases

2 medium heads cauliflower, sliced into florets

1 cup chopped cilantro

2 teaspoons freshly grated lime zest

¼ cup freshly squeezed lime juice

2 tablespoons extra virgin olive oil

1 teaspoon sea salt

Equipment: Food processor

———————————————

Makes: 8 (1 cup) servings
Prep time: 10 minutes

1. Working in batches, add 2 to 3 cups of cauliflower to a food processor and pulse until fine. Transfer to a large mixing bowl. Stir in the cilantro, lime zest, lime juice, olive oil, and salt. Cover and refrigerate until ready to cook, for up to 1 week.

2. To cook, add desired amount of cilantro-lime cauliflower rice to a skillet over medium heat and cook for 5 to 6 minutes or until softened.

Instant Pot Method

1. Prepare an ice bath if you're not serving the cauliflower rice right away. Otherwise, proceed to step 2.

2. Add 1 cup of water to the Instant Pot and insert the silicone trivet that came with your Instant Pot. Press Sauté and bring the water to a boil, about 2 to 3 minutes.

3. Once water is boiling, press Cancel and place the steamer basket with cauliflower florets on top trivet. This will keep the cauliflower from being submerged in the water and becoming soggy.

4. Secure lid and close vent valve. Press Steam for 1 minute.

5. After 1 minute, press the Quick Pressure Release button and remove the lid.

6. If not serving right away, transfer cauliflower to the ice bath for 2 minutes.

7. Drain cauliflower in a colander and transfer to a food processor with the cilantro, lime zest, lime juice, olive oil, and salt. Pulse until cauliflower florets are fine and resemble rice. Work in two batches if needed.

8. Transfer to a large bowl and cover. Serve immediately or refrigerate until ready to serve.

Lemon Parsley Vinaigrette

This bright and tangy lemon-herb vinaigrette pulls double duty as both a dipping sauce for focaccia and a salad dressing. It is made with heart-healthy olive oil and vitamin C–rich fresh lemon juice.

⅔ cup extra virgin olive oil

⅓ cup freshly squeezed lemon juice

½ cup firmly packed fresh parsley leaves

1 tablespoon raw honey

1 garlic clove

½ teaspoon fresh thyme leaves

½ teaspoon sea salt

⅛ teaspoon freshly ground black pepper

Equipment: High-speed blender or food processor, 8-ounce mason jar

1. Combine all of the ingredients in a blender and pulse on high until the parsley is thoroughly chopped.

2. Pour into an 8-ounce mason jar and label it.

Keeps well in the refrigerator for up to 2 weeks.

Makes: ~ 1 Cup
Prep time: 10 minutes

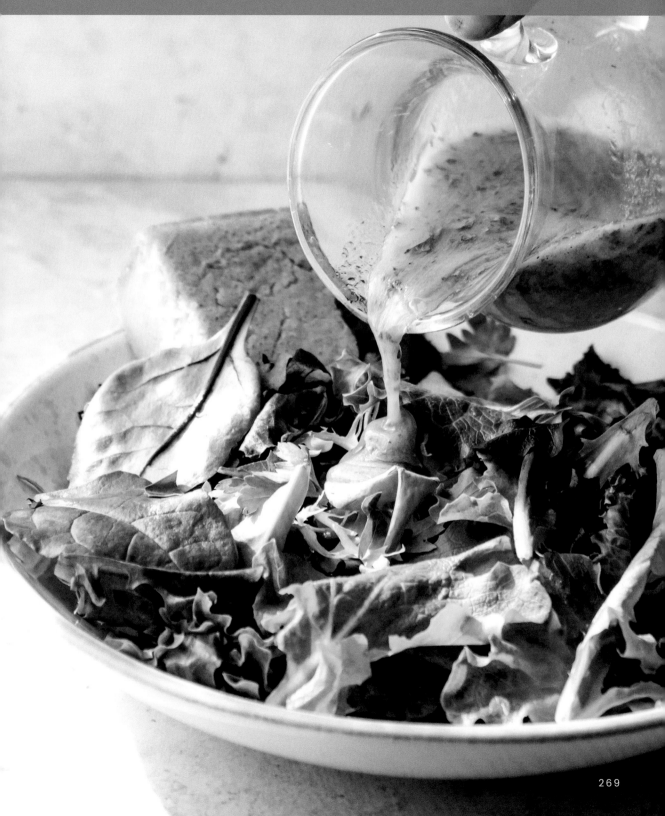

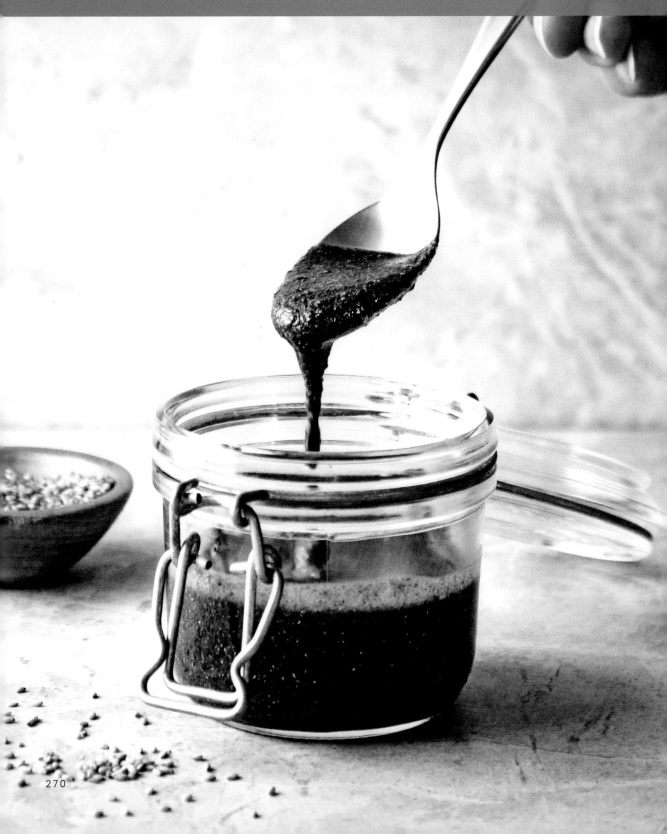

Sesame Thyme Drizzle

This recipe was inspired by a popular Middle Eastern spice mix called za'atar. What I love about it is its anti-inflammatory properties, mainly from the high content of thyme. Sumac, a tart berry (which here can be substituted with lemon peel) is loaded with vitamin C. Cumin and coriander are wonderful digestive aids. I hope you will fall in love with this versatile drizzle, which goes well with pretty much everything!

¼ cup sesame seeds, toasted

¼ cup ground cumin

¼ cup ground coriander

¼ cup ground sumac or ground dried lemon peel

¼ cup ground thyme

1 teaspoon fine sea salt

¾ cup extra virgin olive oil

Equipment: High-speed blender or food processor

1. Combine the sesame seeds, cumin, coriander, sumac, thyme, and salt in a coffee or spice grinder. Pulse several times until the sesame seeds and herbs are well combined.

2. Transfer the mixture to a mason jar and pour the olive oil over it until covered by ½ inch. Stir until thoroughly combined. Add additional oil for a thinner drizzle.

Store at room temperature.

Keeps well at room temperature for up to 2 months.

Makes: 1 cup, ~16 (1 tablespoon) servings
Prep time: 5 minutes

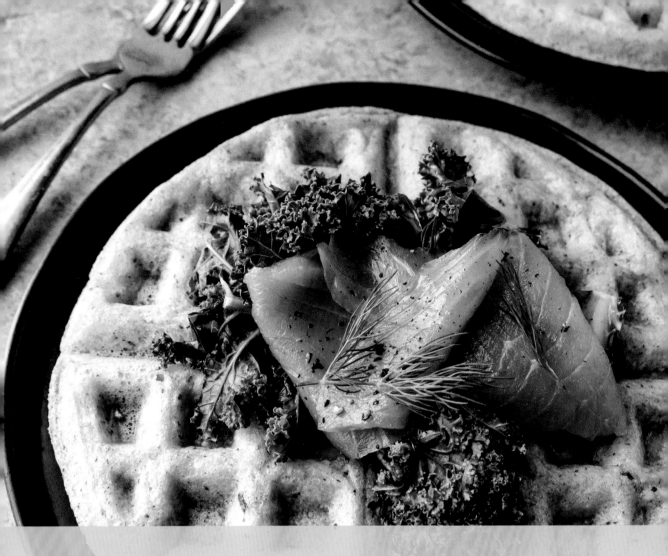

Salmon & Chives Over Waffles

These savory waffles are egg- and dairy-free without sacrificing the texture. They crisp up on the outside while staying fluffy and chewy on the inside. The savory batter has built-in buttery ghee and chive flavor while flax seed adds a boost of fiber and phytoestrogens. Topped with heart-healthy salmon and sautéed kale, you won't miss the eggs with this filling breakfast.

Half of each Belgian-style waffle is a serving, leaving room for leftovers. Slice into triangles and freeze in an airtight container for easy reheating.

For the Waffles

1 cup Bob's Red Mill Gluten-Free 1-to-1 Baking Flour

1½ cups unsweetened almond milk

5 tablespoons melted ghee, plus more for greasing

1 tablespoon minced fresh chives

2 teaspoons freshly ground flax seed

1 teaspoon aluminum-free baking powder

1 teaspoon sea salt

For the Topping

1 tablespoon extra virgin olive oil

1 cup fresh chopped kale

2 ounces smoked salmon

2 tablespoons chopped fresh dill

Pinch of sea salt

Freshly ground black pepper

Equipment: Waffle maker, medium (10-inch) skillet

Waffles:

1. Preheat a waffle maker according to manufacturer's directions and lightly grease with ghee.

2. Meanwhile, in a large bowl, stir together the ingredients for the waffle batter.

3. Pour ⅔ cup of the waffle batter onto the hot waffle maker and spread it evenly, leaving ½ inch around the perimeter. Close the lid and allow the waffle to cook for 6 to 7 minutes or until fully cooked. Repeat the process with remaining batter.

4. While the waffles cook, in a skillet, heat the olive oil over medium heat. Add the kale and sauté for 3 to 5 minutes. Season with salt and pepper.

5. Serve the waffles hot, topped with salmon, sautéed kale, and fresh dill.

Skillet Method (pancakes):

1. Heat a large griddle or pan over medium heat and grease with ghee. Allow the pan to get very hot, about 2 minutes.

2. Pour ½ cup of the batter onto the pan and cook for 4 minutes or until bubbles form and begin to pop on the surface of pancakes. Flip with a spatula and cook for 3 to 4 minutes more. Repeat with the remaining batter. Serve hot, topped with salmon, sautéed kale and dill.

Serves: 4
Prep time: 10 minutes
Cooking time: 20 minutes
Total time: 30 minutes

Avocado Sprout Smoothie

Broccoli sprouts are packed with a wonderful substance called sulforaphane, a powerful antioxidant that supports detoxification in the liver and has anticancer properties. They pair wonderfully with creamy, healthy fat-packed avocado and bright, fresh citrus.

1 large avocado, peeled, pitted, and chopped

1 cup firmly packed raw broccoli sprouts

¼ cup freshly squeezed lime or lemon juice

2 scoops collagen powder

2 tablespoons flax seed

⅛ teaspoon sea salt

Water

Equipment: Blender

1. Place all of the ingredients in the blender. Top it up with water until all the ingredients are well covered.

2. Blend until silky smooth. Drink right away.

Serves: 2
Prep time: 5 minutes
Blending time: 1 minute
Total time: 6 minutes

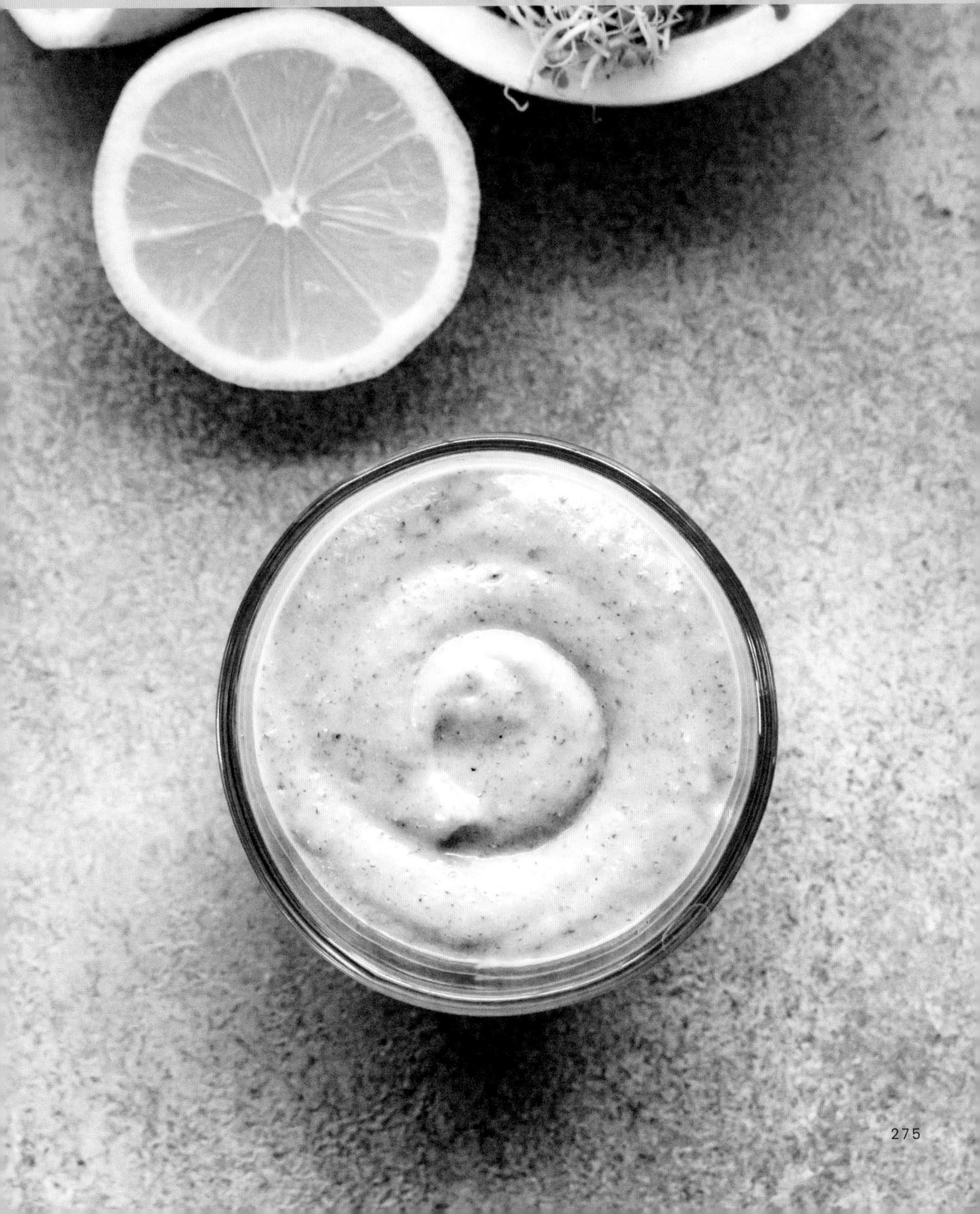

Farmer's Wife's Breakfast

This recipe was inspired by the formidable woman who served many of these breakfasts at one of the best farmers' markets ever, in San Rafael, Marin County, California—the Farmer's Wife. Feel free to modify the patties by replacing half of the lamb with ground pork, bison, beef, chicken, or turkey. Experiment with different herbs, spices, or even fruit that resonate with you and help you to feel energetically balanced. Try some cumin, nutmeg, and apricots or dried cherries.

For the Patties

1 pound ground beef, lamb, bison, turkey or a combination of any of them

2 tablespoons ground fennel seed

2 tablespoons apple cider vinegar

2 tablespoons coconut aminos

1 teaspoon smoked sea salt

1 tablespoon ghee, divided

For the Salad

2 cups mixed greens, such as arugula, bitter greens, mizuna, baby kale, or baby spinach

2 tablespoons extra virgin olive oil

1 tablespoon freshly squeezed lemon juice

Pinch of sea salt

For the Sides

1 ripe avocado, peeled, pitted, and sliced

1 cup lacto-fermented sauerkraut

½ cup fresh pomegranate seeds (optional)

1. To make the patties, in a large bowl, mix together the meat, fennel seed, apple cider vinegar, coconut aminos, and salt.

2. Using your hands, form the mixture into twelve patties.

3. In a skillet over medium-high heat, heat 1 ½ teaspoons ghee. Place six patties in the hot skillet and fry for 4 minutes or until brown. Flip and fry for 3 minutes more. Transfer the cooked patties to a plate. Set aside. Add the remaining ghee to the skillet and fry the remaining patties.

4. To make the salad, in a medium bowl, toss the greens with the olive oil, lemon, and salt until well coated.

5. To serve, divide the salad between two plates and top each with two patties, half the avocado, sauerkraut, and pomegranate seeds. Store the remaining patties for the next day's breakfast.

Patties keep well in the refrigerator for up to 5 days or in the freezer for up to 3 months.

Equipment: Large (11- or 12-inch) skillet

Makes: 12 patties, 6 (2-patty) servings (refrigerate or freeze the leftovers)
Prep time: 20 minutes
Cooking time: 30 minutes

Fisherman's Breakfast

I absolutely love the combination of avocado and smoked salmon in this delightful savory breakfast. It bursts with flavor and is packed with protein. If you are not a fan of smoked salmon, use cooked salmon instead.

Be sure to use bread that is truly whole grain- and gluten-free. Think breads that contain millet, quinoa, buckwheat flours, and a variety of seeds. Steer clear of breads containing a list of white flours, such as tapioca, rice, potato starch, and gums like xanthan gum, which can be irritating to sensitive digestion. There are also many different varieties of sprouts available. My preference is broccoli sprouts for their content of sulforaphane and support in estrogen detoxification.

4 slices Polish Sourdough Buckwheat Bread (page 254) or store-bought gluten-free bread

4 tablespoons Chimichurri Sauce (page 258)

4 tablespoons Sesame Thyme Drizzle (page 270)

4 to 6 ounces sockeye smoked salmon

1 ripe avocado, peeled, pitted, and sliced

½ cup broccoli sprouts

½ cup lacto-fermented sauerkraut

1. Toast the bread. Spread a layer of the chimichurri sauce onto each piece of toast followed by a layer of sesame thyme drizzle.

2. Evenly distribute the salmon and avocado among the toast and top each piece with sprouts and sauerkraut. Serve immediately.

Serves: 4
Prep time: 15 minutes
Cooking time: 35 minutes

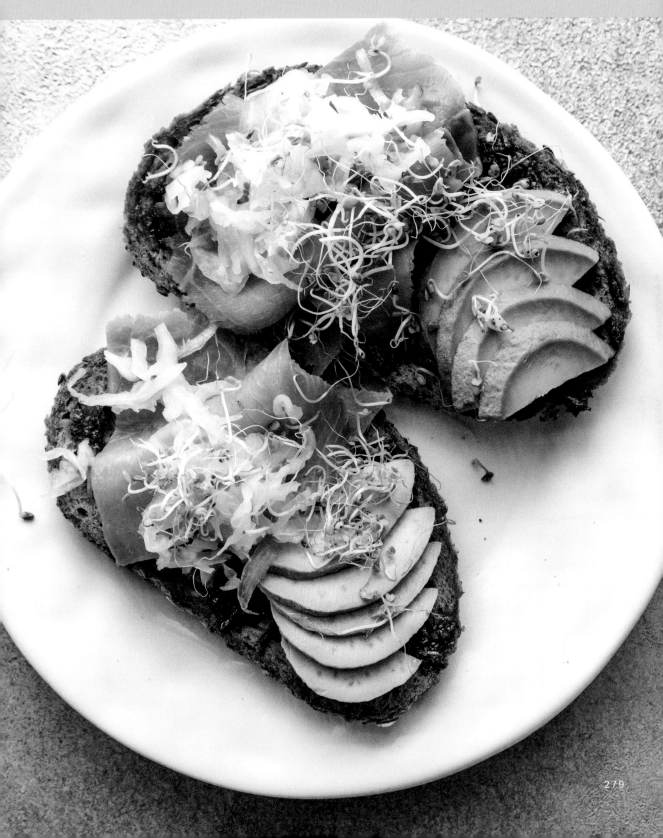

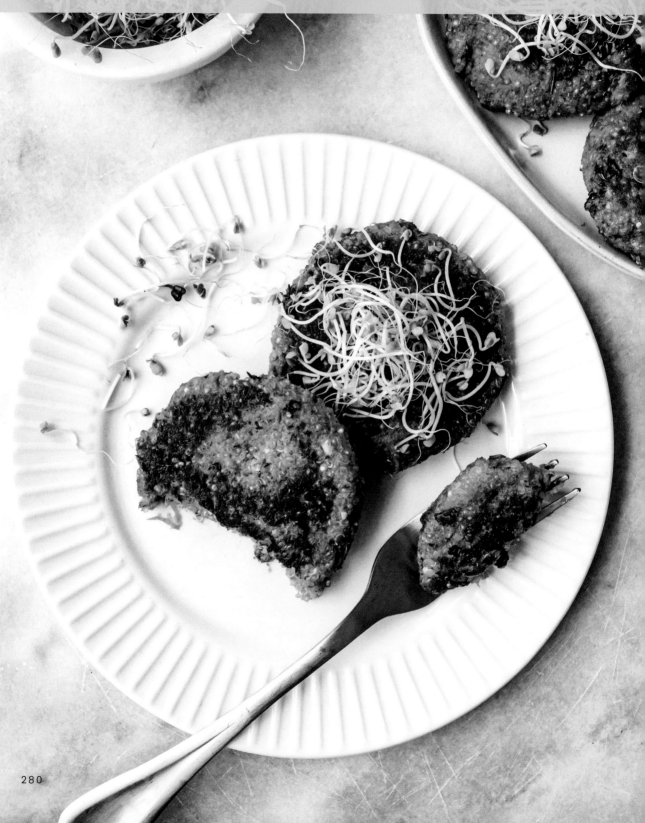

Sweet Potato Quinoa Patties

These patties are a plant-based breakfast that doesn't sacrifice protein or leave you hungry. Sweet potatoes are rich in fiber, which helps to curb hunger and provides sustained energy. Quinoa adds hearty texture and is a terrific plant-based source of protein.

½ cup uncooked quinoa

1 cup peeled, cooked, mashed sweet potatoes

½ cup finely chopped fresh parsley

2 tablespoons freshly ground flaxseed

2 tablespoons Bob's Red Mill Gluten-Free 1-to-1 Baking Flour

2 teaspoons ground turmeric

1½ teaspoons ground cumin

½ teaspoon ground coriander

1 teaspoon minced garlic

1 teaspoon sea salt

¼ teaspoon freshly ground black pepper

3 tablespoons extra virgin olive oil, for cooking, divided

1 cup raw broccoli sprouts

Makes: 8 patties, 4 (2-patty) servings
Prep time: 20 minutes
Cooking time: 20 minutes
Total time: 20 minutes

1. Place the quinoa in a sieve and rinse under cold running water.

2. In a small saucepan combine the rinsed quinoa and 1 cup of water. Bring to a boil, then reduce the heat to low. Simmer, covered, for 15 to 20 minutes, or until quinoa is tender. Turn off the heat and allow quinoa to cool and absorb all the water, 8 to 10 minutes.

3. In a medium mixing bowl, combine the cooled quinoa with the remaining ingredients, except the olive oil and broccoli sprouts, and stir well.

4. In a medium skillet, heat 2 tablespoons of the olive oil over medium heat for 1 minute. Using a ¼ cup measuring cup, scoop the quinoa mixture and, using your hands, form it into 8 patties.

5. Place 4 patties into the pan and cook for 3 to 4 minutes. Gently flip and cook the patties for 3 minutes more.

6. Add the remaining tablespoon of olive oil to the pan and fry the other 4 patties.

7. Serve the patties hot, topped with the broccoli sprouts.

Equipment: Fine-mesh sieve, medium (10-inch) heavy-bottomed skillet

Avocado Cacao Muffins

These muffins are low in added sugar but deliver plenty of chocolate flavor. They're ideal for breakfast, with filling fiber from flax seeds, protein, and plenty of healthy fats to keep you satisfied until lunch.

1 cup blanched almond flour

½ cup Bob's Red Mill Gluten-Free 1-to-1 Baking Flour

½ cup unsweetened cacao powder

2 teaspoons aluminum-free baking powder

½ teaspoon sea salt

2 tablespoons freshly ground flax seeds

⅓ cup mashed avocado

⅔ cup unsweetened almond milk

⅓ cup pure maple syrup

2 teaspoons pure vanilla extract

Equipment: Muffin tin, paper or silicone muffin liners, high-speed blender

1. Preheat the oven to 350°F and line a muffin tin with 6 paper muffin liners.

2. In a medium bowl, combine the almond flour, gluten-free flour, cacao powder, baking powder and salt.

3. In a blender, combine the flax seeds, avocado, almond milk, maple syrup, and vanilla. Blend until smooth.

4. Gradually add the wet ingredients to the flour mixture, stirring until well combined.

5. Divide the batter among the muffin cups, spreading it evenly. You can also tap the tin on the countertop to evenly distribute the batter in the cups. Bake for 30 minutes or until a toothpick comes out clean.

6. Cool in the tin for 30 minutes before serving.

Store in an airtight container in the refrigerator for up to 1 week or freeze for up to 2 months.

Makes: 6
Prep time: 10 minutes
Cooking time: 30 minutes
Total time: 40 minutes

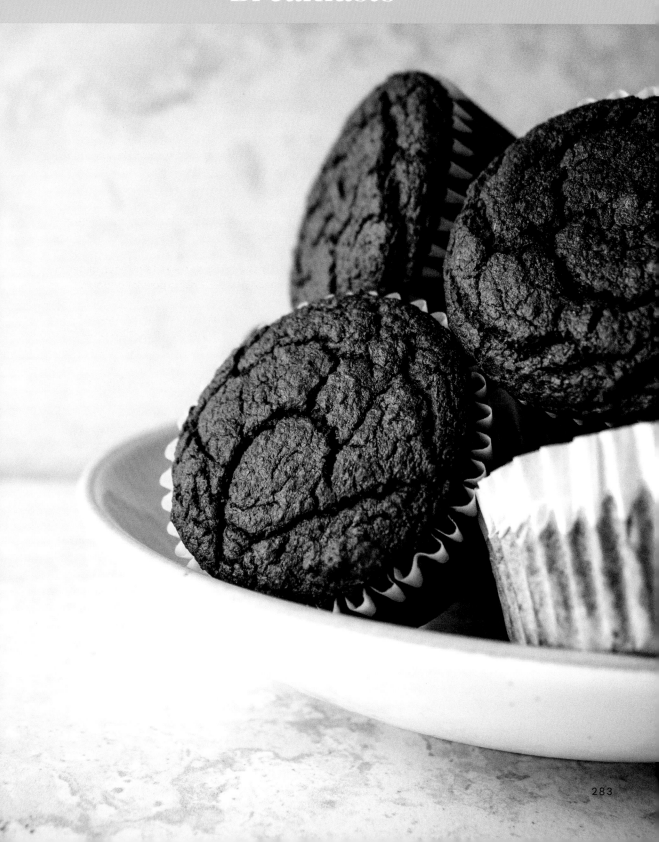

Breakfasts

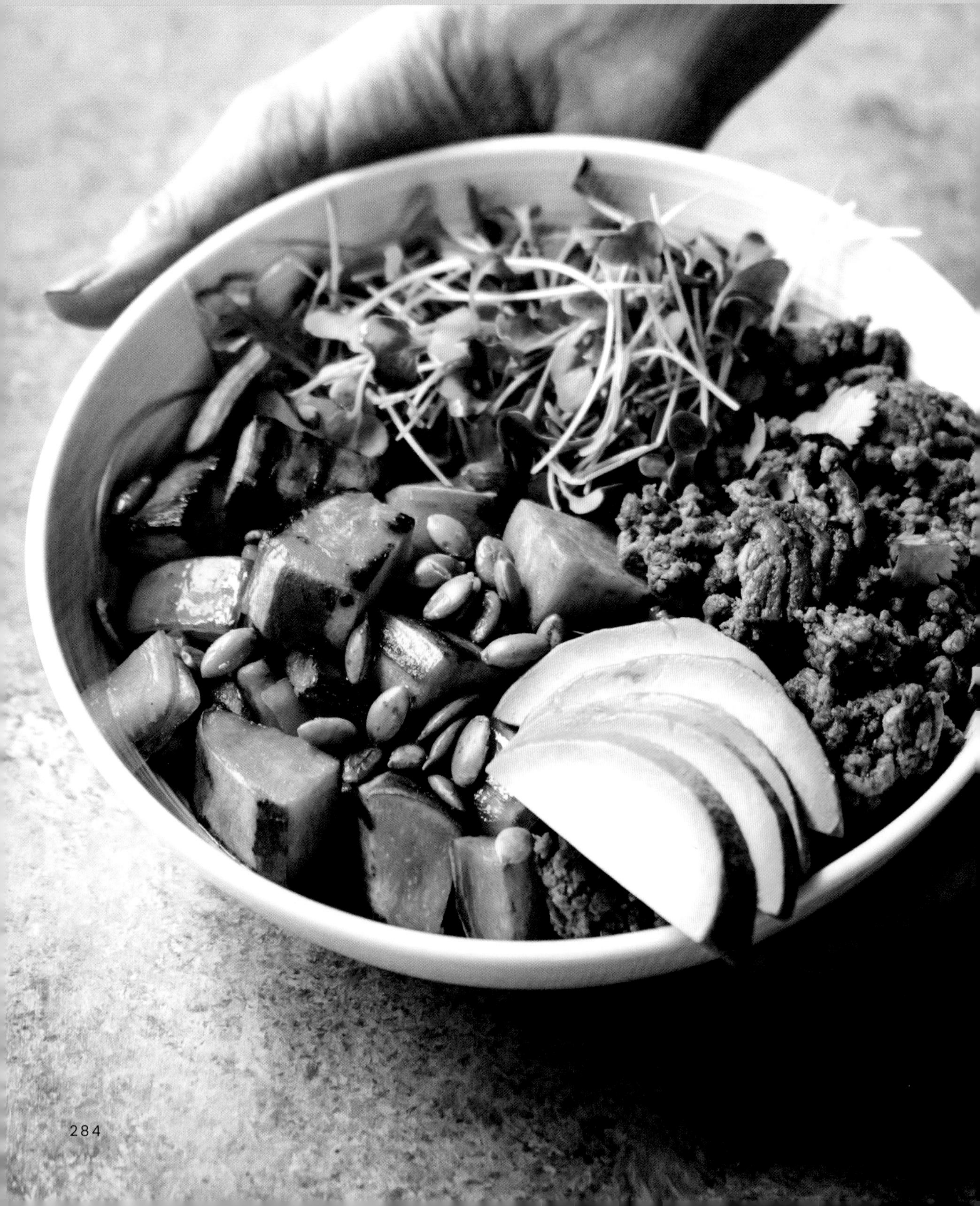

Southwest Breakfast Bowl

For a breakfast bowl high in protein, fiber and antioxidants like beta carotene, reach for this hearty recipe. Fresh avocado adds healthy fats while pumpkin seeds provide a dose of hormone-balancing benefits.

2 tablespoons extra virgin olive oil

2 cups raw diced sweet potatoes

½ cup chopped red onion

½ pound 85% lean grass-fed ground beef or bison

2 teaspoons ground cumin

1 teaspoon ground fennel seed

1 teaspoon sea salt

¼ teaspoon onion powder

⅓ cup chopped fresh cilantro

2 cups microgreens

1 ripe avocado, peeled, pitted, and sliced

4 tablespoons shelled raw pumpkin seeds

Equipment: Medium (10-inch) heavy bottomed skillet

1. Heat the olive oil over medium-high heat in a skillet. Add the sweet potatoes and cook, uncovered, for 10 minutes, stirring occasionally. Add the onion to the skillet and stir. Cover and continue to cook for 10 minutes or until sweet potatoes are tender. Divide between 4 bowls.

2. Return the skillet to the stove over medium heat and add the ground beef. Use a spatula to break up beef into small pieces. Cook for 5 minutes or until browned. Stir in the cumin, fennel, sea salt, and onion powder. Continue to cook for 7 minutes or until beef is completely cooked. Turn off the heat and stir in the cilantro. Divide among 4 bowls alongside sweet potatoes.

3. Add the microgreens, sliced avocado, and pumpkin seeds to each bowl. Serve immediately. Leftovers can be refrigerated in an airtight container and reheated the next day.

Serves: 4
Prep time: 10 minutes
Cooking time: 32 minutes
Total time: 42 minutes

Pineapple Arugula Smoothie

Enjoy the bright, sweet flavor of pineapple with a bit of peppery zing from arugula. Collagen powder benefits your skin, hair, nails, and gut health. Meanwhile, hemp hearts give this smoothie staying power with their healthy fats.

1 cup chopped fresh pineapple

1 cup firmly packed arugula

1-inch piece fresh ginger

¼ cup fresh mint leaves

2 scoops collagen powder

2 tablespoons hemp hearts

3 cups unsweetened almond milk

Equipment: Blender

1. Combine all of the ingredients in a blender and blend until smooth.

2. Divide between 2 glasses and enjoy right away.

Makes: 1 smoothie
Prep time: 5 minutes
Cooking time: 0 minutes
Total time: 5 minutes

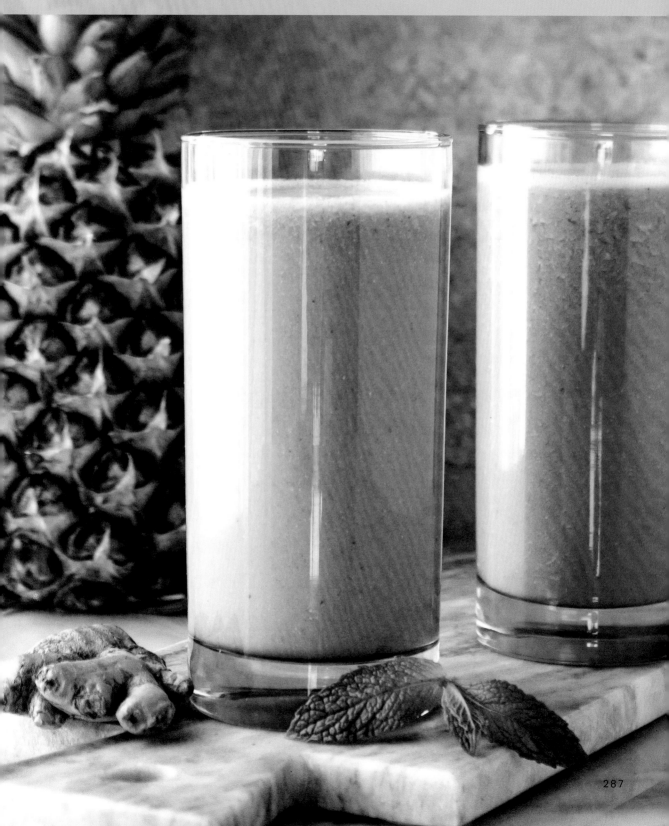

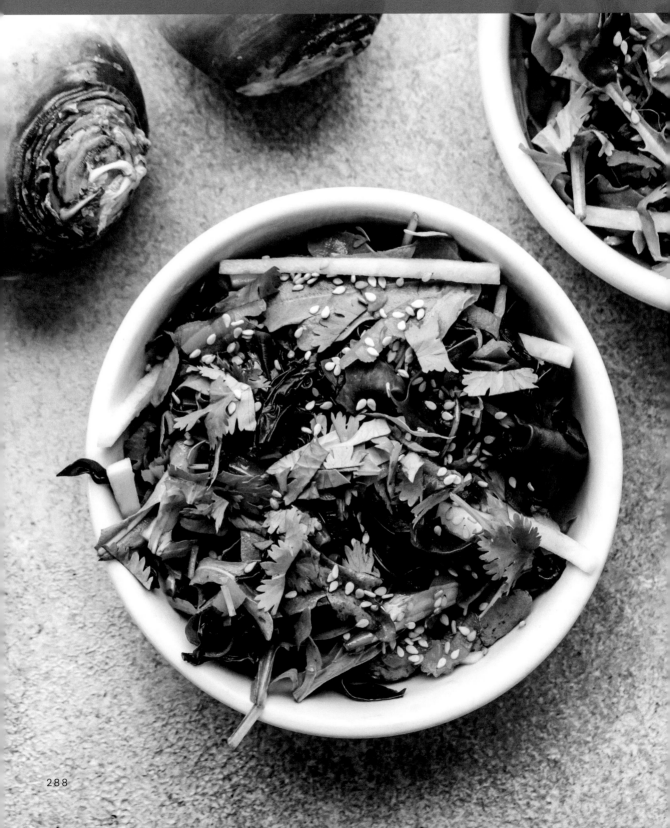

Japanese Powerhouse Salad

This salad is a nutritional powerhouse. Wakame, a readily available seaweed in most health food stores, is high in B vitamins, calcium, magnesium, and iodine. Iodine deficiency can lead to brain fog and breast lumps. It is however not recommended for Hashimoto's patients. Many women have reported feeling energized from this salad. The turnip, a crucifer, is wonderful for liver support and estrogen detoxification.

⅓ cup tightly packed wakame

2 cups firmly packed arugula or bitter greens

1 medium turnip, peeled and sliced to matchsticks

1 medium carrot, grated

2 shallots, thinly sliced

¼ cup chopped fresh cilantro

2 tablespoons black or yellow sesame seeds

For the Dressing

3 tablespoons coconut aminos

2 tablespoons toasted sesame oil

2 tablespoons rice vinegar or apple cider vinegar

Equipment: Medium bowl, large salad bowl

1. In a medium bowl, cover the wakame with room temperature water and soak for about 5 minutes or until rehydrated and soft.

2. In a large salad bowl, place the arugula, turnip, carrot, and shallots. Strain the wakame, discarding the water, and add it to the salad bowl.

3. Place all of the dressing ingredients in a jar, close the lid and shake until well combined.

4. Drizzle the dressing over the salad and toss until the greens are well coated.

5. Sprinkle with cilantro and sesame seeds.

Serve right away.

_____

Serves: 2
Prep time: 20 minutes

Honey Rosemary Pork Chops

Golden-brown pan-seared pork chops satisfy with sweet honey, tangy apple cider vinegar along with herby rosemary and garlic. Serve alongside sauerkraut or Brussels sprouts for a complete meal.

2 tablespoon extra virgin olive oil

3 tablespoon raw honey

3 tablespoons apple cider vinegar

2 tablespoons ghee

2 (8-ounce) bone-in pork chops

¼ teaspoon sea salt

¼ teaspoon freshly ground black pepper

1 teaspoon minced garlic

1 rosemary sprig

Equipment: Medium (10-inch) cast-iron skillet

1. In a small bowl, stir together the olive oil, honey, and apple cider vinegar.

2. In a medium cast-iron skillet, heat the ghee over medium heat for 3 minutes. Pat the pork chops dry with a paper towel and season them with salt and pepper. Add pork chops to skillet and cook for 8 minutes.

3. Flip the pork chops and sear for 2 minutes more. Add the garlic to the pan and cook for 30 seconds.

4. Reduce the heat to medium-low. Pour the honey mixture into the pan and add rosemary. Continue to cook the pork chops for 8 minutes or until they are fully cooked. Occasionally spoon honey mixture from pan onto pork chops. Serve hot.

Serves: 2
Prep time: 5 minutes
Cooking time: 22 minutes
Total time: 27 minutes

Main Dishes

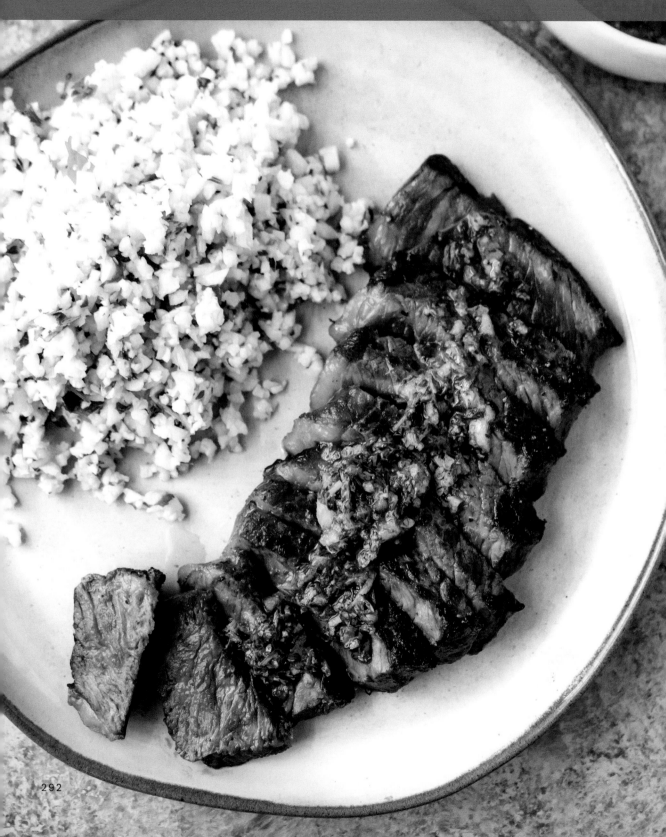

Chimichurri Steak

Strip steak is a versatile cut that is easy to cook. It's tender, affordable and, because of its fat marbling, it's juicy. The rich, meaty flavor of this seared strip steak is balanced with the bright and tangy chimichurri sauce full of vitamin C–rich lemon juice, heart-healthy olive oil, and antioxidant-rich parsley.

2 (6-ounce) strip steaks

½ cup coconut aminos

1 tablespoon toasted sesame oil

1 tablespoon minced ginger

2 teaspoons minced garlic

1 teaspoon extra virgin olive oil

Chimichurri Sauce, for serving (page 258)

Equipment: Medium (10-inch) heavy-bottomed skillet

Serves: 2
Prep time: 10 minutes
Marinating time: 2 hours
Cooking time: 17 minutes
Total time: 2 hours, 27 minutes

1. Place the steaks in a shallow glass dish. Set aside.

2. In a small bowl, stir together the coconut aminos, sesame oil, ginger, and garlic. Pour the marinade over top of the steak, cover, and refrigerate for 2 to 8 hours.

3. Remove the steaks from the marinade and discard marinade. Pat the steaks dry with a paper towel.

4. Lightly grease a medium skillet with the olive oil and heat over medium-high heat for 3 minutes. Place the steaks in the pan and sear for 3 to 4 minutes on each side for medium-rare, or longer if you prefer medium or well-done.

5. Transfer the steaks to a cutting board to rest for 5 minutes before slicing. Serve with chimichurri sauce drizzled over top.

Mediterranean Buckwheat Bowl

The flavors of the Mediterranean come together in one bowl finished with an herb-filled sesame drizzle that adds rich nutty flavor and hormone-balancing sesame seeds. This bowl has a range of flavors and textures, with chewy buckwheat and hearty sautéed vegetables. It makes a great lunch or dinner and can be enjoyed hot or chilled. For this recipe, you'll be using leftovers from the Garlicky Lemon Chicken and the Sesame Thyme Drizzle.

2 tablespoons extra virgin olive oil

½ cup sliced red onion

2 cups chopped kale, ribs removed

1 teaspoon minced garlic

2 cups cooked buckwheat

½ cup chopped fresh parsley

Sea salt and freshly ground black pepper

1 cup shredded Garlicky Lemon Chicken (page 296)

⅓ cup pitted kalamata olives

½ cup broccoli sprouts

¼ cup Sesame Thyme Drizzle (page 270)

2 lemon wedges

1. In a large skillet, heat the olive oil over medium heat. Add the onion and sauté for 5 minutes. Stir in the kale and garlic. Sauté for 3 minutes more.

2. Divide the buckwheat, parsley, and kale mixture between 2 bowls. Season with salt and pepper.

3. Top each bowl with chicken, broccoli sprouts, and olives and drizzle with the Sesame Thyme Drizzle. Serve with a wedge of lemon.

Equipment: Large (12-inch) heavy-bottomed skillet

Serves: 2
Prep time: 10 minutes
Cooking time: 8 minutes
Total time: 18 minutes

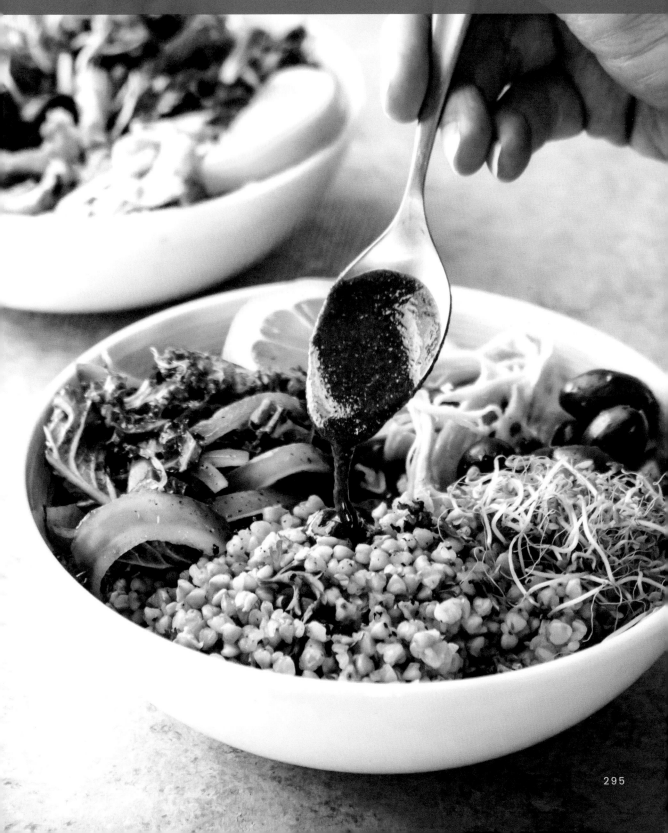

Main Dishes

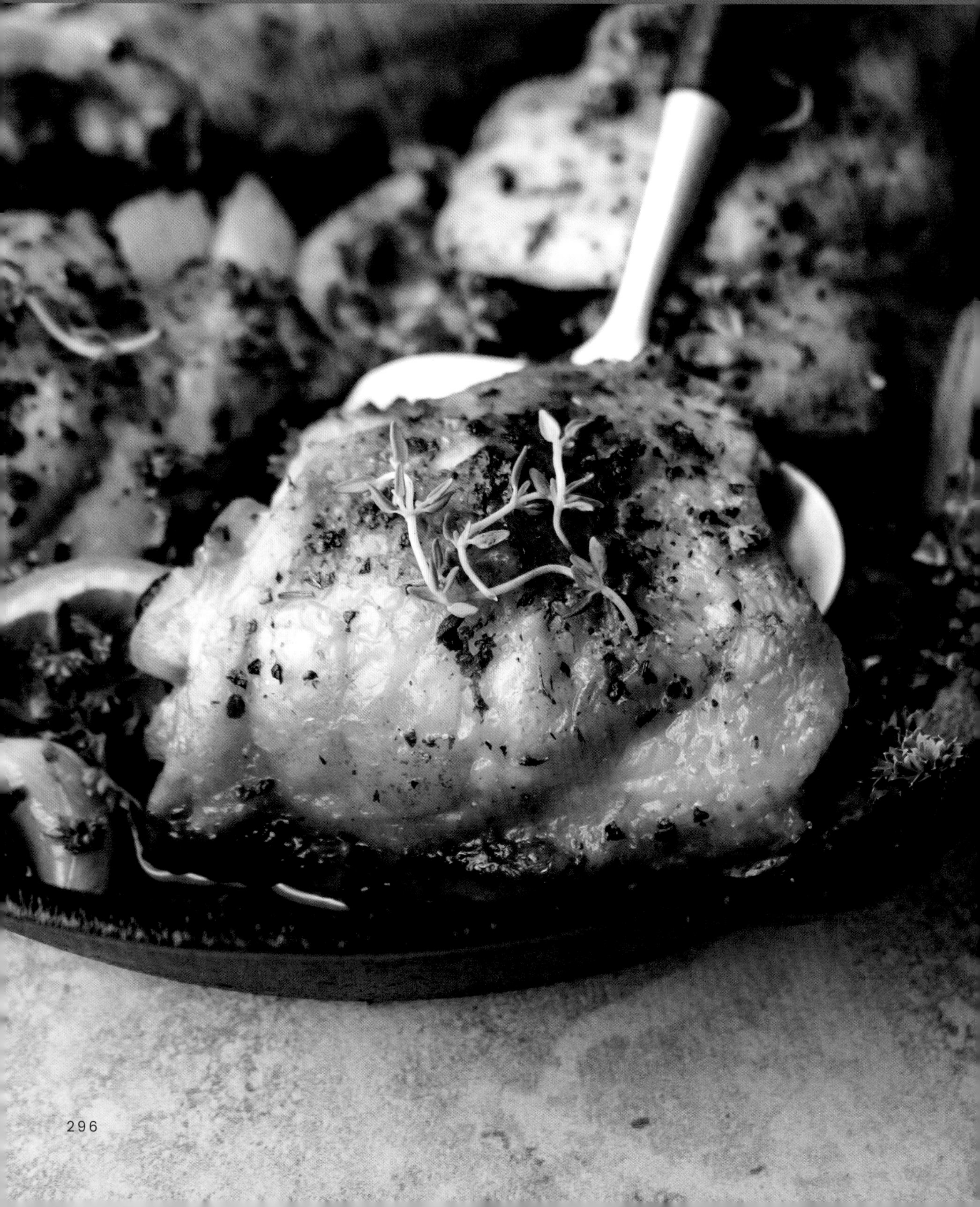

Garlicky Lemon Chicken

This one-pan chicken thigh recipe is full of fresh garlic and lemon juice, which add rich, tangy flavor to the chicken. Roasting the chicken caramelizes the garlic and keeps the meat juicy while the skin turns brown and crisp. Leftover chicken can be shredded and added to soups and salads for a quick dose of protein.

⅓ cup melted ghee, plus more for coating

2 tablespoons freshly squeezed lemon juice

2 teaspoons fresh thyme leaves

1 teaspoon dried oregano, divided

1 teaspoon sea salt, divided

¼ teaspoon freshly ground black pepper, divided

4 bone-in, skin-on chicken thighs

½ lemon, thinly sliced

8 garlic cloves

¼ cup chopped fresh parsley

Equipment: Medium (10-inch) oven-safe skillet

1. Preheat the oven to 425°F and lightly grease a medium skillet with ghee. In a small bowl, stir together the melted ghee, lemon juice, thyme, ½ teaspoon of the oregano, ½ teaspoon of the salt, and ⅛ teaspoon of the black pepper. Transfer the mixture to the skillet.

2. Pat the chicken dry with a paper towel and arrange it, skin side down, in the prepared skillet. Sprinkle the remaining oregano, remaining ½ teaspoon salt, and pepper over the chicken.

3. Tuck the lemon slices and garlic cloves around chicken and roast for 30 minutes or until the chicken skin has become crispy and golden brown. Remove from the oven and spoon the ghee mixture from the skillet over chicken. Return to the oven and roast for 10 minutes more.

4. Remove from the oven, garnish with the parsley, and serve immediately.

Serves: 4
Prep time: 15 minutes
Cooking time: 40 minutes
Total time: 1 hour 15 minutes

Beet and Hummus Sandwich

This vegetable sandwich is a hearty alternative to meat-based entrées without sacrificing the filling texture. The hearty Polish Sourdough Buckwheat Bread brings high protein content and a satisfying feeling. Sliced avocado adds healthy fat, which keeps you satiated. Instead of meat, shredded roasted beets add texture along with their potent liver-detoxing abilities.

2 teaspoons extra virgin olive oil

2 small raw beets, peeled

4 slices Polish Sourdough Buckwheat Bread (page 254) or any store-bought gluten-free bread

⅓ cup Fresh Herb Hummus (page 262)

½ a small avocado, pitted, peeled and sliced

½ cup microgreens, such as broccoli sprouts, peas, or alfalfa

_____

Serves: 2
Prep time: 10 minutes
Cooking time: 45 minutes
Total time: 55 minutes

1. Preheat the oven to 375°F. Rub the olive oil all over the beets. Place on a baking sheet lined with parchment paper and bake for 40 to 45 minutes, or until a fork easily pierces through the beets. Set aside to cool to room temperature.

2. Using a Microplane grater, shred the cooled beets. Spread half of the hummus on one slice of bread. Top with half of the shredded beets, half of the sliced avocado, and half of the microgreens. Place the other slice of bread on top. Repeat with the remaining slices of bread, shredded beets, avocado, and microgreens to create two sandwiches.

Keeps well in a refrigerator, wrapped in parchment paper or in an airtight container. Enjoy within 24 hours.

Equipment: Parchment paper, baking sheet, Microplane Grater

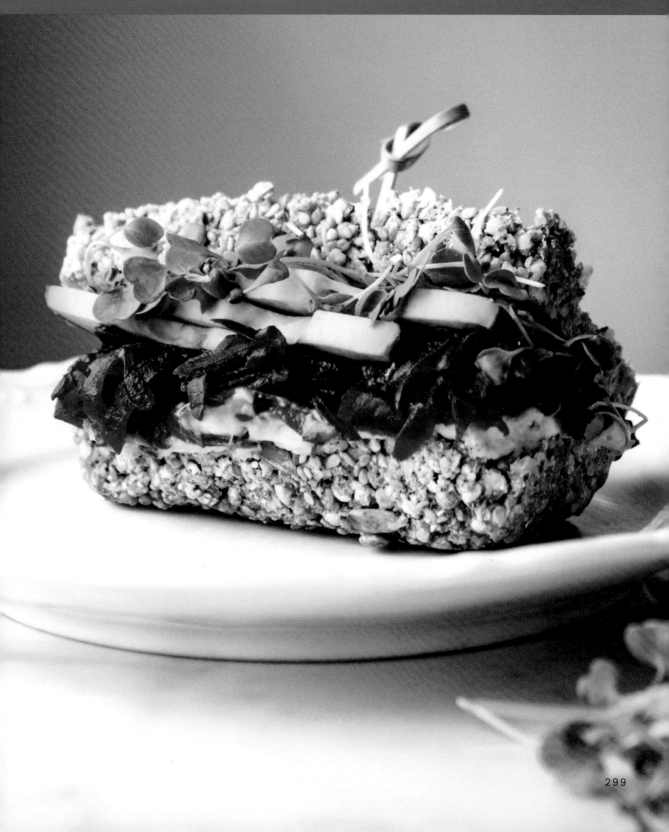

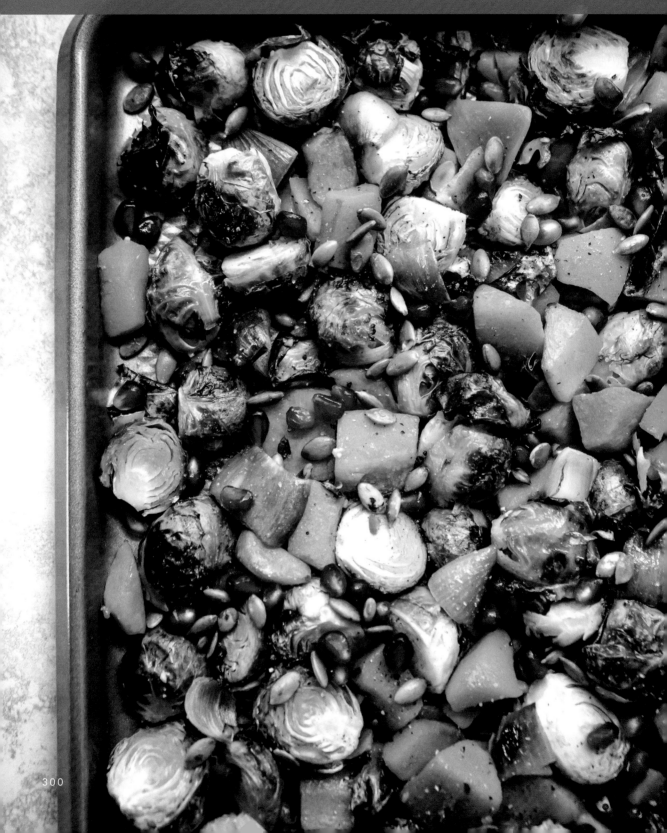

Vegetable Medley with Pomegranate and Pumpkin Seeds

This vegetable medley is hearty enough to enjoy on its own as a plant-based meal or served along-side protein like chicken, steak, or fish. It is full of fiber from Brussels sprouts and butternut squash, with an array of vitamins and antioxidants from tangy pomegranate arils. Pumpkin seeds help balance estrogen levels and add crunchy texture.

1 pound Brussels sprouts, ends cut off and sliced in half

2 cups cubed butternut squash

½ cup chopped shallot or red onion

2 tablespoons extra virgin olive oil, plus more for coating

1 tablespoon raw honey

1 teaspoon minced garlic

1 teaspoon sea salt

⅛ teaspoon freshly ground black pepper

½ cup pomegranate seeds

2 tablespoons raw shelled pumpkin seeds

Equipment: Baking sheet

1. Preheat the oven to 425°F. Lightly grease a baking pan with olive oil. In a large bowl, combine the Brussels sprouts, butternut squash, and onion. Add the oil, honey, garlic, salt, and pepper. Gently stir to coat.

2. Transfer to the prepared baking sheet and spread out into one even layer. Bake for 15 minutes. Gently stir the vegetables and roast for 12 minutes more, or until the vegetables turn golden.

3. Remove the baking sheet from the oven and sprinkle with pomegranate and pumpkin seeds. Serve hot.

Serves: 4
Prep time: 10 minutes
Cooking time: 30 minutes
Total time: 40 minutes

Roasted Pesto Salmon

This no-fuss roasted salmon utilizes pre-prepped ingredients like the nutty Basil Walnut Pesto and Cilantro Lime Cauliflower Rice for a complete meal that's ready in under 30 minutes. Salmon and cauliflower rice are cooked on the same pan for easy cleanup.

The diverse ingredients in this recipe cover a lot of bases in the nutrition department, delivering a ton of fiber, estrogen-clearing benefits of the cruciferous vegetables, vitamin C, plenty of phytonutrients, and healthy protein and fat.

1 pound salmon, sliced into 4 pieces

1 tablespoon extra virgin olive oil

1 teaspoon raw honey

½ teaspoon sea salt

¼ teaspoon freshly ground black pepper

4 cups Cilantro Lime Cauliflower Rice (page 266)

½ cup Basil Walnut Pesto (page 264)

_____

Serves: 4
Prep time: 10 minutes
Cooking time: 14 minutes
Total time: 24 minutes

1. Preheat the oven to 425°F and position the oven rack in the upper third of the oven. Place the salmon pieces on one side of a sheet pan lined with parchment paper, skin side down.

2. In a small bowl, combine the olive oil and honey. Brush the salmon with the oil mixture; season with salt and pepper.

3. Spread the Cilantro Lime Cauliflower Rice on the other half of the pan. Transfer to the oven and roast for 10 minutes.

4. Turn on the broiler and broil the salmon and cauliflower for 3 minutes or until the top of the salmon is caramelized. Remove the pan from the oven and divide the cauliflower rice among 4 bowls. Place a piece of salmon on top of each mound of cauliflower rice and drizzle the Basil Walnut Pesto over top. Serve immediately.

Equipment: Medium baking pan, parchment paper

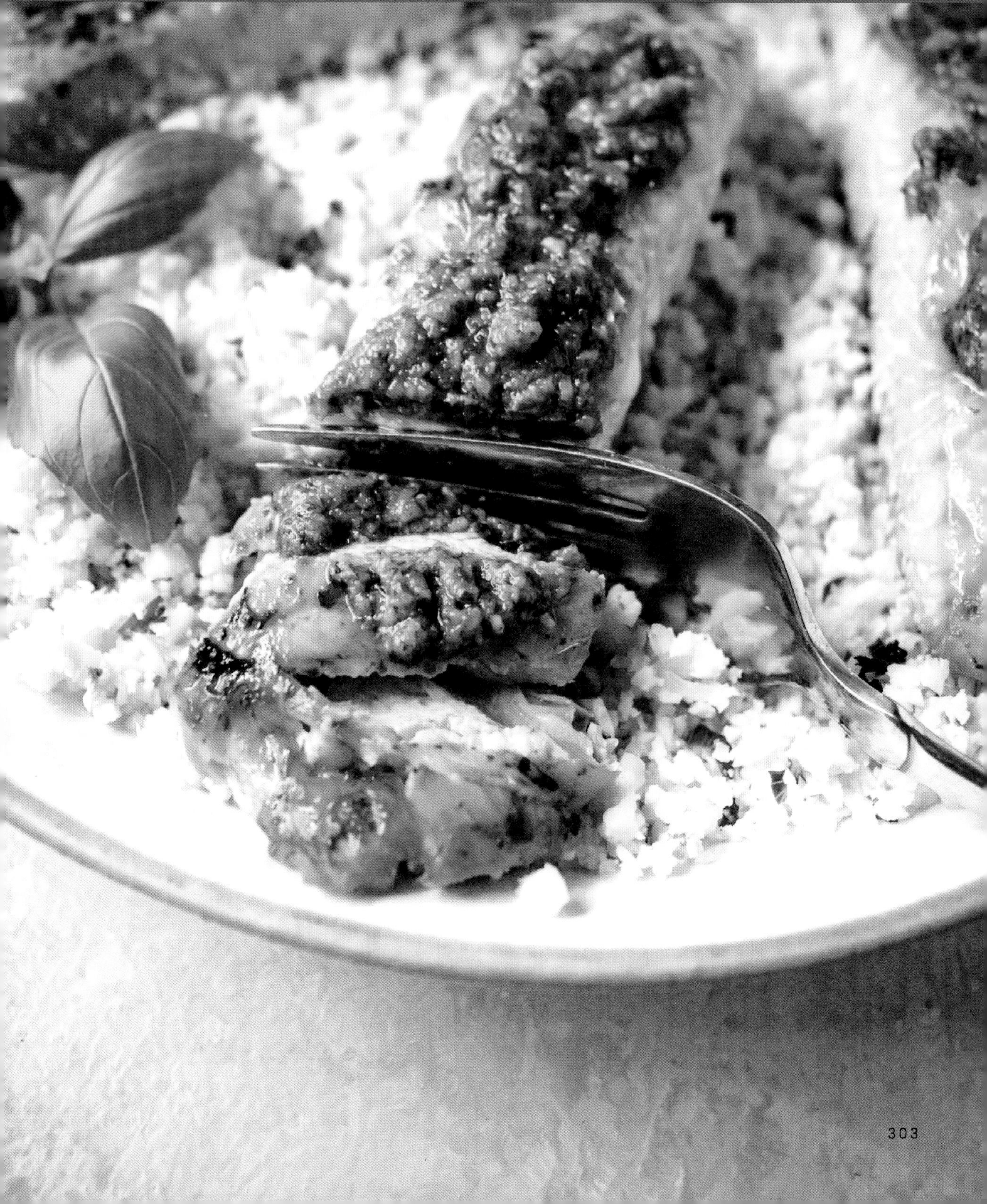

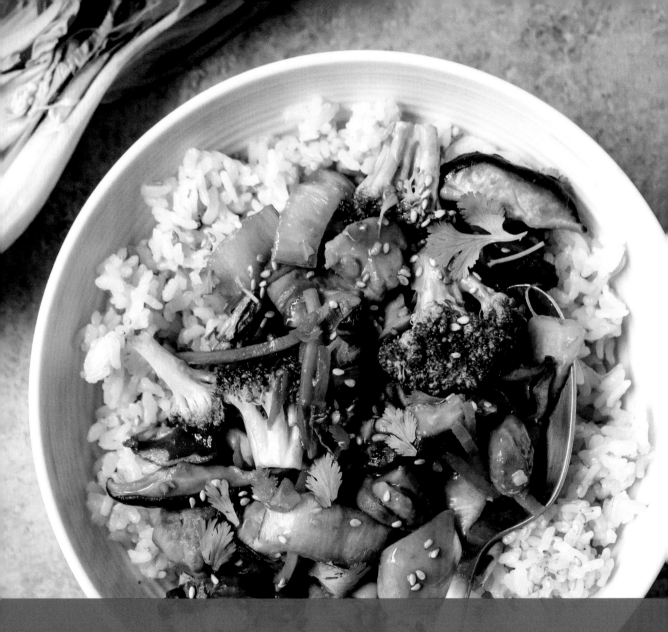

Rainbow Chicken Stir-Fry

If you are craving Asian takeout, this one-pan protein- and veggie-packed stir-fry is sure to satisfy. Stir-fry is my favorite quick meal approach because you can use any leftover vegetables and whip out a dish in under 30 minutes. Coconut aminos are used instead of soy for a lower-sodium sauce that has umami flavor and depth. Brown rice adds plenty of fiber and gives the recipe staying power, keeping you full.

Main Dishes

For the Sauce

½ cup coconut aminos

2 tablespoons toasted sesame oil

2 tablespoons freshly squeezed lime juice

1 teaspoon coconut sugar

1 teaspoon minced garlic

1 teaspoon minced ginger

1 teaspoon rice flour or any gluten-free flour

For the Chicken

1 tablespoon toasted sesame oil

1 pound boneless, skinless chicken thighs, cut into ½-inch cubes

2 cups broccoli florets

1 cup sliced shiitake mushrooms

1 cup chopped bok choy

½ cup shredded carrots

½ cup thinly sliced purple cabbage

2 teaspoons toasted sesame seeds

½ cup chopped fresh cilantro

4 cups cooked brown rice, for serving

1. To make the sauce, in a small bowl combine the sauce ingredients and whisk until the flour is dissolved. Set aside.

2. In a large skillet, heat the toasted sesame oil over medium-high heat for 2 minutes. Add the chicken cubes and cook, stirring occasionally, until browned, about 8 minutes.

3. Add the broccoli, mushrooms, bok choy, carrots, and cabbage. Pour in the sauce and stir to combine. Reduce the heat to medium and simmer for 6 to 8 minutes, until sauce thickens and vegetables are tender.

4. Serve over brown rice and garnish with the sesame seeds and cilantro.

Equipment: Large (12-inch) heavy-bottomed skillet

Serves: 4
Prep time: 10 minutes
Cooking time: 18 minutes
Total time: 28 minutes

Sesame-Ginger Crusted Cod with Asparagus

The crunch of this cod comes from the hormone-balancing sesame-seed coating—no egg or deep-frying necessary. Pieces of cod are baked until cooked through and the sesame seeds are toasted. To round out the dish, asparagus is roasted in ghee.

Cod is a rich source of immune-boosting vitamin D and protein. Look for cod that is wild-caught whenever possible for the highest quality.

2 (6-ounce) cod fillets

½ cup raw sesame seeds

1 teaspoon ground ginger

½ teaspoon sea salt

⅛ teaspoon freshly ground black pepper

6 ounces fresh asparagus, ends trimmed

1 tablespoon melted ghee

2 lemon wedges

Serves: 2
Prep time: 10 minutes
Cooking time: 18 minutes
Total time: 28 minutes

1. Preheat the oven to 400°F and line a baking sheet with parchment paper. Rinse the cod fillets with cold water and pat dry with a paper towel.

2. In a shallow medium bowl, combine the sesame seeds, ginger, salt, and pepper.

3. Place each piece of cod in the sesame mixture and gently press to adhere seeds to the cod. Transfer to the prepared baking sheet with sesame seeds facing up.

4. Add the asparagus to the baking sheet and drizzle with ghee. Bake for 15 minutes or until the flesh easily flakes away when tested with a fork. Gently remove from the pan using a spatula.

5. Serve hot with lemon wedges.

Equipment: Medium baking pan, parchment paper

Main Dishes

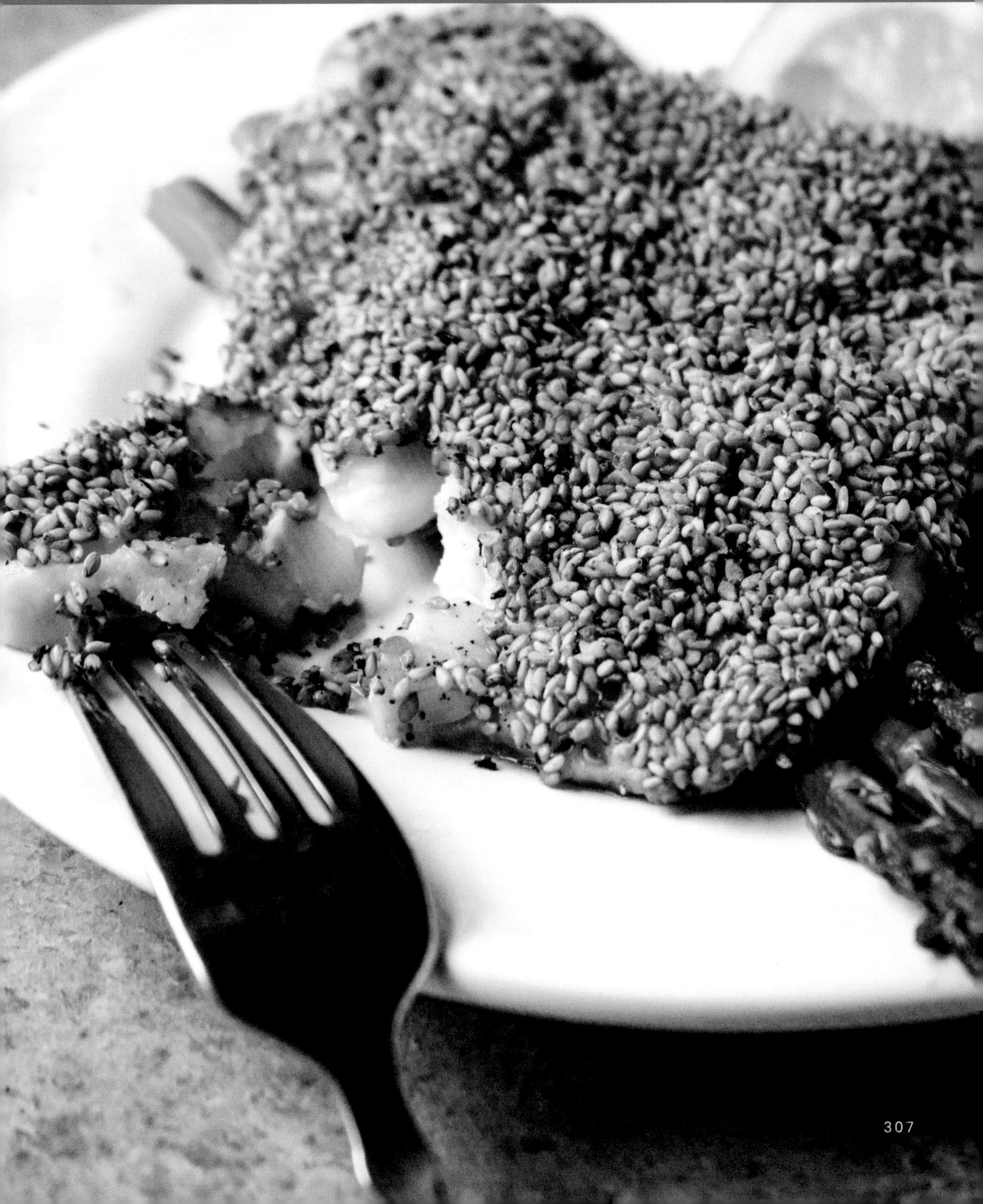

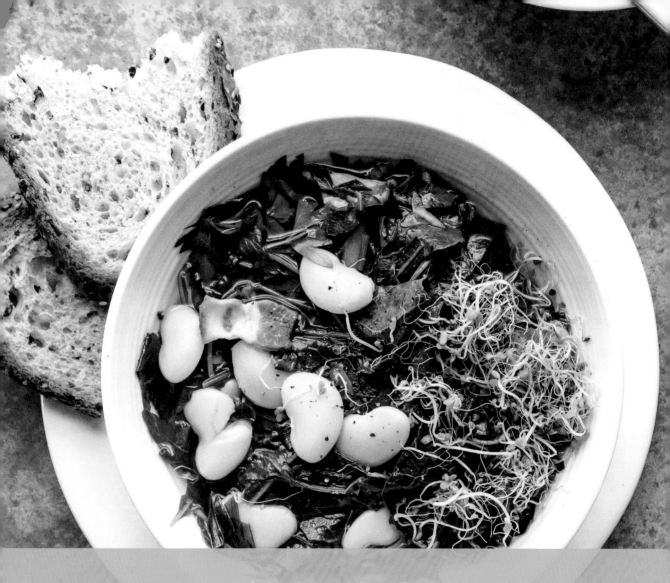

Sardinian Herb Soup
with White Beans

This hearty soup, made in one pot for easy prep and speedy cleanup, is full of tender greens, fragrant herbs, and smoky bacon with creamy white beans adding texture and filling fiber. Fennel seed adds anise aroma and contains hormone-regulating phytoestrogens, which also aids digestion. For this recipe, you can either cook them yourself (see Instant Pot recipe) or use canned beans from a non-BPA can or glass jar.

3 ounces pasture-raised uncured bacon, chopped into 1-inch pieces

1 small bunch flat-leaf parsley, leaves and stems separated; leaves finely chopped and stems coarsely chopped

2 garlic cloves, minced

2 teaspoons fennel seeds

2 quarts Bone Broth (page 260) or store-bought organic chicken stock

1 quart water

4 cups collard greens, chopped

2 cups cooked large white beans (canned beans are OK if from non-BPA can or glass jar)

⅓ cup apple cider vinegar

6 cups baby arugula

½ cup fresh tarragon, chopped

1 teaspoon sea salt

¼ teaspoon freshly ground black pepper

2 cups raw broccoli sprouts

2 tablespoons extra virgin olive oil

Equipment: Large (at least 5-quart) heavy-bottomed pot

1. In a large pot over medium heat, add the bacon and cook, stirring occasionally, until brown, about 5 minutes.

2. Add the parsley stems and cook, stirring often, for 5 minutes or until tender. Add the garlic and fennel and cook for 2 minutes.

3. Stir in bone broth and water. Raise the heat to medium-high and bring to a boil. Add the collard greens, white beans, and parsley leaves. Reduce the heat to low and simmer for 10 minutes.

4. Turn off the heat and stir in the apple cider vinegar, arugula, tarragon, salt and pepper. Allow the arugula to wilt slightly, about 2 minutes. Ladle the soup into bowls and enjoy hot topped with the broccoli sprouts and a drizzle of olive oil.

Instant Pot Method (for the beans):

1 cup dry large white beans, rinsed

2 cups filtered water

1. Add the beans and water to the Instant Pot. Cover and lock the lid and turn the valve to seal. Press the Beans/Chili button (or press Manual for 25 minutes).

2. When the timer goes off, allow the pressure to release naturally for at least 10 minutes. Then turn the valve to release remaining pressure. Remove the lid and drain any excess liquid in the Instant Pot through a colander.

Serves: 4-6
Prep time: 10 minutes
Cooking time: 25 minutes
Total time: 35 minutes

1 tablespoon extra virgin olive oil, plus more for serving

4 strips bacon, chopped

2 teaspoons whole cumin

1 teaspoon ground turmeric

½ teaspoon sea salt, plus more to taste

¼ teaspoon freshly ground black pepper

1 quart Bone Broth (page 260) or store-bought organic chicken stock

1 cup filtered water

1½ cups red lentils, rinsed

1 large carrot, peeled and diced

1 bunch of leafy green vegetables, such as collard greens, kale, or chard, roughly chopped

Juice of ½ lemon, plus more to taste

3 tablespoons chopped fresh cilantro

1 preserved lemon, finely chopped (optional)

Equipment: Large (5-quart or larger) heavy-bottomed pot

Serves: 4
Prep time: 10 minutes
Cooking time: 40 minutes
Total time: 50 minutes

Stove Top Method

1. Add the olive oil and bacon to a large heavy-bottomed pot. Cook on medium-high until the bacon is browned, about 7 minutes.

2. Stir in the cumin, turmeric, salt, and pepper and sauté for 2 minutes.

3. Add the broth, water, lentils, and carrot. Reduce the heat to medium-low and bring to a simmer, then partially cover the pot. Simmer until the lentils are soft, about 30 minutes. Taste and add more salt if necessary.

4. Add the leafy greens and allow them to wilt, about 2 minutes.

5. Stir in the lemon juice, cilantro, and preserved lemon, if using. Ladle the stew into bowls and serve with olive oil for drizzling.

Instant Pot Method

1. Press the Sauté button on an Instant Pot and add the olive oil. Heat for 1 minute. Add the bacon and brown for 5 minutes, stirring occasionally.

2. Stir in the cumin, turmeric, salt, and pepper and sauté for 2 minutes. Press Cancel.

3. Add the bone broth, water, lentils, and carrot. Stir. Lock the lid and close the vent valve. Press Manual setting for 9 minutes.

4. When the timer goes off, press the quick release to release pressure from the Instant Pot. Remove the lid and stir in the greens, lemon juice, cilantro, and preserved lemon, if using. Allow the greens to wilt, about 2 minutes. Ladle the stew into bowls and serve with olive oil for drizzling.

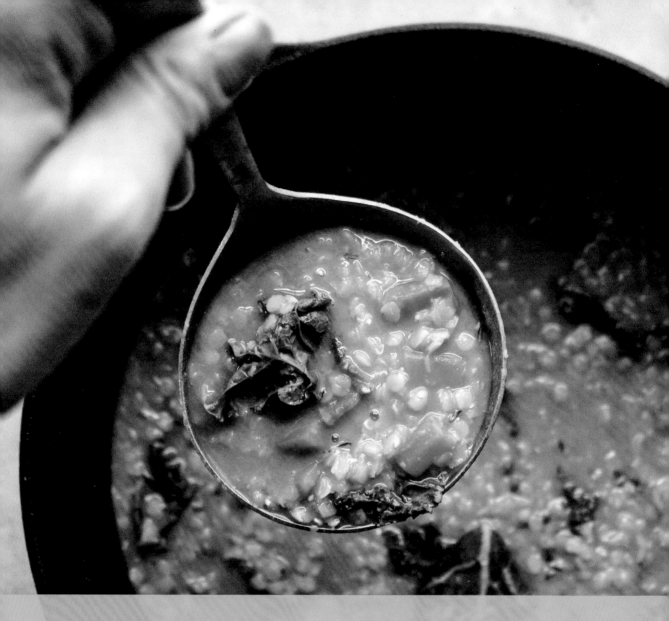

Red Lentil Stew with Greens

This smoky lentil stew is a filling meal on its own, with protein-rich lentils and hearty greens. Bone broth turns the stew into a gut-healing powerhouse, with collagen and amino acids to restore digestive health.

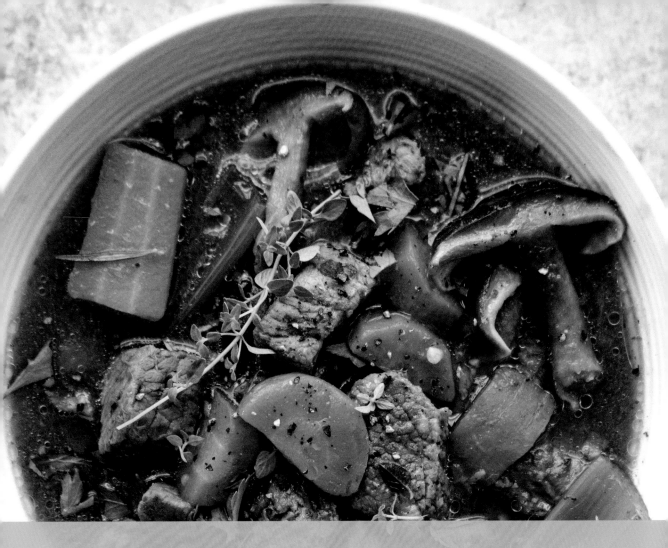

Hearty and Warming
Beef Stew

For a satisfying, protein-rich meal, reach for this hearty bone-broth stew. Bone broth is chock-full of amino acids and collagen, which help restore gut health and protect joints. To save time, this recipe can also be made in the Instant Pot, which cooks the beef to fall-apart-tender in just 25 minutes. You may be surprised by the use of anchovies—they give meat stews a rich, umami flavor and you won't taste them at the end. Rounding out the stew are carrots, celery, and immune-boosting shiitake mushrooms.

1 tablespoon ghee

2 pounds beef stew meat

2 teaspoons minced garlic

2 cups coarsely chopped carrots

2 cups sliced shiitake mushrooms

1 cup coarsely chopped celery

1 cup chopped white onion

2 cups beef bone broth

¼ cup coconut aminos

4 anchovies, minced

1 fresh rosemary sprig

2 fresh thyme sprigs

½ teaspoon sea salt

¼ teaspoon freshly ground black pepper

1 tablespoon gluten-free flour

½ cup chopped fresh flat-leaf parsley, for serving

Equipment: Instant Pot, large (5-quart or larger) heavy-bottomed pot or Dutch oven for stove top method

---

Serves: 4
Prep time: 10 minutes
Cooking time: 2 hours and 15 minutes
Total time: 2 hours and 25 minutes

Stove Top Method

1. In a large pot or Dutch oven, heat the ghee for 2 minutes over medium-high heat. Pat the beef dry using a paper towel. Add the beef to the pot and cook, stirring occasionally, until browned, 8 minutes.

2. Reduce the heat to medium. Add the garlic and sauté for 1 minute. Add the carrots, mushrooms, celery, onion, bone broth, aminos, anchovies, rosemary, thyme, salt, and pepper. Cover and cook for 2 hours, or until the beef is tender.

3. Ladle ½ cup of broth from the pot into a bowl and gradually whisk in the flour. Pour the mixture into the stew and stir. Simmer for 5 minutes or until stew thickens slightly.

4. Ladle stew into bowls and serve hot. Sprinkle the parsley over the top.

Instant Pot Method

1. Heat the ghee on Sauté setting in an Instant Pot. Pat the beef dry using a paper towel. Brown beef, stirring occasionally, in the Instant Pot for 8 minutes.

2. Add the garlic and sauté for 1 minute. Add the carrots, mushrooms, celery, onion, bone broth, aminos, anchovies, rosemary, thyme, salt, and pepper. Secure the lid and close vent valve. Press Manual and set timer for 25 minutes.

3. When the timer goes off, allow pressure to naturally release before opening the vent valve and releasing remaining pressure. Press Cancel. Remove the lid and press Sauté. Ladle ½ cup of broth from the pot into a bowl and gradually whisk in the flour. Pour the mixture into stew and stir. Simmer for 2 minutes or until stew thickens slightly. Press Cancel.

4. Ladle stew into bowls and serve hot, with chopped parsley sprinkled over top.

2 tablespoons extra virgin olive oil

5 cups peeled and cubed sweet potatoes

1 cup chopped celery

1 cup chopped sweet white onion

1 teaspoon minced garlic

2 teaspoons grated ginger

1 teaspoon ground coriander

1 teaspoon ground cumin

3 cups chicken stock

1 teaspoon sea salt

½ cup unsalted and unsweetened creamy cashew or almond butter

2 tablespoons freshly squeezed lime juice

½ cup chopped fresh cilantro, for topping

½ cup chopped raw cashews, for topping

2 cups cooked shredded chicken (optional)

Equipment: Medium (4-quart) heavy-bottomed pot or Dutch oven or Instant Pot, blender

---

Serves: 4
Prep time: 10 minutes
Cooking time: 40 minutes
Total time: 50 minutes

Stove Top Method

1. In a medium heavy-bottomed pot, heat the olive oil over medium heat. Add the sweet potatoes, celery, and onion. Cover and cook for 10 minutes. Add the garlic, ginger, coriander, and cumin. Continue to cook, covered, for 5 minutes more.

2. Stir in the chicken stock and salt. Increase the heat to medium-high and bring to a boil. Reduce the heat to medium-low and simmer, uncovered, for 15 minutes or until the potatoes are tender.

3. Ladle 2 cups of soup into a blender and blend until smooth. Stir the puree back into the soup along with the cashew butter, lime juice, and shredded chicken, if using. Cook for 5 minutes.

4. Ladle into bowls and top with cilantro and cashews.

Instant Pot Method

1. Press Sauté. Heat the olive oil for 1 minute and add the sweet potatoes, celery, onion, garlic, and ginger. Sauté for 3 to 4 minutes, or until the garlic and ginger are fragrant.

2. Stir in the coriander, cumin, chicken stock, and salt. Lock lid and close vent valve. Press Manual button for 10 minutes.

3. When the timer goes off, allow pressure to naturally release before opening the vent valve. Remove the lid and stir in the cashew butter, lime juice, and shredded chicken, if using.

4. Ladle soup into bowls and top with cilantro and chopped cashews.

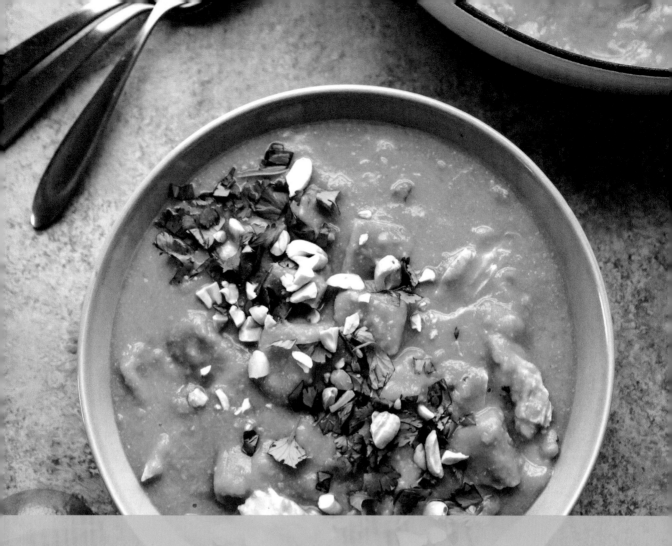

African Sweet Potato Stew

This hearty stew is packed with antioxidant-rich vegetables and protein-rich shredded chicken. Sweet potatoes not only add vitamins and antioxidants, but they are also high in fiber, helping to control hunger. Creamy cashew butter adds texture without using dairy or coconut milk. This recipe is finished with cilantro for a pop of fresh herb flavor. Cilantro is also high in antioxidants and helps cleanse the body of heavy metals that can cause disease. This savory, nutty stew originated in West Africa but is also popular in Central Africa. Different areas of Africa put their own twist on this stew, using different herbs, meat, and vegetables.

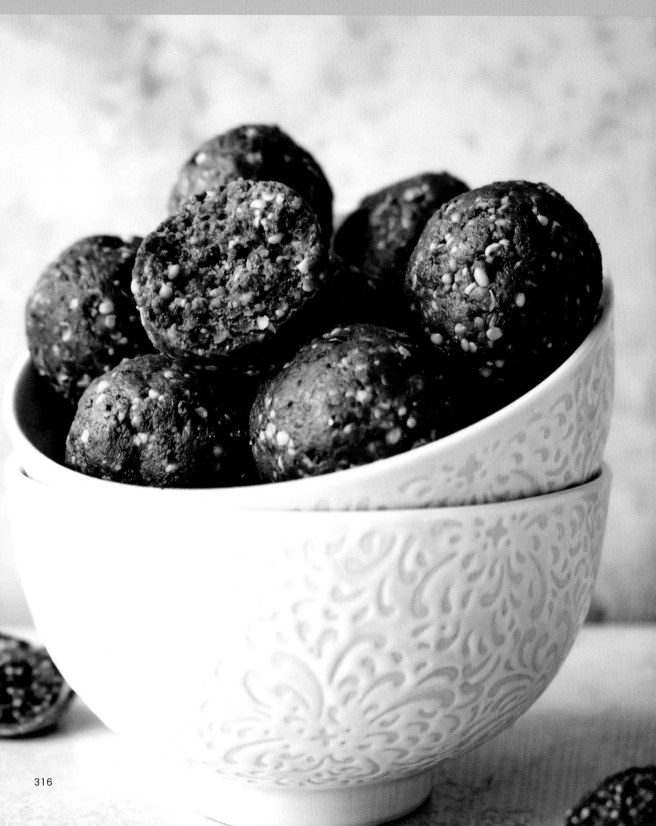

Cacao Fig Bliss Balls

Get your chocolate fix with these two-bite bliss balls. They're made with just five ingredients and need no added sugar. Dried figs add fiber and natural sticky sweetness. Sunflower seed butter and hemp hearts provide a dose of protein and healthy fats.

1 cup dried figs

3 tablespoons raw cacao nibs

½ cup sunflower seed butter

2 tablespoons hemp hearts

Pinch of sea salt

Equipment: Food processor, parchment paper

Makes: ~ 12 balls
Prep time: 10 minutes
Cooking time: 0 minutes
Total time: 10 minutes

1. In a medium glass bowl, add the figs and cover with hot water. Allow to soak for 10 minutes to soften.

2. Drain, discarding the water, and add the figs to a food processor. Blend for 15 seconds or until figs are finely chopped. Add the cacao nibs and pulse 10 to 15 times to break them up.

3. Add the sunflower seed butter and pulse a few more times to combine with the fig mixture.

4. Add the hemp hearts and pulse 2 to 3 times to combine but still leave them visible.

5. Remove the lid from the food processor and scoop out a tablespoon of mixture. Use your hands to form a ball and place it on a plate lined with parchment paper. Repeat with the remaining mixture. Refrigerate the bliss balls for 30 minutes to firm.

6. These keep well in the refrigerator for up to 10 days.

Dong Quai Chocolate Bark

Indulge in a chocolate craving and get the benefits of hormone-balancing seeds with this dark chocolate bark. Dried cranberries add tangy, chewy texture, and dong quai helps regulate hormones.

This recipe is made using a double-boiler; but you don't need any fancy equipment. A medium heat-safe glass bowl placed over a medium saucepan containing simmering water will do the trick. Keep the pieces of chocolate bark in the refrigerator to grab any time a sweet craving strikes. It is especially delicious alongside a hot cup of chai.

12 ounces dark (70% cacao or higher) chocolate chips

½ teaspoon dong quai root powder

1 tablespoon raw sesame seeds

1 tablespoon raw shelled pumpkin seeds

2 tablespoons raw almond slivers

2 tablespoons dried cranberries or cherries

Equipment: Double boiler, small baking sheet (make sure it's small enough to fit into your freezer or refrigerator), parchment paper

1. Melt the chocolate in a double boiler over medium heat, approximately 8 minutes.

2. Once the chocolate is smooth, remove from the heat and stir in dong quai.

3. Line a small baking sheet with parchment paper and pour the chocolate mixture over it. Sprinkle with the sesame seeds, pumpkin seeds, almonds, and dried cranberries. Transfer to the freezer for 30 minutes.

4. Use the tip of a sharp knife to break bark into smaller pieces.

Keeps well in the refrigerator for up to 1 month.

Makes: ~ 10 servings
Prep time: 10 minutes
Cooking time: 8 minutes
Setting time: 30 minutes
Total time: 48 minutes

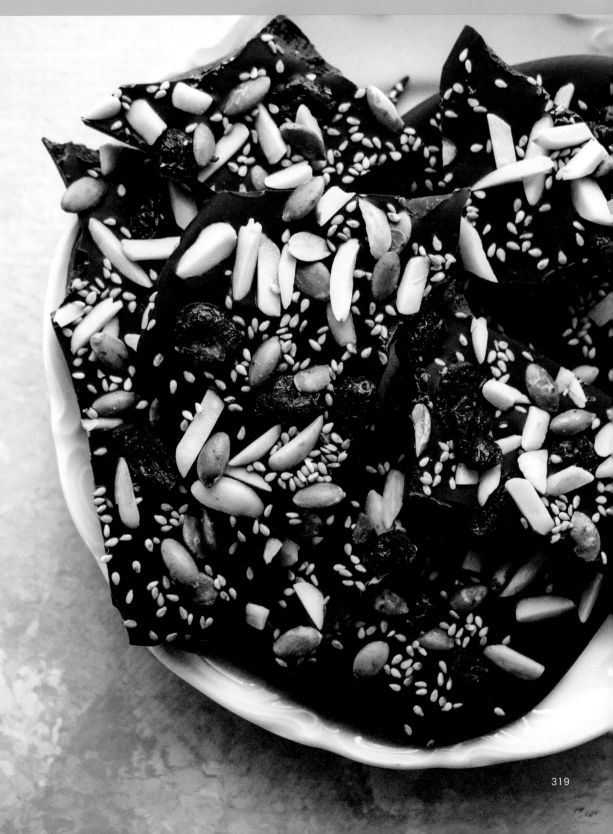

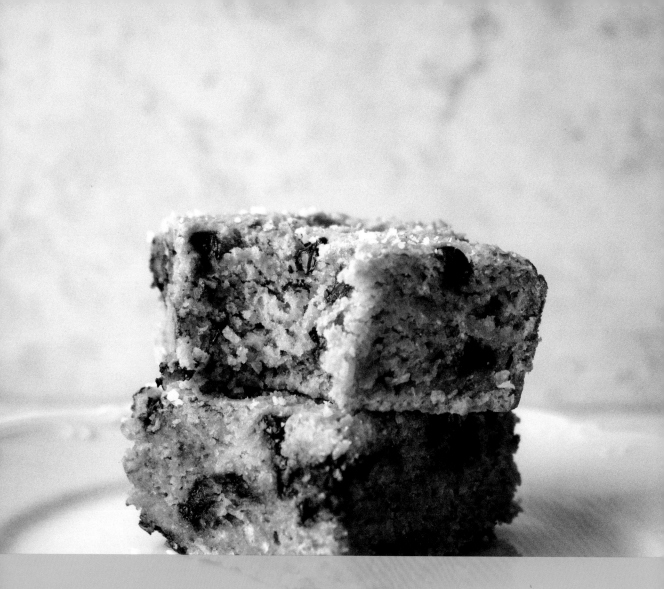

Sweet Potato Bread (Batatada)

I used to go to Macau regularly when I lived in Hong Kong—it's only a 90-minute boat ride to a country with a unique culinary culture that merges Portugese, Chinese, and African food and ingredients. The Batatada is sold on many street corners and each bakery has its own spin on it. What I love about it is the richness, moisture, and the wonderful combination of spices. I've modified the recipe to be free of gluten, dairy, and eggs.

12 ounces unpeeled orange sweet potatoes, cut to ½-inch cubes

2 cups Bob's Red Mill Gluten-Free 1-to-1 Baking Flourr

⅔ cup unsweetened shredded coconut

2 teaspoons ground ginger

2 ½ teaspoons baking powder

¾ teaspoon baking soda

¾ teaspoon sea salt

⅓ to ½ cup packed dark brown sugar, depending how sweet you like it

Zest of 2 limes

2 tablespoons freshly squeezed lime juice

1 medium ripe banana, sliced

¾ cup oat milk (or any other non-dairy unsweetened milk)

2 tablespoons pure vanilla extract

½ cup melted coconut oil, plus more for greasing the pan

⅓ cup dark chocolate shavings or chips (optional)

2 tablespoons shredded coconut, ground to powder

Equipment: 9 x 9-inch baking pan, food processor

1. Preheat the oven to 350°F. Position a rack in the middle of the oven. Grease the baking pan with oil. In a medium glass bowl, place the sweet potatoes, cover with a glass plate and microwave on high for 5 minutes, or until the potatoes are completely tender. Uncover and set aside to cool.

2. In a food processor, combine the flour, coconut, ginger, baking powder, baking soda, and salt. Process until the coconut is finely ground, about 1 to 2 minutes. Transfer to a large bowl.

3. In a food processor, combine the brown sugar, lime zest, and lime juice. Process until well combined, about 30 seconds. Add the sweet potatoes, banana, oat milk, and vanilla; process until completely smooth, about 2 minutes, scraping the bowl as needed.

4. With the machine running, add the melted coconut oil through the feed tube, then process until fully incorporated. Transfer the sweet potato mixture to the bowl with the dry ingredients and gently whisk to combine. Fold in the chocolate shavings.

5. Transfer the batter to the prepared pan and spread evenly. Bake for 30 to 35 minutes or until the cake is golden brown and a toothpick inserted in the center comes out clean. Let cool in the pan on a rack for 30 minutes before slicing into 12 squares. Sprinkle with the ground coconut.

Keep in an airtight container on the kitchen counter for up to 4 days.

Serves: 12
Prep time: 15 minutes
Cooking time: 40 minutes
Total time: 55 minutes

Overnight Berry Chia Pudding

This creamy pudding is made by soaking chia seeds in dairy-free milk until they "bloom," creating a thick pudding that is perfect for breakfast or a healthy snack. Fresh berries add antioxidants and vitamins, turning the pudding into a complete meal. Chia seeds are naturally high in heart-healthy fats and protein. These small seeds help to stabilize blood sugar and prevent insulin spikes.

2 cups unsweetened non-dairy milk, such as oat, cashew, almond, or macadamia milk

2 tablespoons raw honey or pure maple syrup

¼ cup chia seeds

1 cup mixed berries, such as strawberries, blueberries, raspberries, and blackberries

Equipment: 4 (8-ounce) mason jars with lids

1. In a glass bowl, combine the milk, honey, and chia seeds. Divide the mixture among 4 (8-ounce) mason jars and cover with the lids.

2. Refrigerate the pudding at least 4 hours or preferably overnight. Top with berries and additional drizzle of honey and eat it from the jar.

The pudding will keep in the refrigerator for up to 5 days.

Makes: 4 servings
Prep time: 10 minutes
Soaking time: 4 hours
Total time: 4 hours, 10 minutes

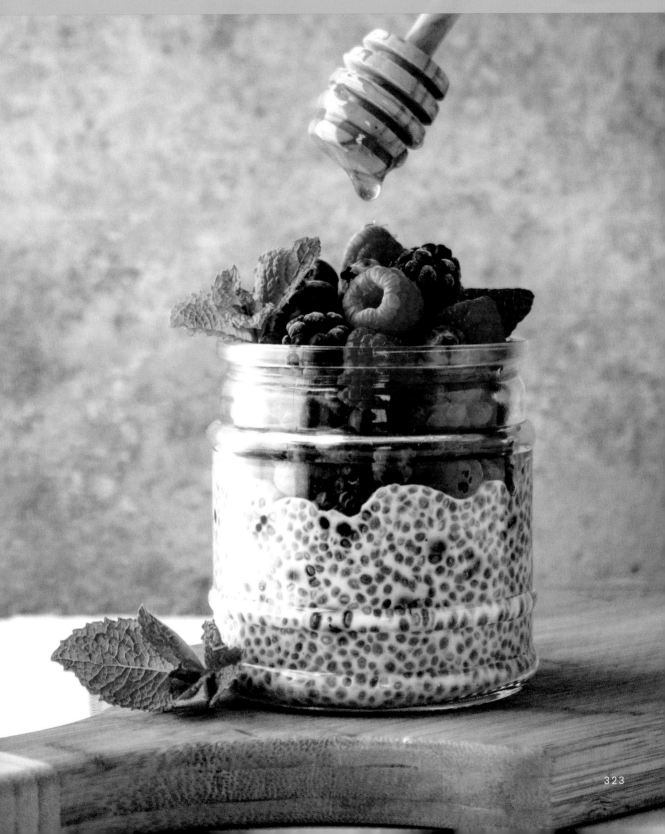

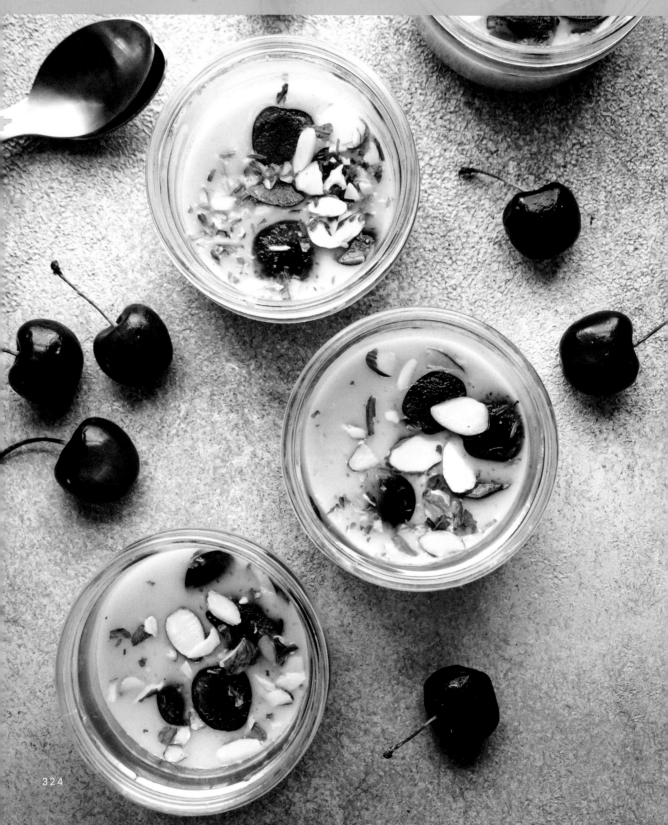

Cherry Almond Pudding

If you crave a little something before bedtime, but want to keep it low in sugar, this recipe might hit the spot. Kudzu root comes from the invasive vine that "ate the South," as it's often referred to by frustrated farmers. Yet it has some wonderful medicinal properties, including helping you fall asleep. Cherries have a similar effect; combining them in this recipe might help you snooze away without being woken up by sugar spikes in the middle of the night.

½ cup unsweetened tart cherry juice

3 tablespoons kudzu root powder

½ teaspoon almond extract

3 tablespoons pure maple syrup

2 cups unsweetened almond milk

½ cup pitted cherries, halved

½ cup raw sliced almonds

Equipment: 4 small (6-ounce) mason jars with lids

1. In a medium saucepan, heat the cherry juice and kudzu over medium heat. Continuously whisk until the kudzu is dissolved, about 2 minutes.

2. Add the almond extract and maple syrup. Gradually whisk in the almond milk. Heat the mixture until boiling, then reduce heat to low. Simmer for 5 minutes.

3. Divide the pudding among 4 small mason jars and cool to room temperature. Seal with the lids and refrigerate for 2 hours. Serve chilled, topped with chopped cherries and sliced almonds.

Serves: 4
Prep time: 5 minutes
Cooking time: 7 minutes
Chilling time: 2 hours
Total time: 2 hours, 12 minutes

Cacao Collagen Smoothie

This dessert-worthy cacao-based smoothie is packed with nutrition, so you can enjoy it guilt-free. Cacao powder and cacao nibs give this a rich chocolate flavor, along with a healthy dose of flavonoids. Collagen adds protein and helps promote gut health, and a simple banana will make this smoothie creamy and indulgent.

1 extra ripe medium frozen banana, cut into chunks

2 cups unsweetened almond milk

2 tablespoons unsweetened cacao powder

2 scoops collagen powder

1 tablespoon cacao nibs plus more for topping

Equipment: Blender

1. Combine all of the ingredients in a blender and blend until smooth and creamy.

2. Divide between 2 glasses and top with more cacao nibs.

Enjoy right away.

Makes: 2 smoothies
Prep time: 5 minutes
Cooking time: 0 minutes
Total time: 5 minutes

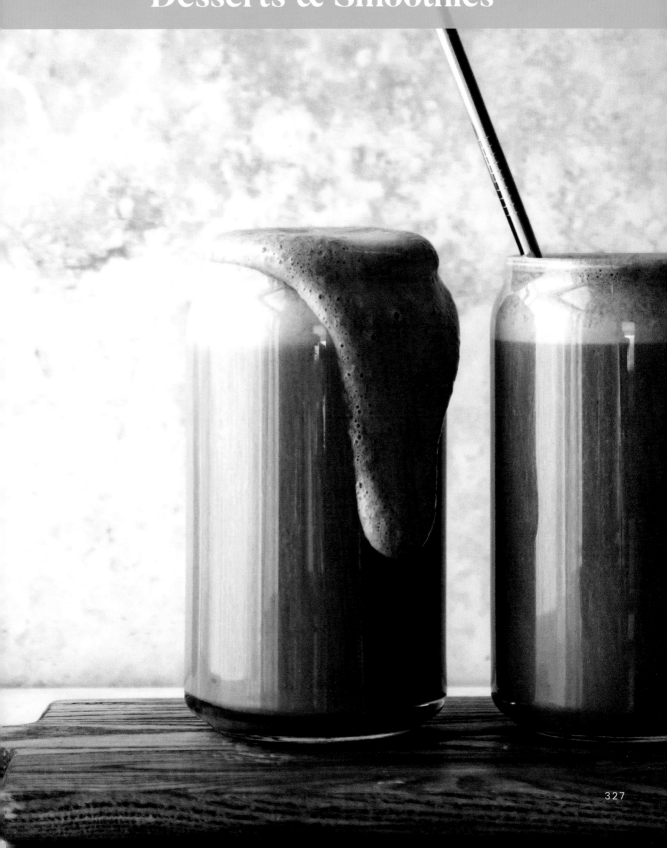

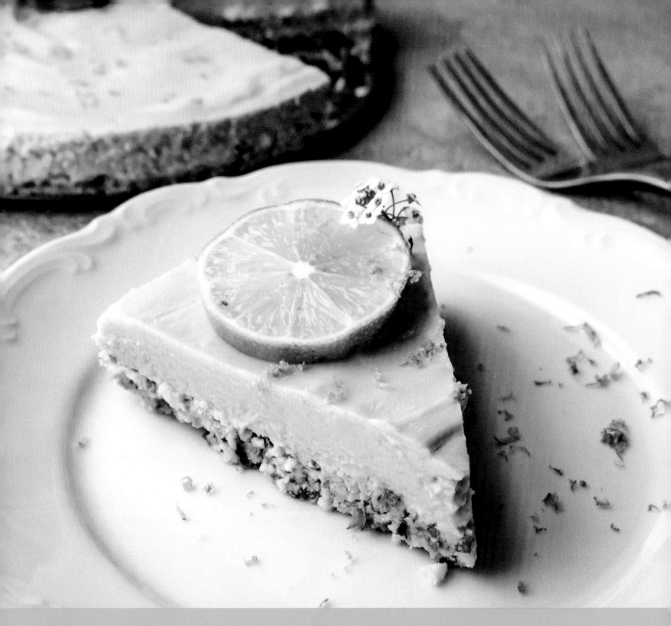

Refreshing Lime Pie

My dear friend Sukaynah, a raw food chef extraordinaire, taught me this recipe.
This rich pie is not only decadent but refreshing and uplifting.

Desserts & Smoothies

For the Crust

2 cups almonds, presoaked for 12 hours, or sprouted almonds

½ cup dried dates, cut into ½-inch pieces

½ teaspoon pure vanilla extract

¼ teaspoon sea salt

For the Filling

1 cup freshly squeezed lime juice (from about 8 limes)

¾ cup amber coconut nectar

¾ cup coconut milk, from a (BPA-free) can or from a Thai young coconut, water with meat blended together

1½ cups peeled, pitted, and sliced avocado

1 tablespoon pure vanilla extract

⅛ teaspoon sea salt

¾ cup coconut oil, melted and cooled

¾ teaspoon apple cider vinegar

Equipment: 8- or 9-inch springform pan, food processor, blender

---

Serves: 8-10
Prep time: 25 minutes
Cooking time: 0 minutes
Total time: 25 minutes

Make the crust

1. Add all of the crust ingredients to a food processor and mix until a coarse texture forms.

2. Grease a springform pan (bottom and sides) with coconut oil. Press the crust into the bottom of the springform pan but not up the sides.

3. Set aside or put in the refrigerator or freezer until you're ready to fill it.

Make the filling

1. In a blender, combine the lime juice, coconut nectar, coconut milk, avocado, vanilla, salt, and apple cider vinegar. Purée until smooth, then add the coconut oil and blend. Adjust for sweetness or tartness.

2. Pour the filling into the prepared crust; tap the pan to bring air bubbles to the surface. Chill in the refrigerator for 8 to 10 hours, until the filling is set.

3. Remove from the springform pan by first running a knife along the inside edge of the pan. Release the side of the springform pan and lower the pie out the bottom of the spring form. Use a wet finger to smooth any indentations.

4. Decorate the pie with edible flowers, coconut, blueberries, and/or lime zest with a little bee pollen. Slice and serve cold.

Store in an airtight container in the refrigerator for up to 5 days.

For the Filling

1 teaspoon ghee

1 pound fresh strawberries, sliced (thawed if frozen)

Zest of 1 lime

2 tablespoons freshly squeezed lime juice

1 tablespoon fresh mint, finely chopped (from about 20 leaves)

1 tablespoon grated ginger

1 teaspoon vanilla powder or extract

2 teaspoons arrowroot or tapioca starch

Pinch of sea salt

For the Topping

1 cup finely shredded coconut flakes

½ cup ghee or coconut oil, melted

¼ cup arrowroot or tapioca starch

1 tablespoon pure maple syrup

½ teaspoon vanilla powder

Pinch of sea salt

Equipment: Medium (8 × 8 or 9 × 9-inch) baking dish or medium (10-inch) cast-iron skillet

1. Preheat the oven to 350ºF. Grease a medium baking dish with the ghee.

2. In a large bowl, combine all of the filling ingredients and toss to evenly coat the strawberries. Transfer the mixture to the prepared baking dish.

3. In a medium bowl, combine all of the topping ingredients. Use your hands to work the ghee into the mixture until it becomes crumbly. Spread the topping evenly over the strawberries.

4. Bake for 30 to 40 minutes or until the topping has browned.

Serves: 4-6
Prep time: 20 minutes
Cooking time: 40 minutes
Total time: 1 hour

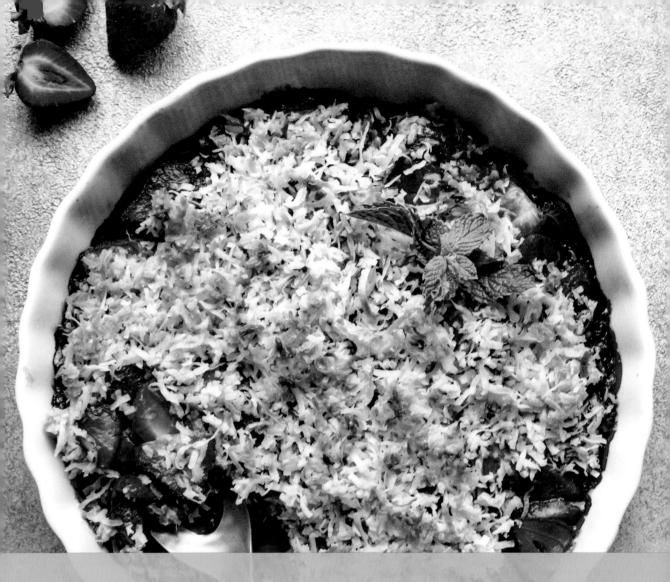

Ginger Mint
Strawberry Cobbler

This healthier cobbler blows conventional desserts out of the water with its bold, ginger and mint-packed flavor. The filling is simple but vibrant, with a combination of strawberries, lime zest and juice, fresh mint, and grated ginger. Meanwhile, a coconut topping adds crunch and tropical flavor.

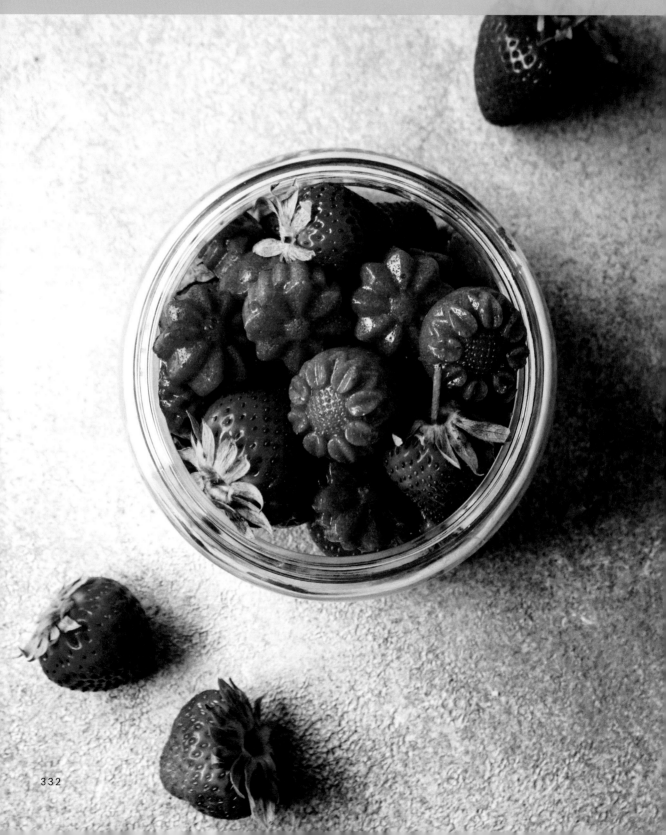

Strawberry Jellies

Here's a great gummy that's much healthier than any conventional treat. You'll only need a handful of ingredients to throw this together, including strawberries, ginger, lime juice, and gelatin. Strawberries deliver antioxidants, while ginger offers anti-inflammatory properties. Gelatin is also a gut-healing ingredient, so you can feel good about snacking on these irresistible gummies.

32 ounces fresh strawberries, hulled (thawed if frozen)

½-inch piece fresh ginger, grated

2 tablespoons freshly squeezed lime juice

3 tablespoons gelatin

Equipment: Food processor or blender, jelly forms or cups

Serves: 6-8
Prep time: 20 minutes
Chilling time: 4 hours
Total time: 4 hours, 20 minutes

1. In a food processor or blender, purée the strawberries, ginger, and lime juice. This should yield approximately 3 cups of strawberry purée.

2. Transfer the purée to a saucepan and warm it, stirring it constantly so you avoid bringing it to a boil, over medium-low heat.

3. When the purée becomes warm to the touch (use your finger to test it), slowly whisk in the gelatin. You can also transfer the mixture to a food processor and pulse to blend.

4. Pour the mixture into a desired form—you can use one large bowl or a number of small dessert bowls.

5. Chill in the refrigerator for at least 4 hours, or until the jelly is firm.

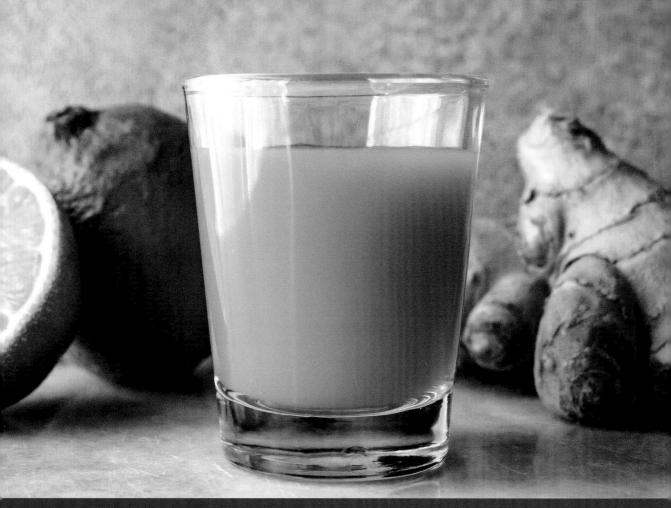

Good Morning Elixir

This drink was inspired by jamu—a traditional herbal drink from Java, an Indonesian island. Sold at every market, jamu is a true pick-me-up, boosting tonic women swear by. Small but frequent doses will go a long way. This recipe taps into the healing powers of turmeric, ginger, and lemon (or lime) and will help lower inflammation, detox the liver, alkalize the body, and get your digestion primed for food. I've had a number of women say that they changed nothing else and this drink has helped them with chronic pain and hot flashes and has helped clear their mind.

You may find this drink too pungent and potent and therefore too intense to drink on an empty stomach. If that's the case, add a little raw honey or pure maple syrup (the less the better) and/or drink it after breakfast (i.e., not on an empty stomach).

This recipe offers an option of using fresh and dried turmeric.

Teas, Lattes, & Drinks

Method 1:
Juicer
(for fresh turmeric)

1½ pounds fresh unpeeled turmeric

1 (3-inch-long) piece of fresh unpeeled ginger

⅓ cup freshly squeezed lime or lemon juice

1. Juice the turmeric and ginger. Add the lime juice and stir.

2. Transfer to a mason jar and label it.

3. Drink a 1-ounce shot once a day. Add a touch of raw honey, if needed.

Equipment: Juicer, large mason jar with lid

_____

Serves: 24; makes 3 cups
Prep time: 5 minutes
Juicing and blending time: 12 minutes
Total time: 17 minutes

Method 2:
Blender and Cheesecloth
(for ground turmeric)

2⅔ cups filtered water

3 tablespoons turmeric powder

1 (3-inch-long) piece of fresh unpeeled ginger, grated

⅓ cup freshly squeezed lime or lemon juice

1. Place all of the ingredients in a blender. Blitz for 2 minutes.

2. Strain into a medium bowl through cheesecloth, squeezing the juice out with your hands.

3. Transfer to a mason jar and label it.

4. Drink a 1-ounce shot once a day. Add a touch of raw honey, if needed.

5. Chill in the refrigerator for at least 4 hours, or until the jelly is firm.

Keeps well in the refrigerator for up to 1 month.

Equipment: Blender, cheesecloth, large mason jar with lid

_____

Serves: 24; makes 3 cups
Prep time: 5 minutes
Juicing and blending time: 7 minutes
Total time: 12 minutes

Raspberry Chia Refresher

4 cups filtered water

1 tablespoon red raspberry leaves

2 tablespoons raw honey

2 tablespoons freshly squeezed lemon juice

¼ cup chia seeds

Equipment: 1-quart mason jar

Serves: 2
Prep time: 5 minutes
Cooking time: 20 minutes
Total time: 25 minutes

1. In a small saucepan, bring the water to a boil. Add raspberry leaves and let steep for 20 minutes.

2. Strain and stir in the honey and lemon juice. Cool to room temperature.

3. Pour into a 1-quart mason jar and stir in the chia seeds. Refrigerate at least 2 hours. Pour into glasses and enjoy.

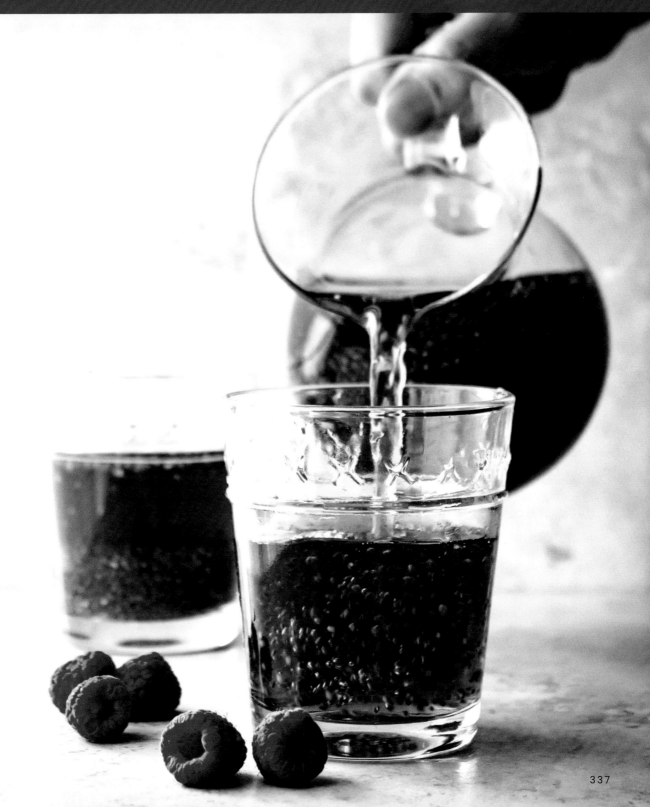

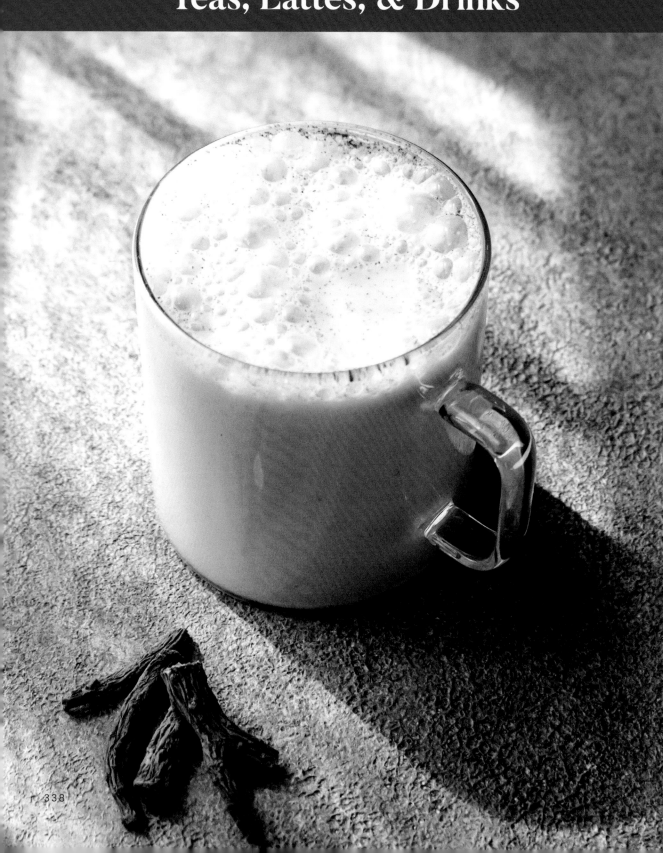

Menopause
Latte

You will be tapping into the healing powers of dong quai (Angelica sinensis), acclaimed in traditional Chinese medicine to help women normalize menopause and experience fewer hot flashes, hormone fluctuations, and low moods.

1½ cups non-dairy milk, such as oat, cashew, almond, or macadamia milk

1 teaspoon dong quai root powder (*Angelica sinensis*)

½ teaspoon ground cinnamon (*Cinnamomum verum*)

1 teaspoon raw honey

_____

Serves: 1
Prep time: 5 minutes
Cooking time: 2 minutes
Total time: 7 minutes

1. In a small saucepan, warm the milk over medium-high heat until almost boiling.

2. Add the dong quai and cinnamon, whisking vigorously. Remove from the heat.

3. Whisk in the honey. Drink warm or chilled.

Keeps well in the refrigerator for up to 1 week.

Mint Matcha Latte

1 cup filtered water

1 tablespoon mint tea leaves

½ cup unsweetened almond milk

1 teaspoon matcha powder

1 tablespoon raw honey

_____

Serves: 1
Prep time: 5 minutes
Cooking time: 5 minutes
Total time: 10 minutes

1. In a small saucepan, bring the water to a boil. Add the mint tea and let steep for a minimum of 5 minutes.

2. While the tea steeps, heat the milk in a small saucepan over medium-high heat until steaming. Vigorously whisk the milk until frothy.

3. Strain the tea, discarding the leaves, and stir in the matcha powder and honey. Pour in frothed milk and enjoy hot.

Teas, Lattes, & Drinks

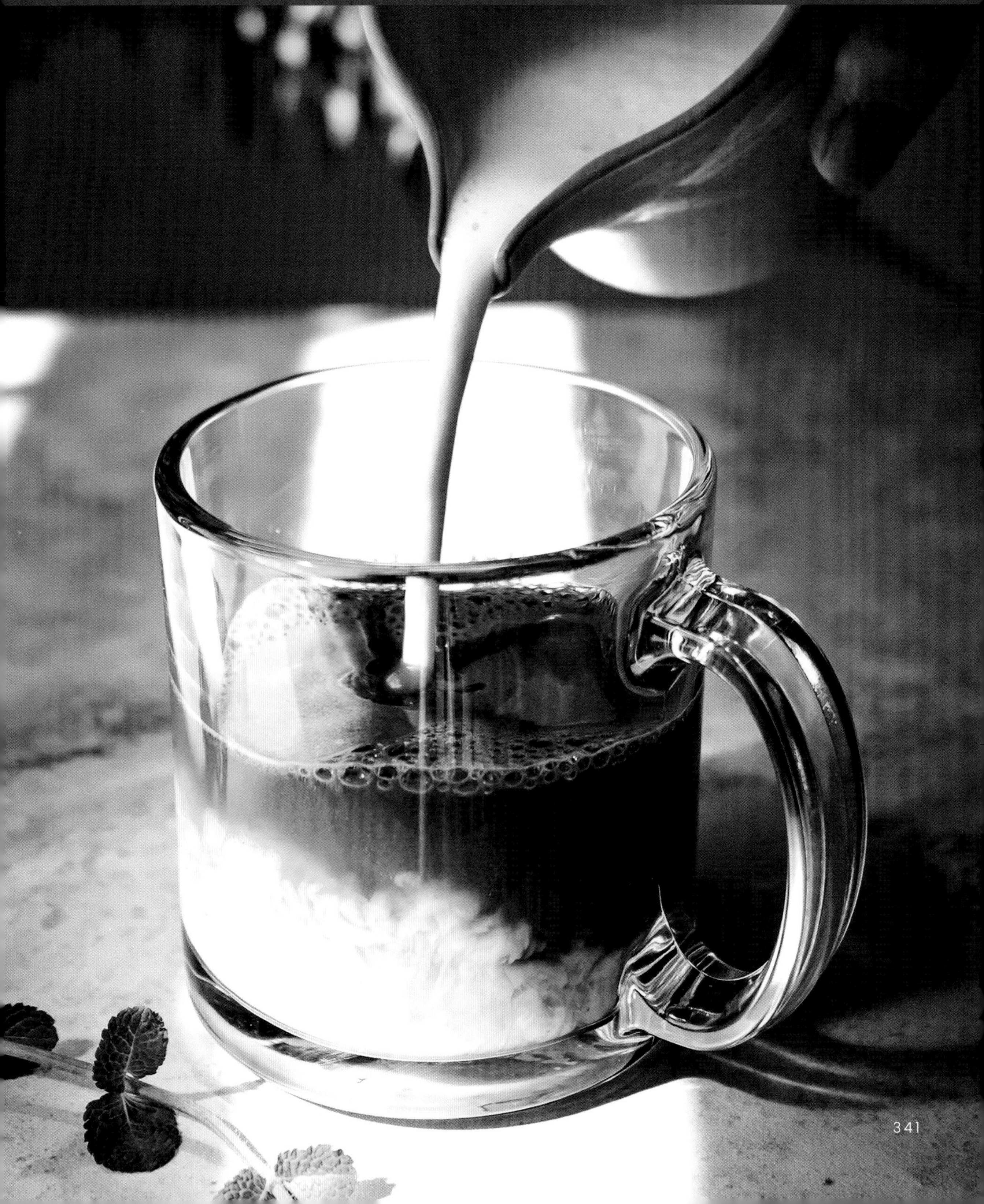

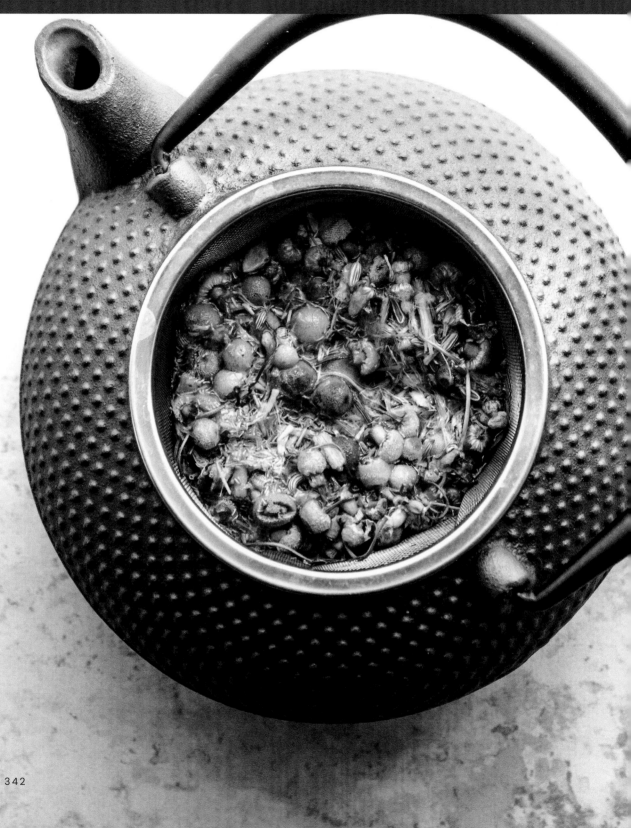

Making Herbal Teas as Infusions and Decoctions

I do not recommend using mass-produced, prepackaged tea bags because they have little medicinal value. Herbs found in tea bags are finely cut so that you can make a quick tea, but that causes them to be oxidized by the time they land on the store shelves. Most tea bags are made with bleached paper or plastic-based sachets, too. For these reasons, and if you want to use herbs for truly therapeutic purposes, I do not recommend using tea bags.

Instead, buy bulk loose herbs and learn to infuse or decoct your own teas. You will never go back to store-bought prepared tea bags again! Making your own is simple and cheaper, too.

How to make an infusion

Infusion is a water extraction method used with herbs that come in the form of leaves, flowers, young barks, and branches.

Makes 1 quart, 4 servings

Use this method with all the infusion recipes listed here.

1. Place the herbs stated in the recipe in a 1-quart mason jar.

2. Pour boiling water over them, close the lid, and let steep for 20 to 30 minutes.

3. Strain and drink 1½ cups a day unless stated otherwise.

If you find the infusion too strong to drink, add a little water.

How to make an decoction

Decoction is a water extraction method used with herbs that come in the form of berries, roots, hardy bark, and branches.

Makes 1 quart, 4 servings

Use this method with all the decoction recipes listed here.

1. Place the herbs stated in the recipe in a medium pot. Pour a quart of cold water over them.

2. Cover and bring to a boil. Reduce the heat to low and simmer for 30 to 40 minutes.

3. Remove from the heat. For best extraction, let the mixture stand on the kitchen counter overnight.

4. Strain and drink 1½ cups a day unless stated otherwise.

If you find the decoction too strong to drink, add a little water.

If you can't find one or two herbs in a recipe, don't worry about it; make it with what you can find.

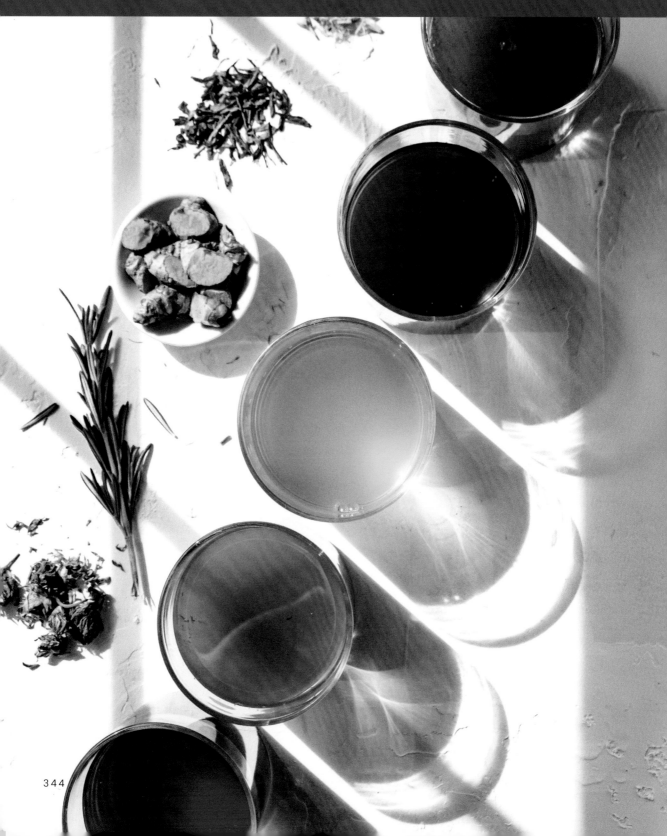

Women's Daily Tea (Infusion)

2 tablespoons red clover
(*Trifolium pratense*)

2 tablespoons red raspberry
(*Rubus idaeus*)

2 tablespoons nettles
(*Urtica dioica*)

1 teaspoon hibiscus
(*Hibiscus rosa-sinensis*)

1 teaspoon licorice root
(*Glycyrrhiza glabra*)

Follow the instructions on
how to make an infusion.

Avoid licorice if you have high blood pressure

Brain Boost Tea (Infusion)

If you need a brain boost, try putting away your
coffee and try this tea.

2 tablespoons peppermint or spearmint
(*Mentha × piperita*)

2 tablespoons gotu kola
(*Centella asiatica*)

1 tablespoons rosemary
(*Salvia rosmarinus*)

Follow the instructions on
how to make an infusion.

Liver Detox Tea (Decoction)

The herbs in this tea are to be reckoned with. They offer a combination of liver detoxification but also regeneration and protection from offensive substances such as alcohol, caffeine, heavy metals, and environmental toxins. Liver health is essential in hormonal health.

1 tablespoon dandelion root (*Taraxacum*) or
burdock root (*Arctium*)

1 tablespoon milk thistle
(*Silybum marianum*)

1 tablespoon turmeric root
(*Curcuma longa*)

1 teaspoon schisandra berry
(*Schisandra chinensis*), crushed

Follow the instructions on
how to make a decoction.

Teas, Lattes, & Drinks

Digestive Tea
(Infusion)

This tea is perfect after a big meal or if you're suffering from IBS or other digestive conditions. The herbs here will help calm your inflammation and rebuild the mucosal lining.

1 tablespoon calendula
(*Calendula officinalis*)

1 tablespoon peppermint
(*Mentha × piperita*)

1 tablespoon chamomile
(*Matricaria chamomilla*)

1 tablespoon plantain
(*Plantago*)

2 teaspoons fennel seed, crushed
(*Foeniculum vulgare*)

1 teaspoon licorice
(*Glycyrrhiza glabra*)

1 teaspoon ginger
(*Zingiber officinale*)

Follow the instructions on how to make an infusion.

Sleepytime Tea
(Infusion)

This is my daily tea before bed. The herbs in this infusion have a dual function. Some calm down the parasympathetic nervous system; helping you quiet the brain and relax your body. Others have a slightly sedative effect to help you fall and stay asleep. California poppy and passionflower are bitter herbs and they will also work on your liver while you sleep. How convenient!

2 tablespoons chamomile
(*Matricaria chamomilla*)

1 tablespoon California poppy
(*Eschscholzia californica*)

1 tablespoon passionflower
(*Passiflora*)

1 tablespoon skullcap (*Scutellaria*)
or lemon balm (*Melissa officinalis*)

1 teaspoon lavender buds
(*Lavandula*)

Follow the instructions on how to make an infusion.

Hot Flash Tea
(Decoction)

This is a wonderful tea that will help with hot flashes by regulating blood sugar levels and increasing the availability of phytoestrogens.

2 tablespoons fenugreek seed
(*Trigonella foenum-graecum*)

2 tablespoons Ceylon cinnamon chips
or finely crushed cinnamon bark (*Cinnamomum verum*)

2 tablespoons tulsi
(holy basil; *Ocimum tenuiflorum*) or red clover (*Trifolium pratense*)

After straining, you may want to
add a touch of raw honey or pure maple syrup.

Follow the instructions on
how to make a decoction.

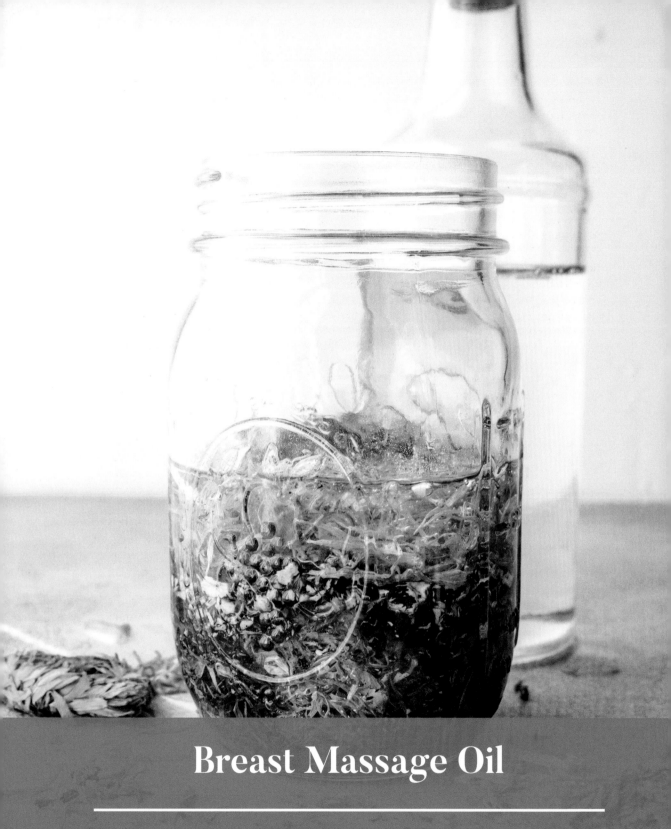

Breast Massage Oil

Personal Care

Use this oil if you experience fibrocystic, lumpy, and painful swollen breasts. The herbs used here have a long folk tradition of moving the lymphatic system and lowering the inflammation in the breast ducts and tissue. Many women report amazing results within days. I've written the recipe in a way that you can decide how much you want to make—you can start with a small batch and then make a big one if you decide that you like it (and also want to gift it to other women). Don't worry if you can't pick fresh flowers and roots—get dried ones. Castor oil will help to bring the herbs deep into the tissue—it's the deepest penetrating oil we know. I like to use jojoba oil too because it is light and highly absorbable, making the absorption of this infusion quick but deep.

If you have not infused oils before, be careful not to fry the herbs! It's common for a beginner to overheat the oil (effectively turning the flowers into fritters!) and make the infusion too fast. The best infusions use little heat and are done over a longer period of time, like the sun method. But I realize that not everyone wants to wait for four weeks, in which case, follow the fast infusion method—it will still generate great results.

1 part dandelion flowers (*Taraxacum*), fresh or dried

1 part calendula flowers (*Calendula officinalis*), fresh or dried

1 part comfrey root (*Symphytum*), fresh or dried

Organic, cold-pressed, and hexane-free castor oil

Organic, cold-pressed jojoba oil

Equipment: Mason jar with lid, slow cooker or double boiler, glass bowl, strainer or cheesecloth

---

Makes: Depends on you
Prep time: 15 minutes
Slow infusion time: 2 to 4 weeks
Fast infusion time: 8 hours

1. Place however many herbs you wish in a mason jar. Pack them down. They will wither and shrink as you infuse them so keep some to add later.

2. Pour the castor oil over the herbs, filling the jar about halfway. Add the jojoba oil, filling the mason jar until the flowers are fully covered. Stir well, packing down the herbs.

3. **Slow infusion method:** Place the jar in the sun and put the lid on. Keep it in a sunny spot (inside or outside) for 2 to 4 weeks. It is ready when the color of the oil changes to deep yellow or orange.

4. **Fast infusion method:** Place the jar, without the lid, in a slow cooker insert (an Instant Pot also has a slow cooker option). Fill up the slow cooker with enough water that it covers most of the mason jar but doesn't spill into it. Set the slow cooker on the lowest setting and heat for 2 hours. Then switch to the Keep warm setting and continue heating for 6 hours more. Keep the slow cooker and the mason jar uncovered to allow the water from the herbs to evaporate.

5. When you see the herbs wither, add more flowers and pack them down.

6. When ready, strain the oil, using a cheesecloth to squeeze out all the goodness, into a bowl.

7. Transfer the massage oil to a glass jar and label it.

Keep at room temperature for up to 3 months. Use daily when you do a breast massage explained on page 176.

PMS Salve

A number of studies show the effectiveness of clary sage and lavender in reducing symptoms of PMS and uterine pain. I've also come to appreciate the deeply anti-inflammatory and antispasmodic effects of the St. John's Wort plant. Combining these beautiful herbs in one simple salve will hopefully give you relief during this time of the month.

2 heaping tablespoons beeswax pellets

¼ cup organic, cold-pressed, and hexane-free castor oil

¼ cup St. John's Wort–infused oil (*Hypericum perforatum*)

20 drops clary sage essential oil

10 drops lavender essential oil

Equipment: Double boiler, 4-ounce glass jar with lid

Makes: 4 ounces
Prep Time: 15 minutes
Stove Time: 20 minutes

1. Melt the beeswax in a double boiler.

2. Add the castor oil and St. John's Wort oil and heat until the beeswax is fully integrated.

3. Remove from the heat and cool for 15 minutes and then add the essential oils.

4. Pour into a glass jar and let cool until solid.

5. Secure the lid and label with the ingredients and date.

6. Apply generously on the uterus (lower part of the abdomen) when painful and swollen.

Keep in a cool, dark place and use within 1 year.

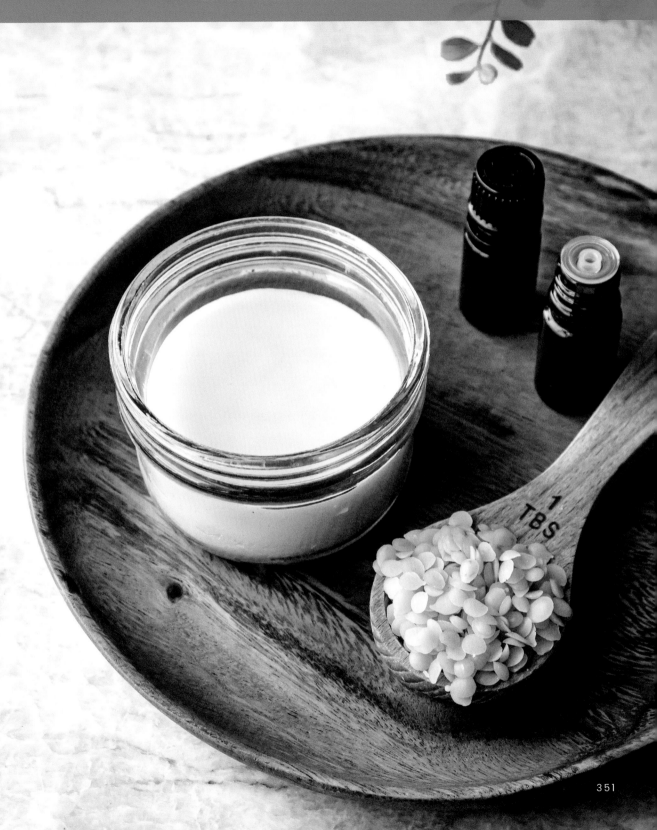

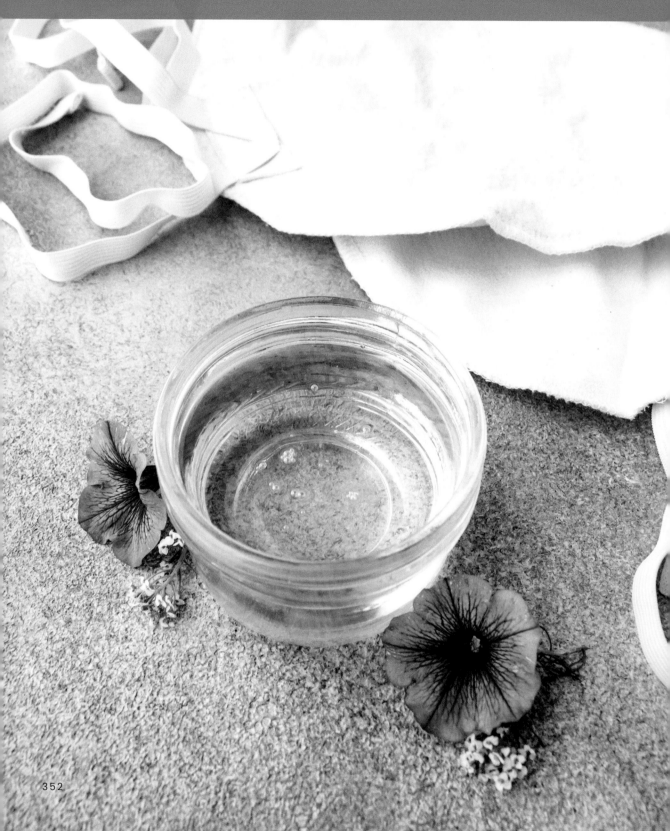

Uterine Oil Pack

This oil is perfect when experiencing painful PMS or ovulation, suffering from fibroids, or when you have swollen and painful breasts.

This recipe is a modification of the castor oil packs many of you are already very familiar with. If you are not, please see page 150 to learn about this powerful method. This recipe is using the organic cotton compress from the Queen of Thrones, but you can make your own using a woolen flannel or washcloth. You can get liquid magnesium from our Wellena store (look for Quick Magnesium). I also like the Ancient Minerals brand.

¼ cup organic, cold-pressed, and hexane-free castor oil

¼ cup liquid magnesium chloride

Cotton compress from Queen of Thrones or woolen flannel or washcloth

Equipment: 4-ounce glass bottle or jar with a lid

_____

Makes: 4 ounces
Prep Time: 15 minutes

1. Pour the castor oil and magnesium into a small bowl and whisk until well combined.

2. Transfer to a glass bottle and label it.

3. Apply generously to the abdomen and cover with the compress.

4. Keep the compress in place for 2 hours or, for best results, leave it on overnight.

Keeps well at room temperature for a year or more.

Thyroid Nodules Oil Pack

This recipe is a modification of the castor oil packs many of you are already very familiar with. If you are not, please see page 153 to learn about this powerful method. I love this recipe and have seen it work with many women. However, topical applications seldom work in isolation. If you are dealing with thyroid nodules, it's essential to also address your diet and detox your liver. Combined with this oil pack, your thyroid will love you. I recommend using a cotton eye mask. I've found it's the easiest way to apply and keep the oil on. You would need to cut the strings or the rubber of the eye mask in order to gently tighten it around your neck.

½ cup organic, cold-pressed, and hexane-free castor oil

20 drops frankincense essential oil

Cotton or flannel eye mask or compress (like the one worn on airplanes)

Equipment: 4-ounce glass bottle or jar with a lid

_____

Makes: 4 ounces
Making Time: 15 minutes

1. Pour the castor oil into the glass bottle. Add the frankincense oil and shake well.

2. Label with the ingredients and date.

3. Apply 1 tablespoon of the oil onto the eye compress and place it at the bottom of the neck (where the thyroid is located). Secure it with the strings or elastic.

4. Wear for 2 hours or, for best results, leave it on overnight.

Keeps well at room temperature for a year or more.

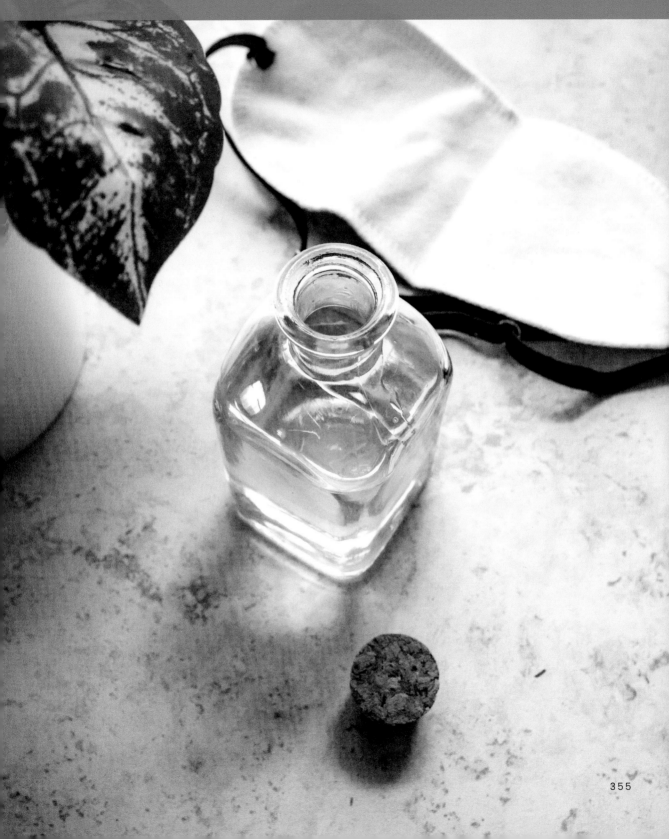

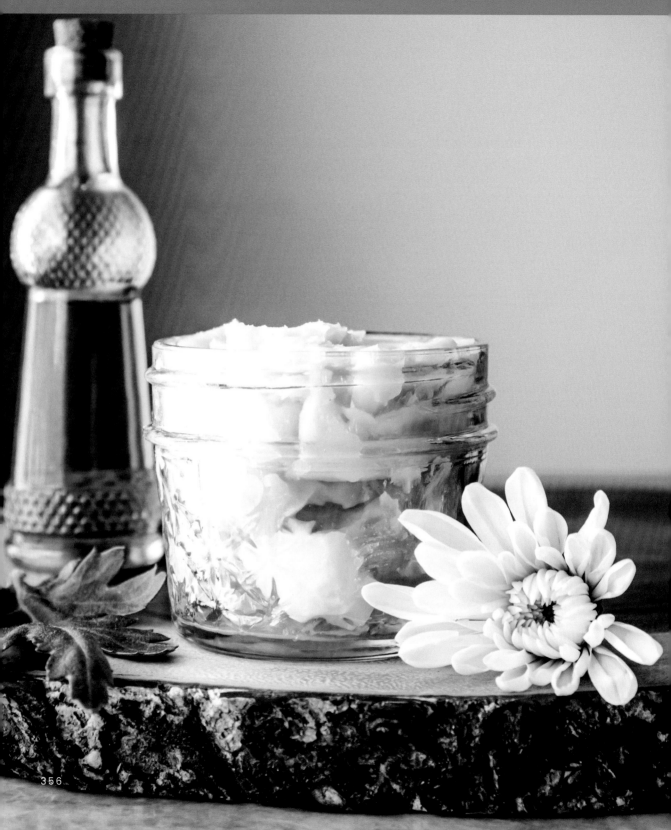

Nourished Skin Salve

Part of getting your estrogen dominance under control is to free yourself from xenoestrogen, or the "foreign" estrogens found in mainstream skin care brands (like the ones you see on TV and glossy magazines). Your skin is a large organ that absorbs whatever you put on it. Changing your body lotions and creams will make an immediate and significant difference. With this recipe, I want to show you how simple, fast, and inexpensive it is to make your own body salve that can replace your mainstream lotions. And if you aren't currently using a lotion for dry skin, many women, especially when going into peri- and menopause, will suddenly have dry skin. This salve will help.

3 tablespoons unrefined shea butter

3 tablespoons lanolin

3 tablespoons organic, cold-pressed, and hexane-free castor oil

5 drops myrrh essential oil (optional)

5 drops patchouli essential oil (optional)

5 drops geranium essential oil (optional)

Equipment: Double boiler, 4-ounce glass jar with lid

1. In a double boiler, place the shea butter, lanolin, and castor oil. Heat until all the ingredients become liquified.

2. Remove from the heat and transfer to a jar to cool for 10 minutes and then stir in the essential oils.

3. Cool completely before securing the lid. Label with the ingredients and date.

Store at room temperature, and use within 1 year.

Makes: 4 ounces
Prep Time: 25 minutes

All-Purpose Cleaner

You can use this cleaner in the bathroom and the kitchen, to clean the oven or fridge, and to wipe down all the surfaces around the house. My house keeper was reluctant at first to use this "hippy spray," as she called it. After a few months, she told me that not only had she started using it with all her other clients (who also loved it), but it most likely also helped her with all her allergies, dry skin, and constant headaches.

2 cups water

1½ cups distilled white vinegar

½ cup rubbing alcohol (70% ethanol)

20 to 30 drops essential oils of choice (lemon, thyme, lavender, oregano, clove, rosemary)

Equipment: 1-quart/32-ounce recycled glass spray bottle

_____

Makes: 1 quart
Making time: 5 minutes

1. Combine all of the ingredients in a spray bottle, shake well, and start cleaning.

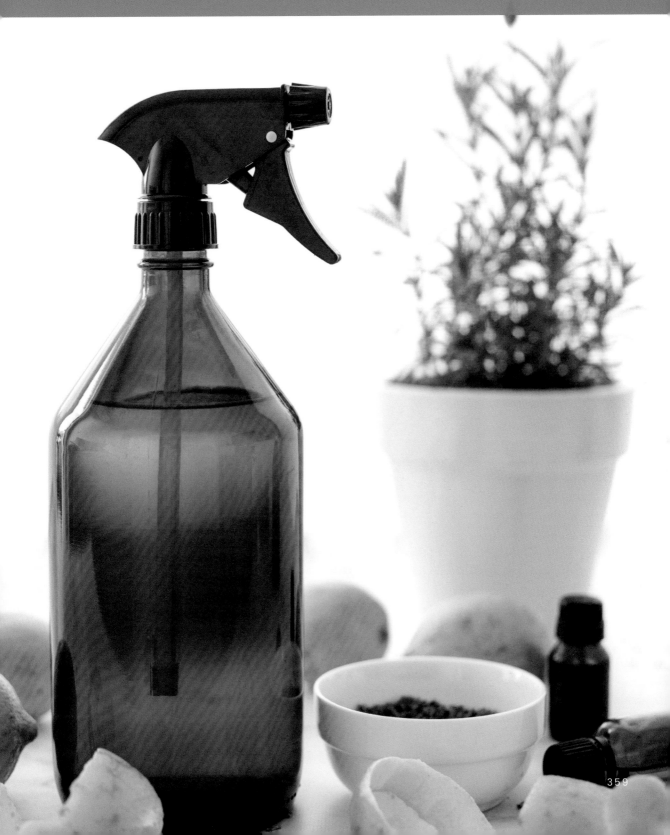

OVERCOMING ESTROGEN DOMINANCE

Supplements and Herbs Guide

Supplement Brands We Recommend

Supplements are an unregulated industry, therefore quality ranges from top-notch to junk. We have formulated many of the supplements mentioned in this book to help you get better quicker, by trusting what you put in your body will help heal. You can find our supplements on wellena.com. If you feel compelled to support our line, my team and I would be forever grateful.

Wellena

wellena.com

B Maximus
Before and After Meal Bitters
Betaine HCl with Pepsin
Brocco Power (Sulforaphane)
Calcium D-glucarate
Chromium Complete
Collagen Complete
Digestive Bitters (Before Meal, After Meal)
Digestive Enzymes
DIM
E Maximus
Fiber Complete
FibroSupport
Gluco Maximus
GLA Maximus
Inflammavail
Insulo Support
Magnesium Citrate
Magnesium Replenish
ProgestPure
Quick Magnesium
Sleep Restore
Vitamin B_6 Liquid

Vitamin C Burst
Wise Women's Balance
Zinc Complete

Other supplements and brands I would recommend:

Megasporebiotics for spore-based probiotics
Pure Encapsulations (Note: they are now owned by Nestlé)
Thorne Research
Douglas Labs (Note: they are now owned by Nestlé)
Designs for Health
Gaia's PlantForce Liquid Iron (recommended for vegetarians)
Floradix's Iron + Herbs (recommended for vegetarians)
HerbPharm (herbal tinctures)
Paleovalley's Grass Fed Organ Complex
Seeking Health's Ox Bile

Recommended Lab Tests

For the most updated labs and discounts from these partners, visit us at www.hormonesbalance.com/oed/testing

Self-order:
www.YourLabWork.com/hormonesbalance

- CBC

- Thyroid and Hashimoto's

- Blood sugar levels

- Lipids panel

- Inflammatory markers

- Nutritional panel

- Food intolerances

- Hormone testing (urine)—DUTCH

- Heavy metal exposure

Hormone testing (saliva)—Labrix or ZRT Labs

Genetic testing, hormone panel—StrateGene, Toolbox Genomics

Resources

For most updated resources, go to https://hormonesbalance.com/AllThingsWeLove.

Where to Connect with Us

Website: www.HormonesBalance.com

Facebook: www.facebook.com/hormonesbalance

Instagram: www.instagram.com/hormonebalance

Join our private online community. As an owner of this book, you will get immediate access to our thriving online support group—join us on www.facebook.com/groups/HormoneThrivers.

Products My Team and I Love and Use

For the most current listings, go to https://hormonesbalance.com/allthingswelove/. It's a curated directory of organic, clean, highly sustainably made products we absolutely love and use in our daily lives.

Food

Bread, Gluten-Free

Simple Kneads (online only)
Three Bakers, 7 Ancient Grain
Food for Life, Exotic Black Rice
Northern Bakehouse, Millet and Chia Bread

Julian Bakery, Paleo Almond Bread
Simply Trudy, 100% Grain-Free Bread
Ask about your local gluten-free bakery

Coconut Milk (truly BPA-free)

Native Forest, full-fat
365 Organic Coconut Milk, full-fat

Olive oil

Freshly Pressed Olive Oil Club

Sardines

Crown Prince
Wild Planet

Tea and coffee

Pique teas (we love them all but my favorite is their matcha tea)
Rasa Koffee (Bold, Dirty)

Yogurt, Non-Dairy (grocery store)

Forager's, Plain Cashewgurt
GT's Living Foods, Plain Coconut Yogurt
Kite Hill, Plain Almond Yogurt

Herbs

Your local herbal store (support local trade!)
Frontier (available on Amazon)
Starwest Botanicals (available on Amazon)
Mountain Rose Herbs

Beauty and Personal Care Products

Body Wash

Dr. Bronner's
Hugo Naturals

Cosmetics and Skincare

100% Pure
Alima Pura
Hugo Naturals
Juice Beauty
John Masters Organics
Annmarie Gianni
Mineral Fusion
W3LL PEOPLE
Wellena (our brand)

House cleaning and laundry

Branch Basics

Perfumes

Annmarie Gianni
Kate's Magik

Household

Cookware

Cast Iron and Enameled Cast Iron

Lodge
Le Creuset
Cuisinart
Heuck

Stoneware

Lodge
Corningware
Emile Henry
Le Creuset
The Pampered Chef

Glass

Pyrex
Life Without Plastic
Ball Mason

Stainless Steel

All-Clad
Cuisinart

Essential Oil Diffuser

Marsboy

Hot Beverage Containers

EcoJarz
Sauna
Sunlighten

Air filters

AirDoctor

Water Bottles

Klean Kanteen
Lifefactor

Water Filters

Acqua Tru
Acquasana
Berkey

Bibliography

Introduction

Birth Control Pill

Khalili, H. "Risk of Inflammatory Bowel Disease with Oral Contraceptives and Menopausal Hormone Therapy: Current Evidence and Future Directions." *Drug Saf.* 2016; 39(3): 193–97. doi:10.1007/s40264-015-0372-y. Retrieved from: https://www.ncbi.nlm.nih.gov/pmc/articles/PMC4752384/.

Kaminski, P., Szpotanska-Sikorska, M., and Wielgos, M. "Cardiovascular risk and the use of oral contraceptives." *Neuro Endocrinol Lett.* 2013; 34(7): 587–89. Retrieved from: https://www.ncbi.nlm.nih.gov/pubmed/24464000.

Oinonen, K. A., and Mazmanian, D. "To what extent do oral contraceptives influence mood and affect?" J Affect Disord. 2002; 70: 229–40. Retrieved from: https://www.ncbi.nlm.nih.gov/pubmed/12128235.

Kulkarni, J. (2007). "Depression as a side effect of the contraceptive pill." *Expert. Opin. Drug Saf.* 6, 371–74 10.1517/14740338.6.4.371. Retrieved from: https://www.ncbi.nlm.nih.gov/pubmed/17688380.

Oliveira, C.A.R., et al. "Combined oral contraceptive in female mice causes hyperinsulinemia due to β-cell hypersecretion and reduction in insulin clearance." *The Journal of Steroid Biochemistry and Molecular Biology.* 2019; 190: 54–63. Retrieved from: https://www.ncbi.nlm.nih.gov/pubmed/30923014.

Palmery, M., Saraceno, A., Vaiarelli, A., and Carlomagno, G. "Oral Contraceptives and Changes in Nutritional Requirements." *Eur. Rev.* 2013; 17:1804–13. Retrieved from: https://www.ncbi.nlm.nih.gov/pubmed/23852908.

Westhoff, C. L., Petrie K. A., and Cremers, S. "Using changes in binding globulins to assess oral contraceptive compliance." *Contraception.* 2012; 87(2):176–81. doi:10.1016/j.contraception.2012.06.003. Retrieved from: https://www.ncbi.nlm.nih.gov/pmc/articles/PMC3494777/.

Brighton, J. "Post-Birth Control Syndrome + How to Heal Now." https://drbrighten.com/post-birth-control-syndrome/. Accessed April 11, 2019.

Chapter 2: Why This Is Happening:

Causes of Estrogen Dominance

Soluble Fiber

Gaskins, Audrey J., et al. "Effect of daily fiber intake on reproductive function: the BioCycle Study." *The American Journal of Clinical Nutrition.* 2009; 90(4):1061–9. doi:10.3945/ajcn.2009.27990.

Trauma and breast cancer

Green, Bonnie L., et al. "Trauma history as a predictor of psychologic symptoms in women with breast cancer." *Journal of Clinical Oncology.* March 2000; 18(5): 1084–93.

Bile acids and gut microbiome

Ridlon, Jason M., et al. "Bile Acids and the Gut Microbiome." *Curr Opin Gastroenterol.* May 2014; 30(3): 332–38.

Xenoestrogens

Fucic, A., Gamulin, M., Ferencic, Z., et al. "Environmental exposure to xenoestrogens and oestrogen related cancers: reproductive system, breast, lung, kidney, pancreas, and brain." *Environ Health.* 2012; 11 Suppl 1(Suppl 1):S8. Published 2012 Jun 28. doi:10.1186/1476-069X-11-S1-S8.

Wittliff, J. L., et al. "Xenoestrogens, Estrogens V," *Mosby's Guide to Women's Health,* 2007.

Watson, Cheryl S., Jeng, Yow-Jiun, and Guptarak, Jutatip. "Endocrine disruption via estrogen receptors that participate in nongenomic signaling pathways." *The Journal of Steroid Biochemistry and Molecular Biology,* October 2011; 127(1–2): 44–50; ISSN 0960-0760, 10.1016/j.jsbmb.2011.01.015.

De Coster, Sam and van Larebeke, Nicolas. "Endocrine-Disrupting Chemicals: Associated Disorders and Mechanisms of Action." *Journal of Environmental and Public Health,* Doi: 10.1155/2012/713696

Vitamin D

Aruna Krishnan V., Swami, Srilatha, and Feldman, David. "The potential therapeutic benefits of vitamin D in the treatment of estrogen receptor positive breast cancer." *Steroids.* 2012; 77(11): 1107–12; doi:10.1016/j.steroids.2012.06.005.

Chapter 3: What You Can Do About It:
Natural Solutions for Estrogen Dominance

The Women's Health Initiative (WHI)

Women's Health Initiative. Hormone therapy trials (HT); https://www.whi.org/about/SitePages/HT.aspx.

Side Effects of Progestins

Wood, C., et al., "Effects of estradiol with micronized progesterone or medroxyprogesterone acetate on risk markers for breast cancer in postmenopausal monkeys," Breast Cancer Res Treat 2007; 101(2):125-34.

Liang, Y., et al., "Synthetic progestins induce growth and metastasis of BT-474 human breast cancer xenografts in nude mice," Menopause 2010; 17(5):1040-47.

Ory, K., et al., "Apoptosis inhibition mediated by medroxyprogesterone acetate treatment of breast cancer cell lines," Breast Cancer Res Treat 2001; 68(3):187-98.

Papa, V ., et al., "Progestins increase insulin receptor content and insulin stimulation of growth in human breast carcinoma cells," Cancer Res 1990; 50(24):7858-62.

Progestins increase the risk of breast cancer

Rossouw, J., et al., "Risks and benefits of estrogen plus progestin in healthy postmenopausal women: Principal results from the Women's Health Initiative randomized controlled trial," JAMA 2002; 288(3):321- 33.

Fournier, A., et al., "Breast cancer risk in relation to different types of hormone replacement therapy in the E3N-EPIC cohort," Int Jour Cancer 2005; 114(3):448-54.

Porsch, J., et al., "Estrogen-progestin replacement therapy and breast cancer risk: the Women's Health Study (U.S.)," Cancer Causes Control 2002; 13(9):847- 54.

Chapter 4: Restore Your Gut

Microbiome and estrogen-related cancers

Plottel CS, Blaser MJ. Microbiome and malignancy. *Cell Host Microbe.* 2011;10(4):324–335. doi:10.1016/j.chom.2011.10.003
Retrieved from: https://www.ncbi.nlm.nih.gov/pmc/articles/PMC3264051/

Medical Xpress. Researchers review the microbiome and its possible role in cancers. Updated October 21, 2011. https://medicalxpress.com/news/2011-10-microbiome-role-cancers.html. Accessed April 9, 2019.

Beta-glucuronidase and estrogen

Skar V, Skar AG, Stromme JH. Beta-glucuronidase activity related to bacterial growth in common bile duct bile in gallstone patients. *Scandinavian Journal of Gastroenterology*. 1988;23(1):83–90. Retrieved from: https://www.ncbi.nlm.nih.gov/pubmed/3344403

Low estrogen and post- menopause

Li JY, Chassaing B, Tyagi AM, et al. Sex steroid deficiency-associated bone loss is microbiota dependent and prevented by probiotics. *Journal of Clinical Investigation*. 2016;126(6):2049–2063. doi:10.1172/JCI86062 https://www.jci.org/articles/view/86062

Serino M, Blasco-Baque V, Nicolas S, Burcelin R. Far from the eyes, close to the heart: dysbiosis of gut microbiota and cardiovascular consequences. *Curr Cardiol Rep*. 2014;16(11):540. doi:10.1007/s11886-014-0540-1 Retrieved from: https://www.ncbi.nlm.nih.gov/pmc/articles/PMC4194023/

Baker L, Meldrum KK, Wang M, Sankula R, Vanam R, Raiesdana A, Tsai B, Hile K, Brown JW, Meldrum DR. The role of estrogen in cardiovascular disease. *J Surg Res*. 2 003;115:325–344. doi: 10.1016/S0022-4804(03)00215-4. Retrieved from: https://www.ncbi.nlm.nih.gov/pubmed/14697301

Lizcano F, Guzmán G. Estrogen Deficiency and the Origin of Obesity during Menopause. *Biomed Res Int*. 2014;2014:757461. doi:10.1155/2014/757461 Retrieved from: https://www.ncbi.nlm.nih.gov/pmc/articles/PMC3964739/

Ley RE, Turnbaugh PJ, Klein S, Gordon JI. Microbial ecology: human gut microbes associated with obesity. *Nature*. 2006;444:1022–1023. doi: 10.1038/4441022a Retrieved from: https://www.ncbi.nlm.nih.gov/pubmed/17183309/

Low microbiome diversity and breast cancer

Goedert JJ, Jones G, Hua X, et al. Investigation of the association between the fecal microbiota and breast cancer in postmenopausal women: a population-based case-control pilot study. *Journal of the National Cancer Institute*. 2015;107(8):djv147. Published 2015 Jun 1. doi:10.1093/jnci/djv147 Retrieved from: https://www.ncbi.nlm.nih.gov/pubmed/26032724

Estrobolome and breast cancer

Kwa M, Plottel CS, Blaser MJ, Adams, S. The Intestinal Microbiome and Estrogen Receptor–Positive Female Breast Cancer. *Journal of the National Cancer Institute*. 2016; 108(8):djw029. Published 2016 April 22. doi.org/10.1093/jnci/djw029 Retrieved from: https://academic.oup.com/jnci/article/108/8/djw029/2457487

Shapira I, Sultan K, Lee A, Taioli E. Evolving concepts: how diet and the intestinal microbiome act as modulators of breast malignancy. *ISRN Oncol*. 2013;2013:693920. Published 2013 Sep 25. doi:10.1155/2013/693920 Retrieved from: https://www.ncbi.nlm.nih.gov/pmc/articles/PMC3800670/

Endometriosis and gut bacteria

Bailey MT, Coe CL. Endometriosis is associated with an altered profile of intestinal microflora in female rhesus monkeys. *Human Reproduction*. 2002; 17(7):1704–1708.10.1093/humrep/17.7.1704 Retrieved from: https://www.ncbi.nlm.nih.gov/pubmed/12093827

Baker JM, Al-Nakkash L, Herbst-Kralovetz MM. Estrogen-gut microbiome axis: physiological and clinical implications. *Maturitas*. 2017; 103:45–53. doi: 10.1016/j.maturitas.2017.06.025.https://www.ncbi.nlm.nih.gov/pubmed/28778332

Puca J, Hoyne GF. Microbial dysbiosis and disease pathogenesis of endometriosis, could there be a link?. *Allied J Med Res*. 2017;1(1):1-9. Retrieved from: http://www.alliedacademies.org/articles/microbial-dysbiosis-and-disease-pathogenesis-of-endometriosis-c ould-therebe-a-link-6652.html

Microbiome and PCOS

Lindheim L, Bashir M, Münzker J, Trummer C, Zachhuber V, Leber B, et al. Alterations in Gut Microbiome Composition and Barrier Function Are Associated with Reproductive and Metabolic Defects in Women with Polycystic Ovary Syndrome (PCOS): A Pilot Study. 2017; *PLoS ONE* 12(1): e0168390. https://doi.org/10.1371/journal.pone.0168390

Betaine HCL

Nutrition Review. Gastric Balance: Heartburn Not Always Caused by Excess Acid. 2018. https://nutritionreview.org/2018/03/gastric-balance-heartburn-caused-excess-acid.

Kines K, Krupczak T. Nutritional Interventions for Gastroesophageal Reflux, Irritable Bowel Syndrome, and Hypochlorhydria: A Case Report. Integrative Medicine: A Clinician's Journal. 2016;15(4):49-53.

Llorente C, Jepsen P, Inamine T, et al. Gastric acid suppression promotes alcoholic liver disease by inducing overgrowth of intestinal Enterococcus. Nature Communications. 2017;8:837. doi:10.1038/s41467-017-00796-x.

Cellini M, Santaguida MG, Virili C, et al. Hashimoto's Thyroiditis and Autoimmune Gastritis. Frontiers in Endocrinology. 2017;8:92. doi:10.3389/fendo.2017.00092.

Esplugues JV, Barrachina MD, Beltrán B, Calatayud S, Whittle BJR, Moncada S. Inhibition of gastric acid secretion by stress: A protective reflex mediated by cerebral nitric oxide. Proceedings of the National Academy of Sciences of the United States of America. 1996;93(25):14839-14844.

Digestive Enzymes

Röder PV, Wu B, Liu Y, Han W. Pancreatic regulation of glucose homeostasis. Experimental & Molecular Medicine. 2016;48(3):e219-. doi:10.1038/emm.2016.6.

Carabotti M, Scirocco A, Maselli MA, Severi C. The gut-brain axis: interactions between enteric microbiota, central and enteric nervous systems. Annals of Gastroenterology : Quarterly Publication of the Hellenic Society of Gastroenterology. 2015;28(2):203-209.

Fiber

Dukas L, Willett WC. Association between physical activity, fiber intake, and other lifestyle variables and constipation in a study of women. Am J Gastroenterol. 2003 Aug;98(8):1790-6.

Galvez J, Rodriguez-Cabezas ME. Effects of dietary fiber on inflammatory bowel disease. Mol Nutr Food Res. 2005 Apr 19.

Collagen

Zdzieblik D, Oesser S, Gollhofer A, König D. Improvement of activity-related knee joint discomfort following supplementation of specific collagen peptides [published correction appears in Appl Physiol Nutr Metab. 2017 Nov;42(11):1237]. Appl Physiol Nutr Metab. 2017;42(6):588-595. doi:10.1139/apnm-2016-0390

König D, Oesser S, Scharla S, Zdzieblik D, Gollhofer A. Specific Collagen Peptides Improve Bone Mineral Density and Bone Markers in Postmenopausal Women-A Randomized Controlled Study. Nutrients. 2018;10(1):97. Published 2018 Jan 16. doi:10.3390/nu10010097

Proksch E, Schunck M, Zague V, Segger D, Degwert J, Oesser S. Oral intake of specific bioactive collagen peptides reduces skin wrinkles and increases dermal matrix synthesis. Skin Pharmacol Physiol. 2014;27(3):113-119. doi:10.1159/000355523

Chapter 5: Detox Your Liver

B vitamins

Welzel TM, Katki HA, Sakoda LC, et al. Blood folate levels and risk of liver damage and hepatocellular carcinoma in a prospective high-risk cohort. *Cancer Epidemiol Biomark* Prev. 2007;16(6):1279–82. Retrieved from: https://www.ncbi.nlm.nih.gov/pubmed/17548697

D-Limonene

Bodake HB, Panicker KN, Kailaje VV, Rao KV. Chemopreventive effect of orange oil on the development of hepatic preneoplastic lesions induced by N-nitrosodiethylamine in rats: an ultrastructural study. *Indian Journal of Experimental Biology.* 2 002; 40(3): 245-51.Retrieved from: https://www.ncbi.nlm.nih.gov/pubmed/12635690

Sun J. D-limonene: safety and clinical applications. *Alternative Medical Review.* 2007; 12(3): 259-264. Retrieved from: https://www.ncbi.nlm.nih.gov/pubmed/18072821.

Selenium

Espinoza SE, Guo H, Fedarko N, et al. Glutathione peroxidase enzyme activity in aging. *J Gerontol A Biol Sci Med Sci.* 2008;63(5):505–509. Retrieved from: https://www.ncbi.nlm.nih.gov/pmc/articles/PMC2964084/

Flax seed

Horn-Ross PL, Hoggatt KJ, Lee, MM. Phytoestrogens and Thyroid Cancer Risk *Cancer Epidemiology Biomarkers & Prevention.* 2002; 11(1): 43-49. Retrieved from: http://cebp.aacrjournals.org/content/11/1/43.article-info

Petit HV, Small JA, Palin MF, Giguère A, Santos GTD. Effects of flax seed supplementation on endometrial expression of ISG17 and intrauterine prostaglandin concentrations in primiparous dairy cows submittedtoGnRH-basedsynchronizedovulation.*CanadianJournalofAnimalScience*. 2007; 87:343-352. https://doi.org/10.4141/CJAS06017

Phipps WR, Martini MC, Lampe JW, Slavin JL, Kurzer MS. Effect of flax seed ingestion on the menstrual cycle. *Journal of Clinical Endocrinol Metabolism.* 1993;77:1215–1219. Retrieved from: https://www.ncbi.nlm.nih.gov/pubmed/8077314

Bergman JM, Thompson LU, Dabrosin C. Flax seed and its lignans inhibit estradiol-induced growth, angiogenesis, and secretion of vascular endothelial growth factor in human breast cancer xenografts in vivo. *Clinical Cancer Research.* 2007; 13(3):1061–7.10.1158/1078-0432.CCR-06-1651 Retrieved from: https://www.ncbi.nlm.nih.gov/pubmed/17289903

Broccoli sprouts (sulforaphane)

Li Y, et al. Sulforaphane, a Dietary Component of Broccoli/Broccoli Sprouts, Inhibits Breast Cancer Stem Cells. *Clinical Cancer Research.* 2010; 16(9): 2580-2590; DOI: 10.1158/1078-0432.CCR-09-2937. Retrieved from: http://clincancerres.aacrjournals.org/content/16/9/2580.short

Pomegranates

Sreeja S., Santhosh Kumar T.R., Lakshmi B.S., Sreeja S. Pomegranate extract demonstrates a selective estrogen receptor modulator profile in human tumor cell lines and in vivo models of estrogen deprivation. *Journal of Nutritional Biochemistry.* 2012;23:725–732. doi: 10.1016/j.jnutbio.2011.03.015. Retrieved from: https://www.ncbi.nlm.nih.gov/pubmed/21839626

NAC, estrogen metabolism and cancer prevention

Zahid M, Saeed M, Ali MF, Rogan EG, Cavalieri EL. N-acetylcysteine blocks formation of cancer-initiating estrogen-DNA adducts in cells. Free Radic Biol Med. 2010;49(3):392-400. doi:10.1016/j.freeradbiomed.2010.04.028

Cavalieri EL, Rogan EG. Unbalanced metabolism of endogenous estrogens in the etiology and prevention of human cancer. J Steroid Biochem Mol Biol. 2011;125(3-5):169-180. doi:10.1016/j.jsbmb.2011.03.008

Chapter 6: Balance Your Blood Sugar

How much sugar is OK?

U.S. Department of Health and Human Services and U.S. Department of Agriculture. Dietary Guidelines for Americans, 2005. 6th Edition, Washington, DC: U.S. Government Printing Office, January 2005. Retrieved from: https://health.gov/dietaryguidelines/dga2005/document/default.htm

Coffee and blood sugar levels

Pizziol A, Tikhonoff V, Paleari CD, et al. Effects of caffeine on glucose tolerance: a placebo-controlled study. *Eur J Clin Nutr*. 1998;52(11):846-849. doi:10.1038/sj.ejcn.1600657

Insulin resistance

Aguilar M . Prevalence of the Metabolic Syndrome in the United States, 2003-2012. *JAMA*. 2015; 313 (19):1973. http://jamanetwork.com/journals/jama/fullarticle/2293286

Artificial sweeteners

Pepino MY, Tiemann CD, Patterson BW, Wice BM, Klein S. Sucralose affects glycemic and hormonal responses to an oral glucose load. *Diabetes Care*. 2013;36(9):2530–2535. doi:10.2337/dc12-2221 Retrieved from: https://www.ncbi.nlm.nih.gov/pubmed/23633524

Mohamed B. Abou-Donia, Eman M. El-Masry, Ali A. Abdel-Rahman, Roger E. McLendon & Susan S. Schiffman (2008) Splenda Alters Gut Microflora and Increases Intestinal P-Glycoprotein and Cytochrome P-450 in Male Rats, *Journal of Toxicology and Environmental Health,* Part A, 71:21, 1415-1429, DOI: 10.1080/15287390802328630. Retrieved from: https://www.ncbi.nlm.nih.gov/pubmed/18800291

Berberine

W. Chang, et al. Berberine as a therapy for type 2 diabetes and its complications: From mechanism of action to clinical studies. *Biochem Cell Biol*. 2015 Oct;93(5):479-86. doi: 10.1139/bcb-2014-0107

Yin J, Xing H, Ye J. Efficacy of berberine in patients with type 2 diabetes mellitus. *Metabolism*. 2008;57(5):712-717. doi:10.1016/j.metabol.2008.01.013

Ming J, Xu S, Liu C, Liu X, Jia A, Ji Q. Effectiveness and safety of bifidobacteria and berberine in people with hyperglycemia: study protocol for a randomized controlled trial. Trials. 2018;19:72. doi:10.1186/s13063-018-2438-5.

Dong H, Wang N, Zhao L, Lu F. Berberine in the Treatment of Type 2 Diabetes Mellitus: A Systemic Review and Meta-Analysis. Evidence-based Complementary and Alternative Medicine : eCAM. 2012;2012:591654. doi:10.1155/2012/591654.

Wang H, Zhu C, Ying Y, Luo L, Huang D, Luo Z. Metformin and berberine, two versatile drugs in treatment of common metabolic diseases. Oncotarget. 2018;9(11):10135-10146. doi:10.18632/oncotarget.20807.

Chromium picolinate

N. Susksomboon, et al., Systematic review and meta-analysis of the efficacy and safety of chromium supplementation in diabetes. *J Clin Pharm Ther*. 2014 Jun;39(3):292-306. doi: 10.1111/jcpt.12147

Chen S, Jin X, Shan Z, et al. Inverse Association of Plasma Chromium Levels with Newly Diagnosed Type 2 Diabetes: A Case-Control Study. Nutrients. 2017;9(3):294. doi:10.3390/nu9030294.

Diabetes Education. A scientific review: the role of chromium in insulin resistance. Diabetes Education. 2004;Suppl:2-14. https://www.ncbi.nlm.nih.gov/pubmed/15208835.

Inositol

Nordio M, Proietti E. The combined therapy with myo-inositol and D-chiro-inositol reduces the risk of metabolic disease in PCOS overweight patients compared to myo-inositol supplementation alone. Eur Rev Med Pharmacol Sci. 2012;16(5):575-81.

D'Anna R, Santamaria A, Giorgianni G. Myo-inositol and melatonin in the menopausal transition. Gynecol Endocrinol. 2017;33(4):279-282. doi: 10.1080/09513590.2016.1254613.

Chapter 7: Amplify Your Healing with
These Foundational Supplements

Mineral content of apples

Paul Bergner. *The Healing Power of Minerals and Trace Elements*. Boulder, CO: North American Institute of medical Herbalism, 2003. 33-34. http://www.medherb.com/gathering/Minerals0803-wo-photo.pdf

Magnesium

Renea L. Beckstrand, PhD, RN, CCRN, CNE and Jann S. Pickens, BS, RN. Beneficial Effects of Magnesium Supplementation. *Journal of Evidence-Based Complementary and Alternative Medicine*. 2011, Oct;16 (3): 181-189. doi: 10.1177/2156587211401746

Dong JY, Xun P, He K, Qin LQ. Magnesium intake and risk of type 2 diabetes: meta-analysis of prospective cohort studies. Diabetes Care. 2011;34(9):2116-22. doi: 10.2337/dc11-0518.

Boyle NB, Lawton C, Dye L. The Effects of Magnesium Supplementation on Subjective Anxiety and Stress—A Systematic Review. Nutrients. 2017;9(5):429. doi:10.3390/nu9050429.

Abbasi B, Kimiagar M, Sadeghniiat K, Shirazi MM, Hedayati M, Rashidkhani B. The effect of magnesium supplementation on primary insomnia in elderly: A double-blind placebo-controlled clinical trial. Journal of Research in Medical Sciences : The Official Journal of Isfahan University of Medical Sciences. 2012;17(12):1161-1169.

Gröber U, Schmidt J, Kisters K. Magnesium in Prevention and Therapy. Nutrients. 2015;7(9):8199-8226. doi:10.3390/nu7095388.

Vitamin C

Hirofumi Henmi, Toshiaki Endo, Yoshimitsu Kitajima, et al. Effects of ascorbic acid supplementation on serum progesterone levels in patients with a luteal phase defect. Fertility and Sterility. 2003 Aug;80(2):459-461. doi:10.1016/S0015-0282(03)00657-5

Zhang S, Hunter DJ, Forman MR, et al. Dietary carotenoids and vitamins A, C, and E and risk of breast cancer. J Natl Cancer Inst. 1999;91(6):547-556. (PubMed)

Michels KB, Holmberg L, Bergkvist L, Ljung H, Bruce A, Wolk A. Dietary antioxidant vitamins, retinol, and breast cancer incidence in a cohort of Swedish women. Int J Cancer. 2001;91(4):563-567. (PubMed)

Vitamin B Complex

Kennedy DO. B Vitamins and the Brain: Mechanisms, Dose and Efficacy—A Review. Nutrients. 2016;8(2):68. doi:10.3390/nu8020068.

Sauberlich HE. Interactions of thiamin, riboflavin, and other B-vitamins. Ann N Y Acad Sci. 1980;355:80-97.

Chen YB, Wang YF, Hou W, et al. Effect of B-complex vitamins on the antifatigue activity and bioavailability of ginsenoside Re after oral administration. Journal of Ginseng Research. 2017;41(2):209-214. doi:10.1016/j.jgr.2016.03.006.

Nutrition's dynamic duos. Harvard Health Publishing: Harvard Health Letter. 2009. https://www.health.harvard.edu/newsletter_article/Nutritions-dynamic-duos

Dong H, Pi F, Ding Z, et al. Efficacy of Supplementation with B Vitamins for Stroke Prevention: A Network Meta-Analysis of Randomized Controlled Trials. Chang AYW, ed. PLoS ONE. 2015;10(9):e0137533. doi:10.1371/journal.pone.0137533.

Jabbar A, Yawar A, Waseem S, Islam N, Ul Haque N, Zuberi L, Khan A, Akhter J. Vitamin B_{12} deficiency common in primary hypothyroidism. J Pak Med Assoc. 2008;58(5):258-61.

Zinc

Berger A. What does zinc do? BMJ : British Medical Journal. 2002;325(7372):1062.

Zinc Fact Sheet for Consumers. National Institutes of Health. 2016. https://ods.od.nih.gov/factsheets/Zinc-Consumer/

Jinno N, Nagata M, Takahashi T. Marginal zinc deficiency negatively affects recovery from muscle injury in mice. Biol Trace Elem Res. 2014;158(1):65-72. doi: 10.1007/s12011-014-9901-2. Epub 2014 Feb 4.

Favier AE. The role of zinc in reproduction. Hormonal mechanisms. Biol Trace Elem Res. 1992;32:363-82.

Jamilian M, Foroozanfard F, Bahmani F, et al. Effects of Zinc Supplementation on Endocrine Outcomes in Women with Polycystic Ovary Syndrome: a Randomized, Double-Blind, Placebo-Controlled Trial. Biol Trace Elem Res. 2016;170(2):271-8.

Ertek S, Cicero AFG, Caglar O, Erdogan G. Relationship between serum zinc levels, thyroid hormones and thyroid volume following successful iodine supplementation. Hormones. 2010;9(3):263-268

Nishiyama S, Futagoishi-Suginohara Y, Matsukura M, et al. Zinc supplementation alters thyroid hormone metabolism in disabled patients with zinc deficiency. Am Coll Nutr. 1994;13(1):62-7.

Morley JE, Gordon J, Hershman JM. Zinc deficiency, chronic starvation, and hypothalamic-pituitary-thyroid function. Am J Clin Nutr. 1980;33(8):1767-70.

Brandão-Neto J, de Mendonça BB, Shuhama T, Marchini JS, Pimenta WP, Tornero MT. Zinc acutely and temporarily inhibits adrenal cortisol secretion in humans. A preliminary report. Biol Trace Elem Res. 1990;24(1):83-9.

Fodor L, Ahnefeld FW, Fazekas AT. Studies on the glucocorticoid control of zinc metabolism. Infusionstherapie und Klinische Ernahrung. 1975;2(3):210-213

Ghavami-Maibodi SZ, Collipp PJ, Castro-Magana M, et al. Effect of oral zinc supplements on growth, hormonal levels, and zinc in healthy short children. Ann Nutr Metab. 1983;27(3):214-9.

Miletta MC, Schöni MH, Kernland K, Mullis PE, Petkovic V. The role of zinc dynamics in growth hormone secretion. Horm Res Paediatr. 2013;80(6):381-9.

Vitamin D$_3$

Nair R, Maseeh A. Vitamin D: The "sunshine" vitamin. Journal of Pharmacology & Pharmacotherapeutics. 2012;3(2):118-126. doi:10.4103/0976-500X.95506.

Alshahrani F, Aljohani N. Vitamin D: Deficiency, Sufficiency and Toxicity. Nutrients. 2013;5(9):3605-3616. doi:10.3390/nu5093605.

Lemire JM, Archer DC, Beck L, Spiegelberg HL. Immunosuppressive actions of 1,25-dihydroxyvitamin D3: preferential inhibition of Th1 functions. J Nutr. 1995;125(6 Suppl):1704S-1708S. doi: 10.1093/jn/125.suppl_6.1704S.

Kim D. The Role of Vitamin D in Thyroid Diseases. International Journal of Molecular Sciences. 2017;18(9):1949. doi:10.3390/ijms18091949.

Mackawy AMH, Al-ayed Bushra Mohammed, Al-rashidi Bashayer Mater. Vitamin D Deficiency and Its Association with Thyroid Disease. International Journal of Health Sciences. 2013;7(3):267-275.

Muscogiuri G, Altieri B, Penna-Martinez M, Badenhoop K. Focus on vitamin D and the adrenal gland. Horm Metab Res. 2015;47(4):239-46. doi: 10.1055/s-0034-1396893.

Al-Dujaili EAS, Munir N, Iniesta RR. Effect of vitamin D supplementation on cardiovascular disease risk factors and exercise performance in healthy participants: a randomized placebo-controlled preliminary study. Therapeutic Advances in Endocrinology and Metabolism. 2016;7(4):153-165. doi:10.1177/2042018816653357.

Roy S, Sherman A, Monari-Sparks MJ, Schweiker O, Hunter K. Correction of Low Vitamin D Improves Fatigue: Effect of Correction of Low Vitamin D in Fatigue Study (EViDiF Study). North American Journal of Medical Sciences. 2014;6(8):396-402. doi:10.4103/1947-2714.139291.

Kinuta K, Tanaka H, Moriwake T, et al. Vitamin D is an important factor in estrogen biosynthesis of both female and male gonads. Endocrinology. 2000;141(4):1317-24.

Mason C, De Dieu Tapsoba J, Duggan C, et al. Effects of vitamin D supplementation during weight loss on sex hormones in postmenopausal women. Menopause (New York, NY). 2016;23(6):645-652. doi:10.1097/GME.0000000000000600.

Krishnan AV, Swami S, Feldman D. The Potential Therapeutic Benefits of Vitamin D in the Treatment of Estrogen Receptor Positive Breast Cancer. Steroids. 2012;77(11):1107-1112. doi:10.1016/j.steroids.2012.06.005.

Tripkovic L, Lambert H, Hart K, et al. Comparison of vitamin D_2 and vitamin D_3 supplementation in raising serum 25-hydroxyvitamin D status: a systematic review and meta-analysis. The American Journal of Clinical Nutrition. 2012;95(6):1357-1364. doi:10.3945/ajcn.111.031070.

Houghton LA, Vieth R. The case against ergocalciferol (vitamin D_2) as a vitamin supplement. The American Journal of Clinical Nutrition. 2006;84(4): 694-697. doi.org/10.1093/ajcn/84.4.694

DIM (Di-Indolyl-Methane)

Rajoria S, Suriano R, Parmar PS, et al. 3,3'-diindolylmethane modulates estrogen metabolism in patients with thyroid proliferative disease: a pilot study. *Thyroid*. 2011;21(3):299–304. doi:10.1089/thy.2010.0245. Retrieved from: https://www.ncbi.nlm.nih.gov/pmc/articles/PMC3048776/

Patel AR, Spencer SD, Chougule MB, Safe S, Singh M. Pharmacokinetic evaluation and In Vitro–In Vivo Correlation (IVIVC) of novel methylene-substituted 3,3`diindolylmethane (DIM). European Journal of Pharmaceutical Sciences. 2012;46(1-2):8-16. doi:10.1016/j.ejps.2012.01.012.

Wang SQ, Cheng LS, Liu Y, Wang JY, Jiang W. Indole-3-Carbinol (I3C) and its Major Derivatives: Their Pharmacokinetics and Important Roles in Hepatic Protection. Curr Drug Metab. 2016;17(4):401-9.

De Santi M, Carloni E, Galluzzi L, et al. Inhibition of Testosterone Aromatization by the Indole-3-carbinol Derivative CTet in CYP19A1-overexpressing MCF-7 Breast Cancer Cells. Anticancer Agents Med Chem. 2015;15(7):896-904.

Im A, Vogel VG, Ahrendt G, et al. Urinary estrogen metabolites in women at high risk for breast cancer. Carcinogenesis. 2009;30(9):1532-1535. doi:10.1093/carcin/bgp139.

Poornima J, Mirunalini S. Regulation of carbohydrate metabolism by indole-3-carbinol and its metabolite 3,3'-diindolylmethane in high-fat diet-induced C57BL/6J mice. Mol Cell Biochem. 2014 Jan;385(1-2):7-15. doi: 10.1007/s11010-013-1808-2

Thomson CA, Ho E, Strom MB. Chemopreventive properties of 3,3`-diindolylmethane in breast cancer: evidence from experimental and human studies. Nutrition Reviews. 2016;74(7):432-443. doi:10.1093/nutrit/nuw010.

Thomson CA, Chow HHS, Wertheim BC, et al. A randomized, placebo-controlled trial of diindolylmethane for breast cancer biomarker modulation in patients taking tamoxifen. Breast cancer research and treatment. 2017;165(1): 97–107. doi:10.1007/s10549-017-4292-7.

Sulforaphane

Yoshida K, Ushida Y, Ishijima T, et al. Broccoli sprout extract induces detoxification-related gene expression and attenuates acute liver injury. *World J Gastroenterol*. 2015; 21(35): 10091–10103. doi:10.3748/wjg.v21.i35.10091. Retrieved from: https://www.ncbi.nlm.nih.gov/pmc/articles/PMC4572790/

Castro, N. P. et al. Sulforaphane suppresses the growth of triple-negative breast cancer stem-like cells in vitro and in vivo. *Cancer Prev. Res. (Phila.)*1 2,147–158 (2019). Retrieved from: https://www.ncbi.nlm.nih.gov/pubmed/30679159

Li Y, Zhang T, Korkaya H, et al. Sulforaphane, a dietary component of broccoli/broccoli sprouts, inhibits breast cancer stem cells. *Clin Cancer Res*. 2010;16(9):2580–2590. doi:10.1158/1078-0432.CCR-09-2937. Retrieved from: https://www.ncbi.nlm.nih.gov/pmc/articles/PMC2862133/

Riedl MA, Saxon A, Diaz-Sanchez D. Oral Sulforaphane increases Phase II antioxidant enzymes in the human upper airway. Clinical immunology (Orlando, Fla). 2009;130(3): 244-251. doi:10.1016/j.clim.2008.10.007.

Wang L, Tian Z, Yang Q, et al. Sulforaphane inhibits thyroid cancer cell growth and invasiveness through the reactive oxygen species-dependent pathway. Oncotarget. 2015;6(28): 25917-25931.0.1158/1078-0432.CCR-09-2937.

Pawlik A, Słomińska-Wojewódzka M, Herman-Antosiewicz A. Sensitization of estrogen receptor-positive breast cancer cell lines to 4-hydroxytamoxifen by isothiocyanates present in cruciferous plants. European Journal of Nutrition. 2016;55:1165-1180. doi:10.1007/s00394-015-0930-1.

Yanaka A. Daily intake of broccoli sprouts normalizes bowel habits in human healthy subjects. Journal of Clinical Biochemistry and Nutrition. 2018;62(1):75-82. doi:10.3164/jcbn.17-42

Hot water bath triples sulforaphane in broccoli sprouts

Matusheski NV, Juvik JA, Jeffery EH. Heating decreases epithiospecifier protein activity and increases sulforaphane formation in broccoli. *Phytochemistry*. 2004; 65(9): 1273-1281. Retrieved from: https://www.sciencedirect.com/science/article/abs/pii/S0031942204001657

Calcium D-glucarate

Calcium D-glucarate. *Alternative Medicine Review*. 2002; 7(4): 336-339. Retrieved from: https://www.ncbi.nlm.nih.gov/pubmed/12197785

Thorne Research. Calcium-D-glucarate. Alternative Medicine Review. 2002;7(4):336-9.

Walaszek Z. Potential use of d-glucaric acid derivatives in cancer prevention. Cancer Letter. 1990;54(1-2):1-8. doi.org/10.1016/0304-3835(90)90083-A

Zoltaszek R, Kowalczyk P, Kowalczyk MC, et al. Dietary D-glucarate effects on the biomarkers of inflammation during early post-initiation stages of benzo[a]pyrene-induced lung tumorigenesis in A/J mice. Oncology Letters. 2011;2(1):145-154. doi:10.3892/ol.2010.221.

Omega 3 Fatty Acids

Masoumi SZ, Kazemi F, Tavakolian S, et al. Effect of Citalopram in Combination with Omega-3 on Depression in Post-menopausal Women: A Triple Blind Randomized Controlled Trial. Journal of Clinical and Diagnostic Research : JCDR. 2016;10(10):QC01-QC05. doi:10.7860/JCDR/2016/19487.8597.

Simopoulos AP. Omega-3 fatty acids in inflammation and autoimmune diseases. J Am Coll Nutr. 2002;21(6):495-505.

Souza LL1, Nunes MO, Paula GS, et al. Effects of dietary fish oil on thyroid hormone signaling in the liver. J Nutr Biochem. 2010;21(10):935-40. doi: 10.1016/j.jnutbio.2009.07.008

Delarue J, Matzinger O, Binnert C, et al. Fish oil prevents the adrenal activation elicited by mental stress in healthy men. Diabetes Metab. 2003;29(3):289-95.

Levant B. N-3 (Omega-3) Polyunsaturated Fatty Acids in the Pathophysiology and Treatment of Depression: Pre-clinical Evidence. CNS & neurological disorders drug targets. 2013;12(4):450-459.

Beydoun MA, Fanelli Kuczmarski MT, Beydoun HA, et al. ω-3 Fatty Acid Intakes Are Inversely Related to Elevated Depressive Symptoms among United States Women. The Journal of Nutrition. 2013;143(11):1743-1752. doi:10.3945/jn.113.179119.

Vitamin B$_6$

Minihane AM, Vinoy S, Russell WR, et al. Low-grade inflammation, diet composition and health: current research evidence and its translation. *Br J Nutr*. 2015;114(7):999-1012. doi:10.1017/S0007114515002093

Padh H. Cellular functions of ascorbic acid. Biochem Cell Biol. 1990 Oct;68(10):1166-73. 4.

Bioidentical Progesterone (Topical)

Formby B, Wiley TS. Progesterone inhibits growth and induces apoptosis in breast cancer cells: inverse effects on Bcl-2 and p53. Ann Clin Lab Sci. 1998;28(6):360-9.

Leonetti HB, Longo S, Anasti JN. Transdermal progesterone cream for vasomotor symptoms and postmenopausal bone loss. Obstet Gynecol. 1999;94(2):225–228.

Prior JC. Progesterone for Symptomatic Peri-menopause Treatment – Progesterone politics, physiology and potential for peri-menopause. Facts, Views & Vision in ObGyn. 2011;3(2):109-120.

Liu C-Y, Chen L-B, Liu P-Y, Xie D-P, Wang PS. Effects of progesterone on gastric emptying and intestinal transit in male rats. World Journal of Gastroenterology. 2002;8(2):338-341. doi:10.3748/wjg.v8.i2.338.

Sathi, P. , Kalyan, S. , Hitchcock, C. L., Pudek, M. and Prior, J. C. (2013), Progesterone therapy increases free thyroxine levels—data from a randomized placebo-controlled 12-week hot flush trial. Clin Endocrinol, 79: 282-287. doi:10.1111/cen.12128

Curcumin

Chainani-Wu N. Safety and anti-inflammatory activity of curcumin: a component of turmeric (Curcuma longa). J Altern Complement Med. 2003 Feb;9(1):161-8.

Yadav VS, Mishra KP, Immunomodulatory effects of curcumin. Immunopharmacol Immunotoxicol. 2005;27(3):485-97

Araujo CC, Leon LL.Biological activities of Curcuma longa L. Mem Inst Oswaldo Cruz. 2001 Jul;96(5):723-8

Sharma OP. Antioxidant Activity of Curcumin and Related Compounds. Biochem Pharmacol. 1976;46:1013.

Suzuki M, Nakamura T. Elucidation of anti-allergic activities of curcumin-related compounds with a special reference to their anti-oxidative activities. Biol Pharm Bull. 2005 Aug;28(8):1438-43.

Holt PR, Katz S Curcumin therapy in inflammatory bowel disease: a pilot study. Dig Dis Sci. 2005 Nov;50(11):2191-3.

Resveratrol

Chow, H.S., Garland, L.L., Heckman-Stoddard, B.M. et al. A pilot clinical study of resveratrol in postmenopausal women with high body mass index: effects on systemic sex steroid hormones. J Transl Med 12, 223 (2014). https://doi.org/10.1186/s12967-014-0223-0

Poschner, S., Maier-Salamon, A., et al. "Resveratrol and other dietary polyphenols are inhibitors of estrogen metabolism in human breast cancer cells." The Journal of Steroid Biochemistry and Molecular Biology Volume 190, June 2019, Pages 11-18. doi: 10.1016/j.jsbmb.2019.03.001.

Vitamin E

Rizvi S, Raza ST, Ahmed F, Ahmad A, Abbas S, Mahdi F. The Role of Vitamin E in Human Health and Some Diseases. Sultan Qaboos University Medical Journal. 2014;14(2):e157-e165.

Takasaki A, Tamura H, Taniguchi K, et al. Luteal blood flow and luteal function. Journal of Ovarian Research. 2009;2:1. doi:10.1186/1757-2215-2-1.

Chamras H, Barsky SH, Ardashian A, et al. Novel interactions of vitamin E and estrogen in breast cancer. Nutr Cancer. 2005;52(1):43-8.

Doshi SB, Agarwal A. The role of oxidative stress in menopause. Journal of Mid-Life Health. 2013;4(3):140-146. doi:10.4103/0976-7800.118990.

Peeters E, Neyt A, Beckers F, et al. Influence of supplemental magnesium, tryptophan, vitamin C, and vitamin E on stress responses of pigs to vibration. J Anim Sci. 2005;83(7):1568-80.

Mancini A, Di Segni C, Raimondo S, et al. Thyroid Hormones, Oxidative Stress, and Inflammation. Mediators of Inflammation. 2016;2016:6757154. doi:10.1155/2016/6757154.

Yu J, Shan Z, Chong W, et al. Vitamin E ameliorates iodine-induced cytotoxicity in thyroid. J Endocrinol. 2011;209(3):299-306. doi: 10.1530/JOE-11-0030.

Vitamin E Fact Sheet for Health Professionals. National Institutes of Health. 2018. https://ods.od.nih.gov/factsheets/VitaminE-HealthProfessional/#en1

Peralta EA, Brewer AT, Louis S, Dunnington GL. Vitamin E increases biomarkers of estrogen stimulation when taken with tamoxifen. J Surg Res. 2009;153(1):143-7. doi: 10.1016/j.jss.2008.03.030.

Chapter 8: Move Beyond Food Practices

Xenoestrogen chemicals

Fernandez SV, Russo J. Estrogen and xenoestrogens in breast cancer. *Toxicol Pathol.* 2009;38(1):110–122. doi:10.1177/0192623309354108. Retrieved from: https://www.ncbi.nlm.nih.gov/pmc/articles/PMC2907875/

Fucic A, Gamulin M, Ferencic Z, et al. Environmental exposure to xenoestrogens and oestrogen related cancers: reproductive system, breast, lung, kidney, pancreas, and brain. *Environ Health.* 2012;11 Suppl 1(Suppl 1):S8.

Published 2012 Jun 28. doi:10.1186/1476-069X-11-S1-S8. Retrieved from: https://www.ncbi.nlm.nih.gov/pmc/articles/PMC3388472/

Santin AP, Furlanetto TW. Role of estrogen in thyroid function and growth regulation. *J Thyroid Res*. 2011;2011:875125. doi:10.4061/2011/875125. Retrieved from: https://www.ncbi.nlm.nih.gov/pmc/articles/PMC3113168/

Derwahl M., Nicula D. Estrogen and its role in thyroid cancer. *Endocrine-Related Cancer*. 2014;21(5):T273–T283. doi: 10.1530/ERC-14-0053. Retrieved from: https://www.ncbi.nlm.nih.gov/pubmed/25052473

Hutz RJ, Carvan MJ 3rd, Larson JK, et al. Familiar and novel reproductive endocrine disruptors: xenoestrogens, dioxins and nanoparticles. *Curr Trends Endocinol*. 2014;7:111–122. https://www.ncbi.nlm.nih.gov/pmc/articles/PMC4364387/

Toppari J, Larsen JC, Christiansen P, et al. Male reproductive health and environmental xenoestrogens. *Environ Health Perspect*. 1996;104 Suppl 4(Suppl 4):741–803. doi:10.1289/ehp.96104s4741. Retrieved from: https://www.ncbi.nlm.nih.gov/pmc/articles/PMC1469672/

Circadian rhythm

Science Daily. Circadian Rhythm. (Accessed April 10, 2019). https://www.sciencedaily.com/terms/circadian_rhythm.htm

The importance of sleep

González-González A, Mediavilla MD, Sánchez-Barceló EJ. Melatonin: A Molecule for Reducing Breast CancerRisk. *Molecules*. 2018;23(2):336.Published2018Feb6.doi:10.3390/molecules23020336. Retrieved from: https://www.ncbi.nlm.nih.gov/pmc/articles/PMC6017232/

Blue light blockers

Shechter A, Kim EW, St-Onge MP, Westwood AJ. Blocking nocturnal blue light for insomnia: A randomized controlled trial. *J Psychiatr Res*. 2017;96:196–202. doi:10.1016/j.jpsychires.2017.10.015. Retrieved from: https://www.ncbi.nlm.nih.gov/pmc/articles/PMC5703049/

Melatonin

Buscemi N, Vandermeer B, Pandya R, et al. Melatonin for Treatment of Sleep Disorders: Summary. 2004. In: AHRQ Evidence Report Summaries. Rockville (MD): Agency for Healthcare Research and Quality (US); 1998-2005. 108.

Reduction of inflammation and edema

Kennedy DA. Evidence for the topical application of castor oil. *International Journal of Naturopathic Medicine*. 2012; 5: 1-2. Retrieved from: http://intjnm.com/evidence-for-the-topical-application-of-castor-oil/

Via prostaglandin EP3 receptors, increased bowel movement, improved OATT, digestion, and absorption

Arslan GG, Eşer I. An examination of the effect of castor oil packs on constipation in the elderly. *Complementary Therapies in Clinical Practice*. 2011;17(1):58-62. doi: 10.1016/j.ctcp.2010.04.004. Epub 2010 May 18. Retrieved from: https://www.ncbi.nlm.nih.gov/pubmed/21168117

Tunaru S, Althoff TF, Nüsing RM, Diener M, Offermanns S. Castor oil induces laxation and uterus contraction via ricinoleic acid activating prostaglandin EP3 receptors. *Proc Natl Acad Sci USA*. 2012;109(23):9179–9184. doi:10.1073/pnas.1201627109 Retrieved from: https://www.ncbi.nlm.nih.gov/pubmed/22615395

Glutathione preserving, liver depuration

Kennedy D and Keaton D. Evidence for the Topical Application of Castor oil: A Systematic Review. CCNM. Presentation 2010 AANP

Biofilm breakdown, improve microbiome

Badaró MM, Salles MM, Leite VMF, Arruda CNF, Oliveira VC, Nascimento CD, Souza RF, Paranhos HFO, Silva-Lovato CH. Clinical trial for evaluation of Ricinus communis and sodium hypochlorite as denture cleanser.J Appl Oral Sci. 2017 May-Jun; 25(3):324-334.

Salles MM, Badaró MM, Arruda CN, Leite VM, Silva CH, Watanabe E, Oliveira Vde C, Paranhos Hde F. Antimicrobial activity of complete denture cleanser solutions based on sodium hypochlorite and Ricinus communis—a randomized clinical study.J Appl Oral Sci. 2015 Nov-Dec; 23(6):637-42.

Walker SC1, Trotter PD2, Swaney WT2, Marshall A3, Mcglone FP4. C-tactile afferents: Cutaneous mediators of oxytocin release during affiliative tactile interactions? Neuropeptides. 2017 Aug;64:27-38. doi: 10.1016/j.npep.2017.01.001. Epub 2017 Jan 19.

Rebounding

Cogoli A. Changes observed in lymphocyte behavior during gravitational unloading. ASGSB Bull. 1991 Jul;4(2):107-15. https://www.ncbi.nlm.nih.gov/pubmed/11537173

Chapter 12: Fibroids Protocol

Occurrence

Baird DD, Dunson DB, Hill MC, Cousins D, Schectman JM. High cumulative incidence of uterine leiomyoma in black and white women: ultrasound evidence. Am J Obstet Gynecol. 2003;188(1):100-107. doi:10.1067/mob.2003.99

Causes

Katz TA, Yang Q, Treviño LS, Walker CL, Al-Hendy A. Endocrine-disrupting chemicals and uterine fibroids. *Fertil Steril*. 2016;106(4):967–977. doi:10.1016/j.fertnstert.2016.08.023. Retrieved from: https://www.ncbi.nlm.nih.gov/pmc/articles/PMC5051569/

Kim MH, Park YR, Lim DJ, Yoon KH, Kang MI, Cha BY, Lee KW, Son HY. The relationship between thyroid nodules and uterine fibroids. *Endocrine Journal*. 2010;57:615–621. doi: 10.1507/endocrj.K10E-024. Retrieved from: https://www.ncbi.nlm.nih.gov/pubmed/20467159

Ott J, Kurz C, Braun R, Promberger R, Seemann R, Vytiska-Binstorfer E, Walch K. Overt hypothyroidism is associated with the presence of uterine leiomyoma: A retrospective analysis. *European Journal of Obstetrics Gynecology and Reproductive Biology*. 2 014;177:19–22. Retrieved from: https://www.ncbi.nlm.nih.gov/pubmed/24690197

Kukhtina EG, Solionova LG, Fedichkina TP, Zykova IE. Night shift work and health disorder risk in female workers. *Gigiena i sanitariia*. 2015; 94(5): 86-91. Retrieved from: https://www.ncbi.nlm.nih.gov/pubmed/26625625

Add-on protocol

Santanam N, Kavtaradze N, Murphy A, Dominguez C, Parthasarathy S. Antioxidant supplementation reduces endometriosis-related pelvic pain in humans. *Transl Res*. 2012;161(3):189–195. doi:10.1016/j.trsl.2012.05.001. Retrieved from: https://www.ncbi.nlm.nih.gov/pmc/articles/PMC3484190/

Messailli EM et al. The possible role of zinc in the etiopathogenesis of endometriosis. *Clinical and Experimental Obstetrics & Gynecology*. 2014;41(5):541-546. Retrieved from: https://www.ncbi.nlm.nih.gov/pubmed/25864256

Zhang Y, Cao H, Yu Z, Peng HY, Zhang CJ. Curcumin inhibits endometriosis endometrial cells by reducing estradiol production. *Iran J Reprod Med*. 2013;11(5):415–422. Retrieved from: https://www.ncbi.nlm.nih.gov/pmc/articles/PMC3941414/

Chapter 13: Endometriosis Protocol

Key facts

Parasar P, Ozcan P, Terry KL. Endometriosis: Epidemiology, Diagnosis and Clinical Management. *Curr Obstet Gynecol Rep*. 2017;6(1):34–41. doi:10.1007/s13669-017-0187-1. Retrieved from: https://www.ncbi.nlm.nih.gov/pmc/articles/PMC5737931/

Chapter 14: Fibrocystic and Lumpy Breasts Protocol

Key facts

Chen YY, Fang WH, Wang CC, et al. Examining the Associations among Fibrocystic Breast Change, Total Lean Mass, and Percent Body Fat. *Sci Rep*. 2018;8(1):9180. Published 2018 Jun 15. doi:10.1038/s41598-018-27546-3. Retrieved from: https://www.ncbi.nlm.nih.gov/pmc/articles/PMC6003905/

Causes

Cleveland Clinic. Fibrocystic Breast Changes. https://my.clevelandclinic.org/health/diseases/4185-fibrocystic-breast-changes. Updated April 9, 2014. Accessed April 11, 2019.

Vobecky J, Simard A, Vobecky JS, Ghadirian P, Lamothe-Guay M, Falardeau M. Nutritional profile of women with fibrocystic breast disease. Int J Epidemiol. 1993;22:989–99. Retrieved from: https://www.ncbi.nlm.nih.gov/pubmed/8144312

Brkic M et al. The influence of progesterone gel therapy in the treatment of fibrocystic breast disease. *Open Journal of Obstetrics and Gynecology*. 2016; 6, 334-341. Retrieved from: https://www.scirp.org/journal/PaperInformation.aspx?paperID=66105.

Types of breast tenderness

Prior JC. Ovulatory disturbances: they do matter. *The Canadian Journal of Diagnosis*. 1 997; 14:64-80. Retrieved from: http://www.cemcor.net/files/uploads/Ovulatory_Disturbances_-_They_Do_Matter.pdf

Iodine

Rappaport J. Changes in Dietary Iodine Explains Increasing Incidence of Breast Cancer with Distant Involvement in Young Women. Journal of Cancer. 2017;8(2):174-177. doi:10.7150/jca.17835.

Du D, Li X. The relationship between thyroiditis and polycystic ovary syndrome: a meta-analysis. International Journal of Clinical and Experimental Medicine. 2013;6(10):880-889.

Ghent WR, Eskin BA, Low DA, Hill LP. Iodine replacement in fibrocystic disease of the breast. Can J Surg. 1993;36(5):453-460.

Al-Attas OS, Al-Daghri NM, Alkharfy KM, et al. Urinary iodine is associated with insulin resistance in subjects with diabetes mellitus type 2. Exp Clin Endocrinol Diabetes. 2012;120(10):618-22. doi: 10.1055/s-0032-1323816.

Leung AM, Braverman LE. Iodine-induced thyroid dysfunction. Current opinion in endocrinology, diabetes, and obesity. 2012;19(5):414-419. doi:10.1097/MED.0b013e3283565bb2.

Borage Oil, GLA

Saldeen P, Saldeen T. Women and omega-3 Fatty acids. Obstet Gynecol Surv. 2004;59(10):722-30; quiz 745-6.

Vitamin E

Parsay S, Olfati F, Nahidi S. Therapeutic effects of vitamin E on cyclic mastalgia. *Breast Journal*. 2009;15:510–4. Retrieved from: https://www.ncbi.nlm.nih.gov/pubmed/19614907

Chapter 15: Hot Flashes

Seed rotation

Habib FK, Maddy SQ, Stitch SR. Zinc-induced changes in the progesterone binding properties of the human endometrium. *Acta Endocrinol* (Copenh). 1980 May;94(1):99-106. doi:10.1530/acta.0.0940099

De Wattevill H, Borth R, Gsell M. Effect of dl-α-tocopherol acetate on progesterone metabolism. *Journal of Clinical Endocrinology and Metabolism*. 1948 Nov;8(11):982-92. doi: 10.1210/jcem-8-11-982

Adlercreutz H, Höckerstedt K, Bannwart C, at al. Effect of dietary components, including lignans and phytoestrogens, on enterohepatic circulation and liver metabolism of estrogens and on sex hormone binding globulin (SHBG). *Journal of Steroid Biochemistry*. 1987;27(4-6):1135-44. doi: 10.1016/0022-4731(87)90200-7

Richter D, Abarzua S, Chrobak M, et al. Effects of phytoestrogen extracts isolated from pumpkin seeds on estradiol production and ER/PR expression in breast cancer and trophoblast tumor cells. *Nutr Cancer*. 2013;65(5):739-45. doi: 10.1080/01635581.2013.797000.

Brzezinski A, Debi A. Phytoestrogens: the "natural" selective estrogen receptor modulators?. *Eur J Obstet Gynecol Reprod Biol*. 1999 Jul;85(1):47-51. doi: 10.1016/s0301-2115(98)00281-4

Chapter 16: Amenorrhea (Absent Periods) Protocol

Causes

National Institute of Child Health and Human Development. What causes amenorrhea? https://www.nichd.nih.gov/health/topics/amenorrhea/conditioninfo/causes. Updated January 1, 2017. Accessed April 11, 2019.

Jacobson MH, Mertens AC, Spencer JB, Manatunga AK, Howards PP. Menses resumption after cancer treatment-inducedamenorrheaoccursearlyornotatall.*FertilSteril*. 2015;105(3):765–772.e4. doi:10.1016/j.fertnstert.2015.11.020. Retrieved from: https://www.ncbi.nlm.nih.gov/pmc/articles/PMC4779728/

Ayesha, Jha V, Goswami D. Premature Ovarian Failure: An Association with Autoimmune Diseases. *J Clin Diagn Res*. 2016;10(10):QC10–QC12. doi:10.7860/JCDR/2016/22027.8671. Retrieved from: https://www.ncbi.nlm.nih.gov/pmc/articles/PMC5121739/

Soni S, Badawy SZ. Celiac disease and its effect on human reproduction: review. *Journal of Reproductive Medicine*. 2010; 55(1-2):3-8. Retrieved from: https://www.ncbi.nlm.nih.gov/pubmed/20337200

Glass AR, Dahms WT, Abraham G, Atkinson RL, Ray GA, Swerdloff RS. Secondary amenorrhea in obesity: etiologic role of weight-related androgen excess. 1978; 30(2): 243-244. Retrieved from: https://www.ncbi.nlm.nih.gov/pubmed/680202

Fourman LT, Fazeli PK. Neuroendocrine causes of amenorrhea-an update. *Journal of Clinical EndocrinologyandMetabolism*. 2015;100(3):812–824.doi:10.1210/jc.2014-3344.Retrievedfrom: https://www.ncbi.nlm.nih.gov/pmc/articles/PMC4333037/

Seed rotation

Habib FK, Maddy SQ, Stitch SR. Zinc-induced changes in the progesterone binding properties of the human endometrium. *Acta Endocrinol* (Copenh). 1980 May;94(1):99-106. doi:10.1530/acta.0.0940099

De Wattevill H, Borth R, Gsell M. Effect of dl-α-tocopherol acetate on progesterone metabolism. *Journal of Clinical Endocrinology and Metabolism*. 1948 Nov;8(11):982-92. doi: 10.1210/jcem-8-11-982

Adlercreutz H, Höckerstedt K, Bannwart C, at al. Effect of dietary components, including lignans and phytoestrogens, on enterohepatic circulation and liver metabolism of estrogens and on sex hormone binding globulin (SHBG). *Journal of Steroid Biochemistry*. 1987;27(4-6):1135-44. doi: 10.1016/0022-4731(87)90200-7

Richter D, Abarzua S, Chrobak M, et al. Effects of phytoestrogen extracts isolated from pumpkin seeds on estradiol production and ER/PR expression in breast cancer and trophoblast tumor cells. *Nutr Cancer*. 2013;65(5):739-45. doi: 10.1080/01635581.2013.797000.

Brzezinski A, Debi A. Phytoestrogens: the "natural" selective estrogen receptor modulators?. *Eur J Obstet Gynecol Reprod Biol*. 1999 Jul;85(1):47-51. doi: 10.1016/s0301-2115(98)00281-4

Chapter 17: Irregular Periods Protocol

Symptoms

Rebar R. Evaluation of amenorrhea, anovulation, and abnormal bleeding. [Updated 2018 Jan 15]. In: Feingold KR, Anawalt B, Boyce A, et al., editors. *Endotext*. South Dartmouth (MA): MDText.com, Inc.; 2000.

Causes

Lawson CC, Whelan EA, Lividoti Hibert EN, Spiegelman D, Schernhammer ES, Rich-Edwards JW. Rotating shift work and menstrual cycle characteristics. *Epidemiology*. 2011;22(3):305–312. doi:10.1097/EDE.0b013e3182130016. Retrieved from: https://www.ncbi.nlm.nih.gov/pmc/articles/PMC5303197/

Sanders KA, Bruce NW. Psychosocial stress and the menstrual cycle. *Journal of Biosocial Science*. 1999; 31(3): 393-402. Retrieved from: https://www.ncbi.nlm.nih.gov/pubmed/10453249

Baker FC, Driver HS. Circadianrhythms,sleep,andthemenstrualcycle. *SleepMedicine*. 2007; 8:613-622. Retrieved from: https://www.ncbi.nlm.nih.gov/pubmed/17383933

Jacobson MH, Mertens AC, Spencer JB, Manatunga AK, Howards PP. Menses resumption after cancer treatment-induceddamenorrheaoccursearlyornotatall.*FertilSteril*. 2015;105(3):765–772.e4. doi:10.1016/j.fertnstert.2015.11.020. Retrieved from: https://www.ncbi.nlm.nih.gov/pmc/articles/PMC4779728/

Ayesha, Jha V, Goswami D. Premature Ovarian Failure: An Association with Autoimmune Diseases. *J Clin Diagn Res*. 2016;10(10):QC10–QC12. doi:10.7860/JCDR/2016/22027.8671. Retrieved from: https://www.ncbi.nlm.nih.gov/pmc/articles/PMC5121739/

Arentz S, Abbott JA, Smith CA, Bensoussan A. Herbal medicine for the management of polycystic ovary syndrome (PCOS) and associated oligo/amenorrhoea and hyperandrogenism; a review of the laboratory evidence for effects with corroborative clinical findings. *BMC Complement Altern Med*. 2014;14:511. Published 2014 Dec 18. doi:10.1186/1472-6882-14-511. Retrieved from: https://www.ncbi.nlm.nih.gov/pmc/articles/PMC4528347/

Seed rotation

Habib FK, Maddy SQ, Stitch SR. Zinc-induced changes in the progesterone binding properties of the human endometrium. *Acta Endocrinol* (Copenh). 1980 May;94(1):99-106. doi:10.1530/acta.0.0940099

De Wattevill H, Borth R, Gsell M. Effect of dl-α-tocopherol acetate on progesterone metabolism. *Journal of Clinical Endocrinology and Metabolism*. 1948 Nov;8(11):982-92. doi: 10.1210/jcem-8-11-982

Adlercreutz H, Höckerstedt K, Bannwart C, at al. Effect of dietary components, including lignans and phytoestrogens, on enterohepatic circulation and liver metabolism of estrogens and on sex hormone binding globulin (SHBG). *Journal of Steroid Biochemistry*. 1987;27(4-6):1135-44. doi: 10.1016/0022-4731(87)90200-7

Richter D, Abarzua S, Chrobak M, et al. Effects of phytoestrogen extracts isolated from pumpkin seeds on estradiol production and ER/PR expression in breast cancer and trophoblast tumor cells. *Nutr Cancer*. 2013;65(5):739-45. doi: 10.1080/01635581.2013.797000.

Brzezinski A, Debi A. Phytoestrogens: the "natural" selective estrogen receptor modulators?. *Eur J Obstet Gynecol Reprod Biol*. 1999 Jul;85(1):47-51. doi: 10.1016/s0301-2115(98)00281-4

Chapter 18: Dysmenorrhea and PMS Protocol

Key facts

Cleveland Clinic. Dysmenorrhea. https://my.clevelandclinic.org/health/diseases/4148-dysmenorrhea. Accessed April 12, 2019.

Grandi G, Ferrari S, Xholli A, et al. Prevalence of menstrual pain in young women: what is dysmenorrhea?.*JPainRes*. 2012;5:169–174.doi:10.2147/JPR.S30602.Retrievedfrom: https://www.ncbi.nlm.nih.gov/pmc/articles/PMC3392715/

Causes

Bernardi M, Lazzeri L, Perelli F, Reis FM, Petraglia F. Dysmenorrhea and related disorders. *F1000Res*. 2017;6:1645. Published 2017 Sep 5. doi:10.12688/f1000research.11682.1. Retrieved from: https://www.ncbi.nlm.nih.gov/pmc/articles/PMC5585876/

Zahradnik HP, Breckwoldt M. Contribution to the pathogenesis of dysmenorrhea. *Archives of Gynecology*. 1984;236(2):99–108. Retrieved from: https://www.ncbi.nlm.nih.gov/pubmed/6596911

Ajmani NS, Sarbhai V, Yadav N, Paul M, Ahmad A, Ajmani AK. Role of Thyroid Dysfunction in Patients with Menstrual Disorders in Tertiary Care Center of Walled City of Delhi. *J Obstet Gynaecol India*. 2015;66(2):115–119. doi:10.1007/s13224-014-0650-0. Retrieved from: https://www.ncbi.nlm.nih.gov/pmc/articles/PMC4818825/

Marjoribanks J., Ayeleke R.O., Farquhar C., Proctor M. Nonsteroidal anti-inflammatory drugs for dysmenorrhoea. Cochrane Database Syst. Rev. 2015:CD001751Cd001751. doi: 10.1002/14651858.CD001751.pub3. Retrieved from: https://www.ncbi.nlm.nih.gov/pubmed/26224322

Seed rotation

Habib FK, Maddy SQ, Stitch SR. Zinc-induced changes in the progesterone binding properties of the human endometrium. *Acta Endocrinol* (Copenh). 1980 May;94(1):99-106. doi:10.1530/acta.0.0940099

De Wattevill H, Borth R, Gsell M. Effect of dl-a-tocopherol acetate on progesterone metabolism. *Journal of Clinical Endocrinology and Metabolism*. 1948 Nov;8(11):982-92. doi: 10.1210/jcem-8-11-982

Adlercreutz H, Höckerstedt K, Bannwart C, at al. Effect of dietary components, including lignans and phytoestrogens, on enterohepatic circulation and liver metabolism of estrogens and on sex hormone binding globulin (SHBG). *Journal of Steroid Biochemistry*. 1987;27(4-6):1135-44. doi: 10.1016/0022-4731(87)90200-7

Richter D, Abarzua S, Chrobak M, et al. Effects of phytoestrogen extracts isolated from pumpkin seeds on estradiol production and ER/PR expression in breast cancer and trophoblast tumor cells. *Nutr Cancer*. 2013;65(5):739-45. doi: 10.1080/01635581.2013.797000.

Brzezinski A, Debi A. Phytoestrogens: the "natural" selective estrogen receptor modulators?. *Eur J Obstet Gynecol Reprod Biol*. 1999 Jul;85(1):47-51. doi: 10.1016/s0301-2115(98)00281-4

Borage Oil, GLA

Saldeen P, Saldeen T. Women and omega-3 Fatty acids. Obstet Gynecol Surv. 2004;59(10):722-30; quiz 745-6.

Ockerman P, et al. Evening primrose oil as a treatment of the premenstrual syndrome. Rec Adv Clin Nutr 1986;2:404-405.

Chapter 19 Menorrhagia (Heavy Period) Protocol

Key facts

Gokyildiz S, Aslan E, Beji NK, Mecdi M. The Effects of Menorrhagia on Women's Quality of Life: A Case-Control Study. *ISRN Obstet Gynecol*. 2013;2013:918179. Published 2013 Jul 8. doi:10.1155/2013/918179. Retrieved from: https://www.ncbi.nlm.nih.gov/pmc/articles/PMC3734607/

Seed rotation

Habib FK, Maddy SQ, Stitch SR. Zinc-induced changes in the progesterone binding properties of the human endometrium. *Acta Endocrinol* (Copenh). 1980 May;94(1):99-106. doi:10.1530/acta.0.0940099

De Wattevill H, Borth R, Gsell M. Effect of dl-a-tocopherol acetate on progesterone metabolism. *Journal of Clinical Endocrinology and Metabolism*. 1948 Nov;8(11):982-92. doi: 10.1210/jcem-8-11-982

Adlercreutz H, Höckerstedt K, Bannwart C, at al. Effect of dietary components, including lignans and phytoestrogens, on enterohepatic circulation and liver metabolism of estrogens and on sex hormone binding globulin (SHBG). *Journal of Steroid Biochemistry*. 1987;27(4-6):1135-44. doi: 10.1016/0022-4731(87)90200-7

Richter D, Abarzua S, Chrobak M, et al. Effects of phytoestrogen extracts isolated from pumpkin seeds on estradiol production and ER/PR expression in breast cancer and trophoblast tumor cells. *Nutr Cancer*. 2013;65(5):739-45. doi: 10.1080/01635581.2013.797000.

Brzezinski A, Debi A. Phytoestrogens: the "natural" selective estrogen receptor modulators?. *Eur J Obstet Gynecol Reprod Biol*. 1999 Jul;85(1):47-51. doi: 10.1016/s0301-2115(98)00281-4

Chapter 20: Thyroid Nodules Protocol

Key facts

Cleveland Clinic. Thyroid Nodule. https://my.clevelandclinic.org/health/diseases/13121-thyroid-nodule. Accessed April 12, 2019.

Causes

Manole D., Schildknecht B., Gosnell B., Adams E., Derwahl M. Estrogen promotes growth of human thyroid tumor cells by different molecular mechanisms. *The Journal of Clinical Endocrinology and Metabolism*. 2001;86(3):1072–1077. doi:10.1210/jcem.86.3.7283. Retrieved from: https://www.ncbi.nlm.nih.gov/pubmed/11238488

Chapter 21: Infertility and Miscarriage Protocol

Causes

National Institute of Child Health and Human Development. Infertility and Fertility. https://www.nichd.nih.gov/health/topics/infertility. Updated January 31, 2017. Accessed April 12, 2019.

Quintino-Moro A, Zantut-Wittmann, DE, Tambascia M, da Costa Machado H, Fernandes A. High prevalence of infertility among women with graves' disease and hashimoto's thyroiditis. International Journal of Endocrinology. 2014; vol. 2014, Article ID 982705, 6 pages. Retrieved from: https://www.hindawi.com/journals/ije/2014/982705/

Melo AS, Ferriani RA, Navarro PA. Treatment of infertility in women with polycystic ovary syndrome: approach to clinical practice. *Clinics (Sao Paulo)*. 2015;70(11):765–769. doi:10.6061/clinics/2015(11)09 Retrieved from: https://www.ncbi.nlm.nih.gov/pmc/articles/PMC4642490/

Fadhlaoui A, Bouquet de la Jolinière J, Feki A. Endometriosis and infertility: how and when to treat?. *Front Surg*. 2014;1:24. Published 2014 Jul 2. doi:10.3389/fsurg.2014.00024. Retrieved from: https://www.ncbi.nlm.nih.gov/pmc/articles/PMC4286960/

Rooney KL, Domar AD. The relationship between stress and infertility. *Dialogues Clin Neurosci*. 2018;20(1):41–47. Retrieved from: https://www.ncbi.nlm.nih.gov/pmc/articles/PMC6016043/.

Chapter 22: Cellulite and Hip Fat Protocol

Key facts

Tokarska K, Tokarski S, Woźniacka A, Sysa-Jędrzejowska A, Bogaczewicz J. Cellulite: a cosmetic or systemic issue? Contemporary views on the etiopathogenesis of cellulite. *Postepy Dermatol Alergol*. 2018;35(5):442–446. doi:10.5114/ada.2018.77235. Retrieved from: https://www.ncbi.nlm.nih.gov/pmc/articles/PMC6232550/

Chapter 23: Breast Cancer Protocol

Alpha-Pregnanediol elevated in daughter of women with breast cancer

Trichopoulos D, Brown JB, Garas J, Papaloannou A, MacMahon B. Elevated Urine Estrogen and Pregnanediol Levels in Daughters of Breast Cancer Patients. *JNCI: Journal of the National Cancer Institute*. 1981;67(3):603–606,https://doi.org/10.1093/jnci/67.3.603

Inherited gene mutation

American Cancer Society. Breast Cancer Facts and Figures 2019-2020. Atlanta, GA: American Cancer Society, 2019; National Cancer Institute. Genetics of breast and gynecologic cancers (PDQ®)—health professional version. https://www.cancer.gov/types/breast/hp/breast-ovarian-genetics-pdq, 2019.

BRACA1/2

Struewing JP, Hartge P, Wacholder S, et al. The risk of cancer associated with specific mutations of BRCA1 and BRCA2 among Ashkenazi Jews. *N Engl J Med*. 1997; 336: 1401-8, 1997; Chen S, Parmigiani G. Meta-analysis of BRCA1 and BRCA2 penetrance. *J Clin Oncol*. 2007;25(11):1329-33; Antoniou AC, Cunningham AP, Peto J, et al. The BOADICEA model of genetic susceptibility to breast and ovarian cancers: updates and extensions. *Br J Cancer*. 2008;98(8):1457-66.

National Cancer Institute. Genetics of breast and gynecologic cancers (PDQ®)—health professional version. https://www.cancer.gov/types/breast/hp/breast-ovarian-genetics-pdq, 2019.

Vitamin D

Streb J, Glanowska I, Streb A, et al. The relationship between breast cancer treatment, tumour type and vitamin D level in pre- and postmenopausal women. *Endocrinol Lett*. 2017 Dec;38(6):437-440. https://www.ncbi.nlm.nih.gov/pubmed/29298285

Iodine

Rappaport J. Changes in Dietary Iodine Explains Increasing Incidence of Breast Cancer with Distant Involvement in Young Women. Journal of Cancer. 2017;8(2):174-177. doi:10.7150/jca.17835.

Du D, Li X. The relationship between thyroiditis and polycystic ovary syndrome: a meta-analysis. International Journal of Clinical and Experimental Medicine. 2013;6(10):880-889.

Leung AM, Braverman LE. Iodine-induced thyroid dysfunction. Current opinion in endocrinology, diabetes, and obesity. 2012;19(5):414-419. doi:10.1097/MED.0b013e3283565bb2.

Resveratrol

Ko, Jeong-Hyeon et al. The Role of Resveratrol in Cancer Therapy. *International journal of molecular sciences*. 2017 Dec;18(12):2589. doi:10.3390/ijms18122589

Chapter 24: High Testosterone (PCOS) Protocol

Undiagnosed

March WA, Moore VM, Wilson, KJ, et al. The prevalence of polycystic ovary syndrome in a community sample assessed under contrasting diagnostic criteria. *Hum Reprod*. 2010 Feb;25(2):544-51. doi: 10.1093/humrep/dep399. Epub 2009 Nov 12.

Berberine

W. Chang, et al. Berberine as a therapy for type 2 diabetes and its complications: From mechanism of action to clinical studies. *Biochem Cell Biol.* 2015 Oct;93(5):479-86. doi: 10.1139/bcb-2014-0107

Yin J, Xing H, Ye J. Efficacy of berberine in patients with type 2 diabetes mellitus. *Metabolism.* 2008;57(5):712-717. doi:10.1016/j.metabol.2008.01.013

Chromium picolinate

N. Susksomboon, et al., Systematic review and meta-analysis of the efficacy and safety of chromium supplementation in diabetes. *J Clin Pharm Ther.* 2014 Jun;39(3):292-306. doi: 10.1111/jcpt.12147

Inositol

Nordio M, Proietti E. The combined therapy with myo-inositol and D-chiro-inositol reduces the risk of metabolic disease in PCOS overweight patients compared to myo-inositol supplementation alone. Eur Rev Med Pharmacol Sci. 2012;16(5):575-81.

Minozzi M, Nordio M, Pajalich R. The Combined therapy myo-inositol plus D-Chiro-inositol, in a physiological ratio, reduces the cardiovascular risk by improving the lipid profile in PCOS patients. Eur Rev Med Pharmacol Sci. 2013;17(4):537-40.

Costantino D, Minozzi G, Minozzi E, Guaraldi C. Metabolic and hormonal effects of myo-inositol in women with polycystic ovary syndrome: a double-blind trial. Eur Rev Med Pharmacol Sci. 2009;13(2):105-10.

Index

Recipe Index

Note: Page references in *italics* indicate recipe photographs.

OVERCOMING ESTROGEN DOMINANCE

Notes

Notes